ADOLESCENT PSYCHIATRY

VOLUME V

*DEVELOPMENTAL AND
CLINICAL STUDIES*

Annals of the American Society for Adolescent Psychiatry

ADOLESCENT PSYCHIATRY

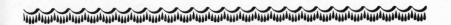

VOLUME V

DEVELOPMENTAL AND CLINICAL STUDIES

EDITED BY

**SHERMAN C. FEINSTEIN
PETER L. GIOVACCHINI**

JASON ARONSON, INC.

NEW YORK

IN MEMORIAM
JUDITH BASKIN OFFER

Healthy children will not fear life if their parents have integrity enough not to fear death.

—Erik Erikson

This volume is dedicated to the memory of our colleague and dear friend, Judith Baskin Offer. The wife of Past–President Daniel Offer, Judy died at the age of thirty-six on May 31, 1976.

In the long struggle with her final illness, Judy and Dan demonstrated the growth and integrity that can be achieved through an honest approach to a difficult reality. All of those who were involved felt inspired by the strength of her conviction that truth should be faced at all times.

Judy was active with the Society since its founding. In collaboration with Dan she had participated in numerous meetings and workshops and had contributed several papers to this publication.

A second year candidate at the Chicago Institute for Psychoanalysis, she attended the University of Michigan, the University of Paris (Sorbonne), and Harvard University. Engaged with her husband in long-term studies of normal adolescence, she was a Research Associate at Michael Reese Medical Center and the University of Chicago. In addition to Dan, she is survived by two children, Tamara and Raphael.

We are honored to publish in this volume the last paper Judy presented. She will be deeply missed by all who knew her.

SHERMAN C. FEINSTEIN
PETER L. GIOVACCHINI

THE AUTHORS

LESTER BAKER is Director, Clinical Research Center, Children's Hospital of Philadelphia.

ANNETTE BARAN is a Psychiatric Social Worker in private practice, Los Angeles, California.

PETER BLOS is on the faculty of the New York Psychoanalytic Institute and the Psychoanalytic Clinic for Training and Research, College of Physicians and Surgeons, Columbia University. He received the 1969 Distinguished Service Award of the American Society for Adolescent Psychiatry.

HILDE BRUCH is Professor of Psychiatry, Baylor College of Medicine, Texas Medical Center, Houston, Texas.

ROBERT A. BURT is Professor of Law, Yale University.

BERTRAM J. COHLER is Associate Professor of Human Development and Education, University of Chicago.

ANDRE P. DERDEYN is Associate Professor of Psychiatry and Pediatrics, and Director of Training in Child and Adolescent Psychiatry, University of Virginia School of Medicine.

JARL E. DYRUD is Professor of Psychiatry and Associate Chairman, Pritzker School of Medicine, University of Chicago.

WILLIAM M. EASSON is Professor and Head, Department of Psychiatry and Behavioral Sciences, Louisiana State University School of Medicine.

AARON H. ESMAN is Chief Psychiatrist, Jewish Board of Guardians, Lecturer, Columbia University School of Social Work, and is on the faculty of the New York Psychoanalytic Institute.

SHERMAN C. FEINSTEIN is Clinical Professor of Psychiatry, Pritzker School of Medicine, University of Chicago, and Director, Child and Adolescent Psychiatry Training Program, Michael Reese Hospital and Medical Center. He is Past President, American Society for Adolescent Psychiatry (1969-1970), and a Managing Editor of this Volume.

WARREN J. GADPAILLE is Adjunct Professor, Department of Psychology, Counseling, and Guidance, University of Northern Colorado.

PETER L. GIOVACCHINI is Clinical Professor of Psychiatry, Abraham Lincoln School of Medicine, University of Illinois, and a Managing Editor of this Volume.

ALAN GOODSITT is Attending Psychiatrist, Psychosomatic and Psychiatric Institute, Michael Reese Hospital and Medical Center, Chicago, Illinois.

ROY R. GRINKER, SR. is Director-Emeritus of the Institute for Psychosomatic and Psychiatric Research and Training, Michael Reese Hospital and Medical Center, and Professor of Psychiatry, Pritzker School of Medicine, University of Chicago.

KATHERINE A. HALMI is Associate Professor of Psychiatry, University of Iowa College of Medicine.

PHILIP S. HOLZMAN is Professor of Psychiatry and Behavioral Science, University of Chicago.

JOE W. KING is Director, Child and Adolescent Service, Timberlawn Psychiatric Center, and Clinical Instructor of Psychiatry, University of Texas Health Science Center, Dallas, Texas. He is President-Elect, American Society for Adolescent Psychiatry (1976-1977).

REUVEN KOHEN-RAZ is on the faculty of the School of Education, the Hebrew University of Jerusalem, and Chief Consultant to the Israel Ministry of Health and the Hadassah Medical Organization, Israel.

LINDA LARSON is Research Social Worker, University of Iowa College of Medicine.

MOSES LAUFER is Director, Brent Centre for the Study of Adolescence, London. He is a staff member of the Hampstead Child Therapy Clinic and Training Analyst, London Institute for Psychoanalysis. He is the 1976 recipient of the William A. Schonfeld Distinguished Award of the American Society for Adolescent Psychiatry.

EDWARD M. LEVINE is Professor of Sociology, Loyola University of Chicago.

RONALD LIEBMAN is Assistant Professor of Child Psychiatry and Pediatrics, University of Pennsylvania School of Medicine.

RICHARD C. MAROHN is Director, Adolescent Program, Illinois State Psychiatric Institute, Attending Psychiatrist, Psychosomatic and Psychiatric Institute, Michael Reese Hospital and Medical Center, and Clinical Assistant Professor, Pritzker School of Medicine, University of Chicago.

DEREK MILLER is Professor of Psychiatry and Chief of the Adolescent Program, Northwestern University School of Medicine.

SALVADOR MINUCHIN is Professor and Director, Division of Child Psychiatry, University of Pennsylvania School of Medicine.

JACK NOVICK is Associate Professor in Psychiatry, Childrens Psychiatric Hospital, University of Michigan Medical School, Ann Arbor, Michigan.

DANIEL OFFER is Director, Institute for Psychosomatic and Psychiatric Research and Training, Michael Reese Hospital and Medical Center, and Professor of Psychiatry, Pritzker School of Medicine, University of Chicago. He was President of the American Society for Adolescent Psychiatry (1972-1973).

JUDITH BASKIN OFFER was Research Associate in Psychiatry, Institute for Psychosomatic and Psychiatric Research and Training, Michael Reese Hospital and Medical Center and the University of Chicago.

LUIZ CARLOS OSORIO is a psychoanalyst in Porte Alegre, Brazil.

REUBEN PANNOR is Director of Community Services, Vista del Mar Child Care Service, Los Angeles, California.

FRANK T. RAFFERTY is Director, Institute for Juvenile Research and Professor of Psychiatry, Abraham Lincoln School of Medicine, University of Illinois, Chicago, Illinois.

MAURICE J. ROSENTHAL is Senior Psychiatric Consultant, Institute for Juvenile Research, and Associate Clinical Professor of Psychiatry, Abraham Lincoln School of Medicine, University of Illinois, Chicago, Illinois.

BERNICE L. ROSMAN is Director of Research, Philadelphia Child Guidance Center.

CHARLES H. SHAIOVA is Attending Psychiatrist, Institute for Psychosomatic and Psychiatric Research and Training, Michael Reese Hospital and Medical Center, and a faculty member, Chicago Institute for Psychoanalysis.

ARTHUR D. SOROSKY is Clinical Assistant Professor of Child Psychiatry, University of California at Los Angeles.

JOHN STEFFEK is Staff Psychiatrist, Institute for Juvenile Research and Assistant Professor of Psychiatry, Abraham Lincoln School of Medicine, University of Illinois, Chicago, Illinois.

HELM STIERLIN is Professor of Psychiatry, University of Heidelberg, Germany.

DAVID B. WATERS is Assistant Professor of Family Medicine and Psychiatry, University of Virginia School of Medicine.

MYRON F. WEINER is Clinical Associate Professor of Psychiatry, University of Texas Health Science Center, and Senior Attending Psychiatrist, Parkland Memorial Hospital.

ROBERT P. WOLENSKY is Assistant Professor of Sociology, University of Wisconsin at Stevens Point.

PREFACE

The *Annals* of the American Society for Adolescent Psychiatry has grown to its fifth volume. As editors, we are pleased and excited with this ever-increasing commitment to the study of the adolescent process and the treatment of the adolescent patient. It is also apparent that such an interest is only minimally concerned with a particular chronological group and extends beyond a preference for a specific age group.

The clinician's desire to know well the adolescent's mind reflects trends that can be considered from various frames of reference. On a macroscopic level one is dealing with a mind that is primarily in a formative state, still evolving, and consequently fluid. A good deal can be accomplished before it consolidates. The adolescent patient stimulates hope and this is helpful for those of us who sometimes feel we are constantly surrounded by misery and hopelessness. When we are successful in the treatment of an adolescent patient, it is especially gratifying. He has the larger part of a life to develop, a life that can now be lived without neurotic constrictions and oppression, in which he can love, do creative work, and experience pleasure. This satisfies our humanistic inclinations.

On a microscopic level, the adolescent reveals facets of character structure that are not so easily discernible in the adult because fundamental elements of the personality have been submerged by defensive superstructures. The relative inflexibility of the adult ego compared to the fluidity of the adolescent's psychic structure prevents us from completely understanding psychic processes, structure building, and adaptive modalities: knowledge which is indispensable for the ultimate understanding of our basic interest, the inner workings, and pathological vicissitudes of the human mind. These pursuits are in keeping with our scientific orientation, but are also syntonic with our humanistic concerns.

This combination of humanistic and scientific perspectives characterizes the medical approach when it is operating at its highest level. For the psychiatrist, psychoanalyst, or any other mental health worker, it is indispensable; it is the essence of our professional identity. Inasmuch as the adolescent stage of life emphasizes both perspectives, it provides us with the opportunity to pursue important elements of our ego-ideal, and— similar to the adolescent's consolidation of his character—our professional character is enhanced.

SHERMAN C. FEINSTEIN
PETER L. GIOVACCHINI

CONTENTS

PART I
ADOLESCENCE: GENERAL CONSIDERATIONS

EDITORS' INTRODUCTION   3

1]   When and How Does Adolescence End:
     Structural Criteria for Adolescent Closure   5
     PETER BLOS

2]   Changing Values: Their Implications for
     Adolescent Development and Psychoanalytic Ideas   18
     AARON H. ESMAN

3]   Discussion of Aaron H. Esman's Chapter   35
     RICHARD C. MAROHN

4]   On Children's Rights and Therapeutic Institutions   39
     DEREK MILLER AND ROBERT A. BURT

5]   Adoption and the Adolescent: An Overview   54
     ARTHUR D. SOROSKY, ANNETTE BARAN,
     AND REUBEN PANNOR

6]   Anomie: Its Influence on Impulse Ridden Youth
     and Their Self-Destructive Behavior   73
     EDWARD M. LEVINE AND CHARLES H. SHAIOVA

7]   College Students in the Fifties:
     The Silent Generation Revisited   82
     ROBERT P. WOLENSKY

8]   Sexuality in Adolescent Males   96
     JUDITH BASKIN OFFER AND DANIEL OFFER

PART II

DEVELOPMENTAL ISSUES: NARCISSISM, PSYCHIC DEVELOPMENT, AND THE ADOLESCENT PROCESS

EDITORS' INTRODUCTION   111

9]   Psychoanalytic Perspectives on Adolescence,
      Psychic Development, and Narcissism   113
      PETER L. GIOVACCHINI

10]   Adolescence: Developmental Phase or Cultural Artifact   143
      WARREN J. GADPAILLE

11]   Filial Obligation in Adolescence: An Orientation   151
      MAURICE J. ROSENTHAL

12]   Parents and Adolescents: Empathy and
      the Vicissitudes of Development   175
      ANDRE P. DERDEYN AND DAVID B. WATERS

13]   The "Juvenile Imposter": Some Thoughts on
      Narcissism and the Delinquent   186
      RICHARD C. MAROHN

14]   Discussion of Dr. Richard C. Marohn's Chapter:
      A Critique of Kohut's Theory of Narcissism   213
      PETER L. GIOVACCHINI

PART III

PSYCHOPATHOLOGY AND ADOLESCENCE

EDITORS' INTRODUCTION   239

15]   A View of Adolescent Pathology   243
      MOSES LAUFER

16]   Depression in Adolescence   257
      WILLIAM H. EASSON

17]   Schizophrenia in Adolescence   276
      PHILIP S. HOLZMAN AND ROY R. GRINKER, SR.

VARIOUS PERSPECTIVES ON ANOREXIA NERVOSA

18]   Anorexia Nervosa   293
      HILDE BRUCH

19]   Narcissistic Disturbances in Anorexia Nervosa   304
      ALAN GOODSITT

20] Input and Outcome of
    Family Therapy in Anorexia Nervosa   313
    BERNICE L. ROSMAN, SALVADOR MINUCHIN,
    RONALD LIEBMAN, AND LESTER BAKER
21] Behavior Therapy in Anorexia Nervosa   323
    KATHERINE A. HALMI AND LINDA LARSON
22] The Significance of the Therapist's Feelings in
    the Treatment of Anorexia Nervosa   352
    BERTRAM J. COHLER

PART IV

PSYCHOTHERAPY OF ADOLESCENCE

EDITORS' INTRODUCTION   387

23] Termination of Treatment in Adolescence   390
    JACK NOVICK
24] Treatment Perspective on Adolescent Runaways   413
    HELM STIERLIN
25] To Tell the Truth in Retrospect   422
    JARL E. DYRUD
26] A Group Approach with the Hapless Adolescent   429
    FRANK T. RAFFERTY AND JOHN C. STEFFEK
27] The Psychoanalysis of Communication in Adolescence   442
    LUIZ CARLOS OSORIO
28] Self-Disclosure by the Therapist to the Adolescent Patient   449
    MYRON F. WEINER AND JOE W. KING
29] Special Education Needs for Adolescents   460
    REUVEN KOHEN-RAZ

CONTENTS OF VOLUMES I-IV   489

INDEX   503

PART I

ADOLESCENCE: GENERAL CONSIDERATIONS

EDITORS' INTRODUCTION

Traditionally, this section deals with the phenomenon of adolescence. For the most part, these explorations concern behavior and movements, and constitute a preamble to our humanistic concerns. We believe they should be of interest to a larger group than therapeutically oriented clinicians.

For the psychotherapist, these chapters also contain much of value that goes beyond the phenomenological. One might say that a benign circle is operating, a sequence of positive feedbacks. Discussions of the general characteristics of adolescence lead to knowledge about the intrapsychic. There is often a movement from the general to the particular, but it is not unidirectional. The more one learns about the specifics of the fluid character structure of the adolescent, the more inferences one can make about wider issues, such as social movements, that can then be systematically investigated.

As repeatedly demonstrated, the intrapsychic and sociological focus are never so closely intertwined as during the developmental stage of adolescence. The impact of what can be called the adolescent movement on our culture has been tremendous. During the past several years, however, it appears to have diminished. Our present culture seems to have a greater influence on adolescents than the reverse. Why this should be is a question that has important implications for all behavioral scientists and lurks behind most of the discussions that follow.

Peter Blos discusses the characteristic of the consolidation aspects of late adolescence by describing four developmental tasks which collaboratively and synergistically lead the individual adolescent into adulthood. He believes that during this phase the predictability of behavior and motivation waxes in constancy and accuracy until a characterological

3

stabilization replaces tentative and arbitrary predictions with what has become the established pattern of individual conduct.

Aaron H. Esman writes that while psychoanalysis originated as a psychology of conflict, with special interest in the conflicts of the oedipus complex, the new breed of patients reveal at least as much weight on the side of developmental disorder as on specific unconscious conflict. Psychoanalysis must be prepared to reexamine some of its general and clinical theoretical assumptions in the light of changes in the social matrix within which it operates.

Derek Miller and Robert A. Burt stress that the decision for residential placement of adolescents should be based not only on symptomatic behavior but also on how successfully that behavior can be contained within the context of human relationships and the general social system. They decry the current trend toward abandoning the rehabilitative promises of the juvenile court and recommend increased efforts toward designing more effective treatment resources.

Edward M. Levine and Charles H. Shaiova discuss the profound social changes experienced by cohesive communities with well-defined, stable social structures and deeply rooted traditional values when they succumb to the forces of urbanization and industrialization. They examine the special significance of this anomic condition for psychoanalytic theory with respect to its implications for ego and superego formation and management of impulse life. Robert P. Wolensky examines the college student of the 1950s and concludes that the "the silent generation" had internalized the value system of their parents and were, therefore, unable to exhibit a distinct generational character.

Arthur D. Sorosky, Annette Baran, and Reuben Pannor review the problems related to the adoption process and consider the issues from the stresses on the adoptive parents, the birth parents, and the adolescent adoptee. The recent interest in the search for biological relatives is considered and the authors report that these experiences have been quite successful in establishing a greater sense of identity and ego integrity in the adoptees as well as an improvement in the relationship with adoptive parents. They recommend that adoption agencies revise their traditional approach to the matters of secrecy and confidentiality.

1] WHEN AND HOW DOES ADOLESCENCE END: STRUCTURAL CRITERIA FOR ADOLESCENT CLOSURE

PETER BLOS

The question of how to conceptualize the termination of the adolescent process has for too long been no question at all, because it was hardly ever asked. Adolescence seemed to be a stage of development one simply outgrows. A widely held opinion tells us that it might linger on indefinitely, in which case people speak of the "eternal adolescent." Such talk is devoid of any biological or psychological reference or meaning. This stricture is a necessary one because normative reference points, in relation to developmental stages and to their sequential order, represent the requisite and essential data for the assessment of normal or pathological conditions at any level of growth. Therapy, research, and social planning depend in equal measure on normative definitions because they constitute the only means by which observations or interventions can become comparative, evaluative, predictive, and purposeful.

We are well acquainted with the milestones of child development formulated somatically, behaviorally, and psychologically. We owe this familiarity to child research and its effort to delineate what is typical or normative in a given stage of development and to define as precisely as possible whatever is characteristic for the beginning or end of a developmental stage.

Admittedly we are much better informed about the entry into adolescence than about its termination. This fact should not surprise us because the onset of adolescence is coincidental with measurable somatic

Address presented to the Third Pan-American Forum for the Study of Adolescence, Mexico City, February 3, 1975.

landmarks, such as primary and secondary sex characteristics as well as growth curves and reliable psychological data. We are familiar with somatic sequences and with the chronological and morphological variations of pubertal maturation within the sequential order of somatic maturation. The latitude of these variations within the limits of normality is well documented. Psychological repercussions to these somatic novelties have also been widely studied. We also know with certainty when the somatic process of puberty has concluded. However, we have no comparable certainty when it comes to psychological changes, their timing, transciency, or stability. The synchronicity between somatic and psychological changes which is quite apparent during the early stage of adolescence fades into disjunction by the time the conclusion of adolescence is reached. This disparity should be reason enough to adjust our terminology and speak of puberty only when we refer to the somatic process and reserve the term adolescence to denote the psychological changes. These latter changes reflect psychic and social adaptations to puberty. While this is generally true, we must not forget that adolescent psychological change does not merely cope with the present somatic event of puberty, but is equally, perhaps more urgently, called upon to integrate the individual's immediate social reality with a still active past and an anticipated future.

Summarily I might say that puberty is an act of nature and adolescence, an act of man, emphasizing the fact that neither the completion of physical growth, the attainment of sexual functioning, nor the social role of economic self-support are reliable indices for the termination of the adolescent process. Additionally, one might be interested in the history of the word "adolescence" which literally means becoming an adult: the word appearing for the first time in the English language in 1430, referring to the period between childhood and adulthood, from fourteen to twenty-five in the male and from twelve to twenty-one in the female.[1] It is obvious from the usage of "adolescence," five centuries ago, that a parallelism between psychological, psychosocial, and physical growth was disclaimed. The usage of the word implied that the adolescent personality reaches adulthood in almost total chronological independence from sexual maturity. Similar observations, especially with reference to college students, have led some investigators to interpose a developmental stage, called "youth" (Keniston 1971) or "late- and post-adolescence" (Blos 1962) between adolescence and adulthood. Erikson (1956) has suggested the term "psychosocial moratorium" to denote this period. I view this extension of preadult life as the terminal stage of adolescence because the typical

6

psychological development of this period, called consolidation, is a direct continuation of the adolescent process. Just as any developmental stage of childhood, if extended beyond its timing or normative limit, generates a pathological nucleus or a manifest disturbance, so adolescence also has its time of closure, be this a normal or a pathological one.

I must examine, a moment longer, the issue of the developmental continuum and the adolescent phases which constitute it. As pointed out earlier, puberty follows a clearly delineated pattern of physical growth. However, in the realm of emotional development of personality and character formation during adolescence we have to rely on inferences from clinical data. These, in their totality, constitute the theory of adolescence, borrowing its basic assumptions from psychoanalytic psychology. Among these we are familiar with the adolescent revival of protolatency or early childhood learnings, predilections and conflicts which are reworked again. These conflicts, including the most crucial and prominent oedipal conflict, are resuscitated by the advent of puberty. This formulation is usually understood as the reexperiencing of a conflict that was settled long ago by identification, repression, and sublimation, thereby establishing latency. Briefly, this outlines the psychoanalytic recapitulation theory of adolescence. It postulates that the oedipus complex was resolved, for better or for worse, at the end of early childood and reappears, essentially unchanged, at puberty when extrafamilial sexual objects are to be sought, found, and gained.

From my therapeutic work with young and late adolescents a more complex picture has emerged. It is apparent that the resolution of oedipal conflict at the end of the phallic phase is normally partial. There remains a suspension of oedipal issues in détente, which nevertheless establishes definitive thresholds of conflictual anxiety, narcissistic vulnerabilities, and idiosyncratic coping styles. We might say that the settlement of the oedipus complex thus achieved was the most effective and developmental one which the ego of the child, at this tender age, could attain. During adolescence, however, a continuation, not only a recapitulation of the oedipal conflict, becomes apparent. What I have found most revealing in observing the fate of this particular childhood conflict at adolescence is the incomplete settlement or the suspended conflict of the reversed, or negative, oedipus complex: the child's love for the parent of the same sex.

Psychoanalytic theory has always emphasized the bifold tendency (one being normally dominant) of infantile object-directed sexuality which culminates in the oedipal constellation. The suspended conflict of this attachment always comes to light in adolescent therapy and presents a formidable obstacle within the context of oedipal transferences. Pubescence, by its very nature, bestows on this highly ambivalent attachment a sexual quality, discernable in fantasies or by dramatization during treatment. Since the resolution of the negative oedipus complex has to be accomplished during the latter part of adolescence, and since the attainment of sexual identity is predicated on this resolution, it is only to be expected that issues of a homosexual nature constitute an inherent aspect of any adolescent psychotheropy or analysis.

The defensive maneuver in relation to the negative oedipus complex often takes the form of a hostile or aggressive attitude toward the parent of the same sex and an obstinate, even obsessive and intractable clinging to the positive or heterosexual component of the oedipus complex. The child's oedipal attachment to the parent of the opposite sex is reactively pushed into the foreground. Observation in adolescent analysis has shown, over and over again, that the boy's oedipal love for his father or the girl's for her mother, remain unreachable, or well defended, for some time. It is no easy task for the therapist to tease out such Janus-faced issues and deal with them therapeutically in accordance with their essential references. Normally, the adolescent is eminently assisted in the resolution of these internal conflicts by the advanced and advancing ego, by a widened social awareness and, particularly, by the psychological support he received and gave as a member of the peer group.

Due to the continuation, not merely the repetition, of childhood conflicts, I propose to extend psychological childhood to the termination of adolescence. In supervision I have found that psychiatrists with training and experience in child therapy use this experience to advantage in adolescent therapy by applying child therapeutic techniques and insights whenever appropriate. Usually, it is a quite arbitrary decision by the therapist—a trial and error approach—as to where typical child therapy should end and adolescent therapy begin. Too often, this decision amounts to nothing more than the peremptory introduction of an adultomorphic model of therapy.

It might seem to you that I have wandered far afield from my essential topic. I can only assure you that everything I have said so far is essentially related to the thoughts I will presently develop. It must be apparent that I intend to formulate normative reference points of development, or psychologically defined criteria, that allows us to draw the demarcation line of adolescent closure. Physical status, sexual status, social status, and cognitive level have all proven to be unreliable indices, even though they avail us of the pursuit of an answer to our original question. The psychological assessment of an individual's developmental status is a most elusive one. Yet, in order to attain a meaningful answer to the question of adolescent closure, it constitutes the indispensible reference point. The ego, Hartmann (1964) once said, is defined by its functions. With reference to the present inquiry, I submit an extension of Hartmann's thought, that it is the degree of coordination and integration of ego functions, old and new, that defines the completion of any developmental stage. In describing and defining developmental stages, the concept of developmental tasks or challenges has been found particularly useful. In what follows, I take this very approach to answer the question of "How?" the termination of adolescence can be determined.

There are, no doubt, phenomenological criteria that have been recognized by both laymen and professionals in their efforts to define the end of adolescence. Notice the gradual decline of the typical adolescent mood swings, which finally reach a point where a state of relative composure is attained. Emotions are now selectively and discriminatively veiled from society and become privileged communications between friend and lover. This capacity of selectively sharing some aspects of the self with either the private or public worlds, without feeling divided or wrenched apart, is a sign of passing or completed adolescence. The attempt to understand oneself renders the need to be always understood, by specific persons or by the larger social order, less urgent, less uncontrollable, and less exacting. This novel characteristic of the consolidation phase, or late adolescence, can also be described by saying that the predictability of behavior and motivation waxes over time in constancy and accuracy until character stabilization has replaced tentative and arbitrary predictions within the established pattern of individual conduct.

If we conceive of character as the automatization of behavior that allows no alternative, then we can point to another typical aspect of adolescent closure. Character formation reaches a condition of definitive stability at the end of adolescence when ego autonomy, allied with the ego ideal, partially and effectively challenges the dominance of the superego. This agency of the mind that reigned supreme during childhood and evoked a continuous struggle between insurrection and submission, attended by feelings of omnipotence or helplessness, guilt or shame, during adolescence undergoes a critical revision within the motivational system. In consonance with the consolidation of the late adolescent personality, it follows that the emergence of a life style, a purposive striving toward reasonably attainable goals, has become feasible if not mandatory. While most adolescents are not offered an abundance of choices and options by the circumstances of their lives, even here a projection of oneself into the future remains indispensable.

To these phenomenological signs of adolescent closure could be added the gradual transformations in personal and communal relationships, in the direction of discriminatory involvements and ultimate commitments both within the private and public realms of individual needs and aspirations. Must I add that the vicissitudes of relationships or their relative liability remains a lifelong concern, causing infinite disruptions and corruptions of personal and communal life everywhere and always? Whenever, in good faith, the consolidation of late adolescence has done its work, the structure of any personality will persist if relatively benign circumstances prevail. With this perhaps pessimistic comment on the human condition, I conclude the discussion of the phenomenological criteria relevant for the determination of adolescent closure and turn to the more reliable and crucial psychological criteria. We find this verified in professional encounters with adolescents who have failed to traverse the developmental terrain of late adolescence. The impact of maturational, developmental, and social mandates leaves these late adolescents with no course but to terminate adolescence in some form of psychopathological accommodation.

When I spoke earlier of developmental tasks and challenges, I was well aware that such entities are isolated only for the purpose of assessment and discussion. I will now present four developmental tasks which, collaboratively and synergetistically, lead the individual adolescent into adulthood.

The Second Individuation Process

It is commonly known that the adolescent must disengage himself from infantile dependencies. Anna Freud (1958) has referred to this as the "loosening of the infantile object ties." Borrowing terminology from Mahler's (1968) research in early childhood I will discuss the second individuation process of adolescence.

Infantile individuation proceeds in relation to the mother. During the separation-individuation phase and by a process of internalization, the mother emerges as a discrete object. In other words, the formation of object- and self-representations establishes the boundary between the internal and the external world. The internalized parents and, through them, the internalized culture, remain relatively unchallenged until puberty. When adolescence occurs, old and familiar dependencies as well as infantile love and hate objects are drawn anew into the emotional life of the developing child. The object disengagement through individuation at the adolescent level does not proceed only in relation to external objects as it did in early childhood, but also in relation to the internalized objects of later childhood. A characteristic cathectic shift which signals this disengagement is seen in the libidinal cathexis of the self, resulting in the proverbial and transient narcissisism of the adolescent. This narcissistic grandeur rarely fails to elicit its counterpart, namely, the sense of nothingness, or helplessness and that of despair or object-loss. These well-known affective states are akin to mania, depression, and mourning. In short, the mood swings of adolescence are a corollary of the second individuation process.

From treatment we know how infantile object attachment appears in numerous disguises; of these the attachment to fantasies and to quasidelusional states deserves our special attention. Their stubborn resistance to being left behind as the price of maturation reflects the wish to enshrine for good those infantile object attachments that have acquired an extraordinary importance for psychological survival. It must be remembered that infantile parental imagos perpetuate the belief in perfection.[2] With the advent of adolescence, this notion is challenged as never before; a critical deidealization, or humanization, of the infantile world order is called for. The reflection of this disillusionment has a more or less devastating effect on the adolescent's sense of self. Even if the parents or their societal representatives are perceived by the adolescent as bad or evil, the polarity of the beneficent and nurturant infantile object always looms in the background of the adolescent's mind as a realizable alternative. Thus, the adolescent strives to contradict Heraclitus' saying that "you can never step twice into the same river."

The conflictual constellation of the second individuation process can be observed most dramatically in certain forms of dramatization. In cases of this kind the internal conflict is experienced as one between the individual and the environment; the conflict is externalized. The developmental reel, so to say, is played backwards. Much of what we see as adolescent rebellion is an attempt to surround the object(s) of love and hate. The imperfections of social institutions become the wholesale target of aggression; they become internalized. As such they are endowed with intentionalities, perpetrating frustration, and humiliation in the adolescent when need for support in the pursuit of self-realization reaches a critical peak. The imperfections of the wider world to which the adolescent turns upon leaving the dependencies of childhood are bound to upset his narcissistic balance. In the narcissistic rage that follows, the adolescent either succumbs to defeatist, sullen resignation (passive aggression), to psychotic regression, or he sets out to shape a perfect world by force. Incapable of resolving the internal state of dependency, the mechanism of externalization is resorted to with the aim of creating a new and perfectly gratifying world; the imperfections of the old have to be eradicated by whatever means will serve this purpose. This resuscitation of infantile narcissism temporarily wards off the disillusionment in self and object by the projection of evil onto social institutions and the concrete as well as the symbolic mandates of society. The student rebellion of recent times has brought these developmental dynamics to my attention through radical students who were my patients. The same dynamics are applicable to other epochs and other social arenas in which the second individuation process is enacted in one form or another.

In order not to be misunderstood I must add here a word of caution. Adolescent maladaptation always points to serious defects, inconsistencies, archaisms, and corruptions in the social order. It takes historical and political astuteness to bring about needed changes; no doubt, some late adolescent rebels have acquired these faculties. To consider all adolescent, radical, reformist activism, be this political or social, as mere projection, externalization, or displacement is nothing but simplistic nonsense. I do not conceive of the revolutionary or activist personality to be developmentally regressed or arrested, taking recourse to the externalization of emotional disharmonies. Behavior alone never renders a reliable assessment of any individual's developmental status nor does it reveal the inner workings of a motivational system. In fact, a valid case could be made for the contributory role which the non-conformist adolescent plays in the renewal of societal patterns.

Ego Continuity

The second task or challenge which the late adolescent has to meet in order to bring the adolescent process to a close is the achievement of *ego continuity*. For the child to survive in the world into which it is born, it needs for many years the support, guidance, and orientation provided by care-taking persons. In this extended psychological ecosystem, the parents function as extensions of the child's ego. Adolescence alters this state radically. During normal adolescence, the growing child cannot but use an advanced cognitive faculty and somatic maturity to gain emotional, moral, and physical independence. This is the period when the adolescent forms an individual past, present, and future. The past is, retrospectively, subjected to a kind of historical reality testing. Here we witness the ascent of self-conscious man who, as never before, has become aware of the unique, yet ordinary, life that lies between birth and death. Existential anxiety cannot be experienced before adolescence; the same is true for the sense of the tragic.

Disturbances in the formation of ego continuity or its clinical pathology are most clearly reflected in cases of a particular reality distortion. In such cases a reality misrepresentation was wilfully inflicted on the child's mind. As a result, the child accepted as real what he was told to be real; thus sacrificing the veracity of his own perception and cognition. This kind of reality distortion is to be kept distinct from psychotic delusion or the contamination by a psychotic parent or primal scene traumatization. The pathogenetic factor lies rather in the unavailability on the conscious level of circumstances the child once shared with others, but was afterwards, by gesture and innuendo, forbidden to acknowledge as real. In such cases, disturbances in reality testing are always a part of the clinical picture. A brief reference to a clinical example shall make this clear.

A seventeen-year-old delinquent boy was brought to me by his maternal uncle because incidents of truancy, shoplifting, forgery of checks, and lying had reached the point of serious legal consequences. The culprit's attitude was one of resignation to the fact that he was "fated to become a criminal." He showed none of the aggressive and defensive indifference nor downright oppositionalism we frequently observe whenever acting out is, at least partially, based on simple impulse discharge. The boy told me that he has no memory of his father because he had lost him while stil an infant. He had never known him; his mother had told him about his father's death.

From the uncle who had taken a fatherly interest in his nephew, I learned a piece of family history that contradicted these facts. Briefly, the father had been sent to prison for embezzlement when the child was six years old. Preceding this event, father and child had lost contact for a few years after the parents' divorce when the patient was three. According to what the mother had told me, the father died in prison and she was a widow. The child accepted this fact and never again asked a question about his father. In his own mind the child had predated the father's death to a time when he was an infant, thus eliminating all possible memory of image and affect. They were both replaced by the sense of being fated to become a criminal, thus resurrecting and rescuing the father image by identification. In fact the father was alive in a prison hospital for the criminally insane. Time does not permit me to go into the labyrinthine search for a lost past. But I must mention that treatment was initiated by my telling the boy the facts about his father's life or, conversely, of his mother's lie. As always in such cases, the patient reacted to this information as if he were told what he had always known, even if unconsciously. With the gradual restoration of his personal history, or ego continuity, the delinquent behavior lost its compulsive character.

It became clear that delinquent acting out in this case was an abortive, maladaptive effort to rescue the integrity of his perception and cognition, even though it was contradicted and declared illusory by the strictures of his environment. A follow-up after ten years presented the following picture: criminal behavior had long since become a matter of the past; besides having built his own personal life and a satisfying career, he had regularly sent to his father those material comforts which, so the son felt, would make his hopeless existence more endurable. From his mother, on the other hand, he had become distant, even though he kept up a perfunctory family tie. I may add that my telling the boy his factual history was based on the assumption that a reality distortion which is willfully imposed from the outside on the child has to be rectified by a rational or truth loving environment of which the therapist is the representative and guardian. Only then could treatment begin and proceed to the child's self-initiated distortions of reality and their dynamic as well as genetic implications.

Residual Trauma

The third challenge or task is related to the concept of residual trauma. I consider it axiomatic that trauma is an inevitable, injurious experience of the infantile period. Whatever the accommodation to or neutralization of these noxious jolts to psychological growth, there remains, nevertheless, at the end of adolescence a residue that challenges the adaptive resourcefulness of the late adolescent. Idiosyncratic vulnerabilities due to residual trauma are part of the human condition. Even heroes and semigods had to live with them: Achilles had his vulnerable heel by which Thetis held him when she dipped the infant into the river Styx to fortify him against mortal injury. Mythology tells us that such extraordinary protection against "the slings and arrows of outrageous fortune," are acquired only during babyhood and youth and never without a minor, accidental miscarriage of the intended absolute invulnerability.

That aspect of trauma that is never resolved nor resolvable, far from being a lamentable impediment, is a universal predicament that provides a driving impetus to its mastery. This persistent impetus propels the late adolescent into a more or less definitive set of commitments of a personal as well as an impersonal nature. The master of traumatic residues proceeds within the scope of those opportunities which societal institutions and social communalities offer, such as training facilities, work associations, ideological affiliations, and intimate relations of various kinds. In this sense, we might speak of a socialization of the residual trauma during late adolescence. This process coincides with the waning intrusion on the motivational system by infantile fantasies and their transposition or relegation to the world of daydream, playfulness, and restorative communality—from bullfighting to reciting poetry. In essence, the residual trauma serves as an organizer which promotes the consolidation of the adult personality and accounts for its uniqueness. The socialization of residual trauma is heralded in therapy whenever the young patient assumes the responsibility for his own life, tolerating a modicum of tension, and ceasing to mourn the death of infantile fantasies and expectancies.

Sexual Identity

I will now discuss the fourth and last challenge in my schema of developmental criteria in relation to adolescent closure, namely *sexual identity*. This concept is distinct from gender identity, which is established early in life.

Formation of sexual identity is predicated on the transmutation of the sex-inadequate component of the sexual drive into a new psychic structure, the ego ideal. What I have in mind is the transmutation of the infantile, narcissistic ego ideal into the adult abstracted and desexualized ego ideal. It is a common experience in adolescent therapy that this forward step is an extraordinarily difficult and slow process; requiring the relinquishment of infantile self- and object-idealizations. An unabated perseverance on infantile aggrandizement precludes the formation of stable, adult object relations. Sexual activity per se is, obviously, no indication of adolescent closure and offers no assurance that sexual identity has been achieved. Formation of sexual identity requires no clinical example, because the many ways in which the failure to transcend this developmental challenge as it manifests itself in psychopathology and in therapy are too well known.

Conclusions

Within the present context, it is impossible to pursue the complexity of this subject any further. However, I want to stress one point, namely, the intrinsic interconnections between sexual identity formation and deidealization of self and object. I am convinced that a review of your own experiences with adolescent patients will provide my proposition with a verifiable self-evidence.

The four structural criteria I have outlined were derived from my work with adolescents because they had served me well over time, and served to order my clinical observations. However, it should be understood that the four developmental challenges or tasks which I have defined represent integral components of a total process. All four act synergistically and in unison; their developmental resolutions are global; one without the other can never bring about a normal termination of adolescence. Due to this interconnectedness of the four challenges, it is possible to gauge, from the assessment of a component aspect, the relative progress toward adolescent closure as a whole. Ultimately, however, it is the integration of the four challenges, or the nodal intersection of the four coordinates that assures us with reasonable certainty that the developmental stage of adolescence has reached termination. I know very well that this formulation is an ideal one, rarely or never encountered in real life, and should be looked at as a schema. Experience tells us that unresolved psychological issues are always bound to remain; it is, however, their stable integration into the adult personality—the work of the consolidation stage—that gives these persistent issues a patterned and rather irreversible structure. The characterological stability, thus attained, signals that adolescence has passed.

NOTES

1. *The Compact Edition of the Oxford English Dictionary,* (1971). Oxford: Clarendon Press.
2. For a detailed discussion see, Blos, P. (1976). The split parental imago in adolesclent social relations, an inquiry into group psychology. *Psychoanalytic Study of the Child:* 31: 7-33.

REFERENCES

Blos, P. (1962). *On Adolescence.* New York: The Free Press of Glencoe.
Erikson, E. H. (1956). The problem of ego identity. *Journal of the American Psychoanalytic Association* 4: 56-121.
Freud, A. (1958). Adolescence. *Psychoanalytic Study of the Child* 16: 225-273.

Hartmann, H. (1964). *Essays on Ego Psychology*. New York: International
  Universities Press.
Keniston, K. (1971). Youth as a stage of life. *This Annual* 1: 161-175.
Mahler, M. S. (1968). *On Human Symbiosis and the Vicissitudes of
  Individuation*. New York: International Universities Press.

2] CHANGING VALUES: THEIR IMPLICATIONS FOR ADOLESCENT DEVELOPMENT AND PSYCHOANALYTIC IDEAS

AARON H. ESMAN

For a psychoanalyst to choose the effects on values of a changing society as a subject of discussion may appear odd, since psychoanalysis is supposed to be a value-free science and the psychoanalyst, one who dispassionately eschews value judgments, seeking only to understand the behavior of patients and to aid them in forming or clarifying their own moral codes. A moment's reflection, however, will dispel any sense of incongruity. Even if this picture be an accurate one, the scientific study of values and their place in human psychology is, as Hartmann (1960), Brierley (1947), and others have shown, surely within our purview. Indeed, those of us who are professionally concerned with adolescents know that the consolidation of values is one of the crucial issues of this developmental phase and is thereby a matter of major scientific interest. I suggest that much of the clinical and social phenomenology of adolescence, particularly of late adolescence, can best be understood in this context.

Beyond this, however, I shall hope to show that psychoanalysis is itself deeply implicated in a value system of its own that significantly influences both theory and practice. I believe that a clear recognition of the psychoanalytic value system is necessary, at this time, to help us to adapt both our theory and our practice to the cultural climate in which we now exist.

Freud (1905) was able to suggest, by quoting a contemporary, that what is moral is self-evident. In the milieu in which he lived and worked, few who cared would have quarreled with such a statement. The social structure was clearly demarcated, the rate of social and technological change was slow and measured, and a long tradition of Judeo-Christian values held sway in

18

Western society. Even though Nietzsche (1882) had recently proclaimed the "death of God," those outside the dominant tradition were generally regarded as inferior, deluded, or degenerate.

Clearly, no one can make such a statement as Freud's today. The "transvaluation of values" of which Nietzsche spoke has set in with a vengeance. Morality itself is no longer self-evident, and is virtually impossible to discern. Certainly it is impossible to set forth generalizations about moral or ethical values in almost any sphere that will not be seriously challenged in some quarters. Even those supposedly immutable values graven into the tables of the law given to Moses on Mt. Sinai are subject to disputation. Consider: the death of God undoes the first commandment; the importation into our Western world of Eastern cults negates the second; ubiquitous profanity in the name of "open communication" blasphemes the third; the appalling scandals around care of the elderly give evidence to the perversion of the fourth; seven days a week shopping centers and weekend atheletic events violate the fifth; war hawks and terrorists who constitute themselves as "liberation armies" make mockery of the sixth; the new sexuality morality as preached by such as Alex Comfort (1972) subverts the seventh; youthful "rip-off" artists who rationalize stealing in the name of social protest transgress the eighth; the disclosure of the Watergate felons and similar perjuries in the name of "national security" defile the ninth; and the ubiquitous envy of the possessions and life-styles of others reduce the tenth to a pietism.

In a brilliant survey of the phenomenon of value change in our time, Trilling (1972) has shown the historical evolution of the decline of "sincerity" and the rise of "authenticity" as dominant attitudes in literature and in social intercourse. Sincerity, he suggests, is concerned with one's relations with other people, and is a value embedded in a stable system of class and personal relationships. Authenticity, on the other hand, seems to reflect a self-oriented system where one is concerned with the fidelity of one's own self-expression regardless of its consequences to others. It suggests, as Trilling says, a primacy of the id in contrast to the superego emphasis in sincerity. Can it be that this change in values parallels the rise in psychoanalytic concern with problems of narcissism, acting out, and the decline of the classical neurosis?

In any case, the value system that lies at the heart of psychoanalysis—the primacy of reason, the acceptance of delayed gratification in the service of future goals, the idea of stable monogamous heterosexual bonds, and a commitment to a lifelong career ("love and work")—each of these values is in question now in the setting of kaleidoscopic social and technological change that puts all of us, to some degree at least, in that state which Toffler (1971) has called "future shock." It is a setting in which one third of all marriages end in divorce, in which monogamy is being replaced by serial marriage, and in which the largest selling book in the United States is titled "Joy of Sex," whose much-praised author explicitly advocates extramarital experiments. It is a setting in which rapid technological change tends towards the obsolescence of technical skills that require either repeated and constant retraining, the frequent shifting of vocational involvements, or precocious retirement. It is a setting in which homosexuality is represented as merely one of a number of possible choices of sexual behavior and bisexuality is widely proposed as the ideal. It is a setting in which children and adults are subjected on television to an unceasing diet of violence, murder, and mayhem that numbs the sensibilities and promotes a cool acceptance of brutality and dehumanization. It is a setting in which the new irrationalities of drug intoxication, spiritual power, and Eastern mysticism are proposed as being of equal value to, indeed of greater value than, traditional Western logic and scientific method; where, indeed, the very enterprise of science is depreciated or at times coopted, as in the current vogue for bio-feedback. It is a setting in which psychosis is represented as a reasonable and healthy response to a sick society and in which we are treated to a return of the myth of the "holy fool." About this, Trilling says:

> No expression of disaffection from the social existence was ever so desperate as this eagerness to say that authenticity of personal being is achieved through an ultimate isolatedness and through the power that this is presumed to bring. The falsities of an alienated social reality are rejected in favor of an upward psychopathic mobility to the point of divinity, each one of us a Christ—but with none of the inconveniences of undertaking to intercede, of being a sacrifice, of reasoning with rabbis, of making sermons, of having disciples, of going to weddings or to funerals, of beginning something and at some point remarking that it is finished.

Finally, it is a setting in which the major traditional sources of cultural values—religion, the tribe or clan, the family, the political establishment—have lost either their credibility or their very essence.

Just twenty years ago, Gardner (1957) made a similar statement at a time to which we now look back with nostalgia as an era of relative stability and simplicity. I can only add that our times are a quantum leap beyond in their complexity and stressfulness.

All this, however, is familiar. I do not aim to deliver a jeremiad, or to declare that "the time is out of joint." Our concerns here are: first, what effects do these sociocultural phenomena have on the process of adolescence in our time and, second, how if at all does this affect the corpus of psychoanalytic ideas?

Regarding the first question, it is my impression that these phenomena have rendered the process substantially more difficult and precarious than it was at other times and places. Offer (1969) has presented evidence that the classical psychoanalytic picture of adolescent turmoil has been overdrawn and that the normal adolescent, at least in the suburbs of Chicago, passes through this phase with minimal psychological disruption. I have no doubt this is so. And yet, can we not see in the recent rise of interest in adolescent psychiatry indirect evidence of an increase in casualties at least among those young people who lie at the far end of the spectrum of vulnerability? Such reports as those of Deutsch and Ellenberg (1973) suggest that those young people who refer themselves to a college mental health service are uniformly suffering from more than adjustment reactions. They show in almost all cases significant and definable long-term psychopathology.

A clinical illustration will highlight some of these issues. I recall an appealing, asthenic, gifted young man who came to me first at seventeen in the throes of recovery from the last in a series of bad LSD "trips." He had become and was still obsessively preoccupied with questions of his own personal worth, with feelings of will-lessness, of mediocrity, and lack of direction. In his last year of high school he was performing in mediocre fashion despite intellectuality and literary talent. He could see little or no purpose in anything he was doing and ruminated at great length on existential questions.

This young man was the first of two products of a marriage that had for years been only nominal. His father, a highly successful professional, had withdrawn emotionally from the family in growing disaffection from an increasingly alcoholic wife. It was impossible to say which began first, the alcoholism of the one or the disengagement of the other, but by the time Jonathan turned to me the two were equally extensive. The father came home only to sleep and the mother was drunk when she was not engaged in maintaining a face to the community. Jonathan and his two-years-younger brother prepared their own meals—irregular and at times dangerously inadequate—and cared for their own part of the house. They were essentially unsupervised and received virtually no emotional support from either parent. Jonathan's deep craving for nurturance from his mother and direction from his father was, and remains, one of the most poignant aspects of his psychology.

It was clear that Jonathan's extensive experiments with hallucinogens, undertaken in the company of peers of generally similar background, represented a pathetic quest for the meaning, purpose, and affectivity he could not derive from his parents or from society. Frightened by his recent experiences, however, he gave up drugs—permanently, it developed—and turned to psychotherapy. With its support he succeeded in finishing his year at school and gaining admission to a new experimental college with high academic expectations but little or no structure.

There, his passivity and lack of direction again asserted themselves, so that within a few months he was devoting most of his time to playing poker and ruminating about his inability to study. He turned to the college counseling service, but the counselor's exhortations and confrontations failed to modify Jonathan's behavior. Again, failing to complete his second term academic contract he withdrew and returned to therapy with me. I have seen Jonathan for two years now. The first year he worked in a family business and lived—at nineteen—with a girl with whom he began a liaison at college and who out of her own desperation and clinging dependency had followed him to New York. He was a relatively passive partner in this affair, resentful of the burdens she imposed on him and emotionally disaffected from her as his father had been from his wife. Yet, Jonathan was unable to express his resentments or detach himself because of his fear of destroying her by any aggressive or assertive act. Chronically short of funds, he occasionally participated in marijuana deals in order to raise money with no evident feelings of guilt or conflict.

This year he has returned to college, attending a local university while living in the family home, now occupied by his divorced father and his paramour who live as man and wife though unmarried. Essentially the same pattern of emotional detachment exists among them as did while the mother was present. Jonathan used this move as the occasion to divest himself of his girlfriend. Now, however, deprived of regular sexual activity, he has at times been drawn to the easily available homosexual outlets, has occasionally cruised homosexual areas, and has toyed with the idea of joining the "gay lib" group at his university. He minimizes conflict about this, contending that one way is as good as another, and his deep shame is evidenced by the hesitation and obvious reluctance with which he discusses these matters in therapy.

Now twenty, Jonathan has yet to commit himself to a career goal. He would like to be a writer, but he sees no economic future in it and, since he enjoys the luxury that his affluent father has provided for him, he feels no calling to a vocation that may be economically precarious. Alternatively, he toys with entering his father's profession, but retards that possibility as a cynical compromise with the bourgeoisie.

Jonathan exemplifies, I believe, many of the problems besetting the contemporary adolescent as he struggles through what we have thought to be universal developmental issues—the maturation of sexual identity, the commitment to vocation, and the consolidation of values. A decade or more ago Jonathan might not have turned to homosexuality to deal with his heterosexual deprivation. In the current climate, however, in which homosexuality is not only tolerated but valued as an expression of authenticity in the face of hypocritical bourgeois moralism, Jonathan found social support for this turn. I do not state here whether I consider this to be good, bad, or anything else, but I am certain that it is a different situation which makes adolescent consolidation of sexual role and object-choice a more diffuse and less defined process than hitherto.

In his earlier childhood, Jonathan was deprived of any credible source of ethical values or existential meaning. At its best, the modern family has great difficulty in the face of gradually dwindling functions, crumbling social supports, and the growing sense of ethical relativity. Increasingly, therefore, young people turn outside the family for such values and sources of meaning—traditionally, at least for the more thoughtful among them— to art, literature, music, philosophy, and political ideology. Most recently, however, they have turned in large numbers to mystical and exotic religious sects and gurus that offer a sense of certainty, prefabricated and usually puritanical moral codes, and a system of restrictions that repress those drive impulses that may be found threatening (Johnson 1975). Intellectual-ly unable to accept this sort of solution, Jonathan felt unanchored, unsure of his values, awash in a sea of moral relativism.

The tenuousness of Jonathan's emotional commitment—to ideals as well as to people—was of course a reflection and an extension of his parents' lack of commitment to him as a person: they were not so much hostile to him as they were indifferent and detached. His father, seen as a moderately benign but unsupporting figure, had been always remote and unavailable. His mother related to Jonathan as a would-be personification of her unfulfilled aspirations, demanding high levels of performance and expecting of him rigid adherence to her haut-bourgeois way of life, offering him in return little warmth, affection, or tenderness. Jonathan's capacity for passion was stunted, his affectivity blunted, and his ability to engage

23

himself deeply with anyone or anything curtailed. His only true love was literature which early became a source of solace, and, through writing, a means for discharging some of his feelings of loneliness and muted rage.

No doubt, young men like Jonathan have been with us for generations. The fragmented family is not an invention of our time, and anomie was not born in 1945 with the impact of the atomic bomb. I would suggest, however, that there are many more such young men and that Jonathan's is the typical pathology of our time, as the oft reported decline of the classical neurosis in psychoanalytic and psychotherapeutic practices would suggest. Certainly the recent upsurge of interest in problems of the self, evidenced by the work of Kohut (1971), Kernberg (1970, 1974), and others would seem to bear this out. Our usual patient is not the hysterical young woman or the obsessive compulsive young man. Our usual patient is the bewildered, undirected, vaguely dissatisfied, passive, sexually undifferentiated youth of either gender for whom our task is less often the resolution of unconscious conflict than the repair of disordered development.

As I have pointed out, Jonathan's family is fragmented. In other ways, however, it is typical of the family of our era—the small nuclear family of parents and two sibs—as it has evolved in the face of urbanization, mobility, generational separation, the extrusion of the elderly, and the decline of the house servant and hired hand. I believe that this phenomenon has contributed significantly to the shape of adolescence. By focusing the child's early object relations on only two significant figures it has intensified oedipal conflicts and, equally, the struggle to overcome and emerge from them that is characteristic of the early and middle adolescent years. The young person's repudiation of his parental ties—and, with it the sense of loss and need for reattachment—is raised to a higher pitch by the intensity of the early attachments and the absence of alternative objects in the form of grandparents, benevolent uncles and aunts, wise handymen, and so forth. It is, of course, possible to sentimentalize the extended family of the past, but I have the distinct impression that the relatively rootless, isolated nuclear family of our time is often a pressure cooker of intense and potentially explosive object ties that generates a centrifugal force for its young members or, alternatively, cements them into passivity with unresolved bonds that cripple their autonomy. Equally, the absence of significant parent surrogates depletes the store of alternative sources of nurturance and emotional support for those, who, like Jonathan, have parents that cannot or will not support them.

Paradoxically, further difficulties confront our young people in the very process of differentiating themselves from the familial matrix. The increasing technological complexity of our culture has led to an almost indefinite extension of the process of becoming that defines adolescence. Higher education, once the prerogative of a select few, is now virtually a requirement for any but a dead-end menial occupation. As a result, hundreds of thousands of young people are impressed into the college treadmill who have no particular interest in learning in its own right, but are maintained thereby in a fully or semidependent state far beyond the time of their physical maturity. It seems clear to me, at least, that the latent resentment engendered by this situation was one factor that contributed to the campus rebellions of the late 1960s. Now, of course, many of these young people are confronted with the spectre of unemployment after their graduation, raising to an even higher pitch the sense of meaninglessness and futility of the whole enterprise. College counselors with whom I have met speak of a pervasive aura of depression, particularly among students in the community colleges, generating at the same time the dogged grade-grubbing that is now seen as the one possible way out of the morass. But of meaning, of a sense of intellectual adventure, of the joy of learning, little, I gather, is to be seen on the campuses of today.

The sexual revolution and the new feminism represent an additional clutch of factors that, in my view, serve to complicate the consolidation processes of late adolescence. A whole new set of demands and expectations has arisen that, at least for the middle-class urban adolescent, offer further opportunity for the undermining of self-esteem. Our young men now expect themselves not only to be potent in the pursuit of their own sexual pleasure but to satisfy their partners by providing them with the invariable orgasm that sexual equality demands. Failure to meet these expectations—or fear of such failure—has generated a sharp increase in potency complaints among young men, as documented by Ginsberg, Frosch, and Shapiro (1972), among others.

Conversely, many of those young women who have been convinced by Sherfey (1966) and others that orgasm—and multiple orgasm at that—is their sexual due on every occasion of intercourse regard any deviation from this pattern as a sign of failure, deficiency, frigidity on their parts or sexual incompetence on the part of their partners. Ignorant of the variabilities of sexual potential, of the irregularities of rhythms and rates of excitement and discharge within the normal range of variation, they conceive of sexual performance as a natural phenomenon in which learning, practice, and experience play no role. This mystique of the orgasm may interfere seriously with the integration of sexuality into a synthesis of body and mind, promoting its use as a tool of interpersonal conflict, and tending to divorce it from its affective correlates. Thus we have such a new Don Giovanni as a certain egregious magazine publisher, cataloguing his conquests of over two thousand women as though this were a proud achievement rather than a pathetic confession of affective incapacity. Gagnon (1974) has said that among contemporary adolescents, sex has become "like MacDonald's hamburgers," by which I assume he means that it is easy to get, cheap, and essentially tasteless.

In addition, the revolution of rising female expectations has served to raise the level of the traditional battle of the sexes to a full-scale war, with intense suspicion and mutual fears of exploitation and status challenge. (For evidence, see virtually any novel written by a young woman in the past five years.) The atmosphere of hostility is a veritable breeding ground for problems of potency and sexual dissatisfaction. Can this be the source of the outpouring of literature that seeks to promote technical solutions to the joylessness of sex?

The new sexuality and women's liberation have made great contributions to society in freeing it of some of its accretions of hypocrisy and inequity. For many young people they have been truly liberating influences. But for many—again, the vulnerable ones—they seem to have added additional stresses to the developmental process.

I would suggest then that the effects of the sociocultural and technological phenomena I have referred to earlier has been to make the process of maturation more difficult than it has ever been before. I believe that Offer (1969) was correct in suggesting that most adolescents will develop ego-coping capacities that will enable them to get through the process with relative success. Unfortunately, the proportion of those who will falter along the way has grown.

Adolescence is at best a period of major developmental stress in which support is needed from various sources to promote optimal maturation. I suggest that our society does not now offer such support for many of our young people, that the traditional institutions of our society are increasingly failing to function in ways that can provide such support, and that the more vulnerable members of the group passing through this phase are manifesting signs of this failure in increasing psychopathology. There is, I believe, in all times and places a scale of vulnerability to adaptive failure. In an ordered society with clear structure and functioning institutions the developmental support offered will place the line high on the scale, while in a situation such as I have described the line will be further down the scale and more will succumb. The essence of the pathology will doubtless be similar—the same fundamental conflicts and developmental issues will be involved—but the outward forms will be shaped by the available social conditions and cultural norms. Perhaps there is, as Heilbroner (1975) has suggested, in the end no great difference between the crowds of youthful pilgrims to the Astrodome seeking salvation from the Guru Maharaji and the throngs that have gone to Lourdes or the shrine of Guadelupe with the same hopes. It is equally true, however, that there is a direct correlation between the numbers seeking salvation at such shrines and the level of disturbance in the social fabric. It is precisely those young people who cannot turn for solace—or for meaning—to the traditional social institutions that are following the siren song of the new gurus. Others, surely at the far end of the scale of vulnerability, are swelling the ranks of adolescent suicides, whose numbers have, as Hendin (1975) and others have pointed out, grown dramatically over the past ten or fifteen years.

Now, in our second question—What does all this imply for our body of theoretical ideas and their application?—the latter area, that of clinical application, is easier to discuss. I have pointed out elsewhere (Esman 1972), as have others, that psychoanalytic clinical theory, and most particularly its judgments of what Anna Freud (1965) calls "normality and pathology" are deeply rooted in a framework of culturally determined values. I recall, for example, that in my childhood the subject of divorce was generally spoken of *sotto voce,* and the general view was that any divorced person, particularly a divorcee, was thereby degraded and pathological. Though somewhat gross, this picture would, I think, apply to our own evaluative notions which have until recently included the tacit assumption that one who is over thirty and unmarried was suspect, that one who is unable to sustain a marriage once entered was probably immature, and that one who, married, elected to remain childless was reluctant to assume adult responsibilities. Yet in the current socio-culturo-economic scene such judgments, perhaps valid in some cases, cannot possibly be held general or regarded as accurate guides to clinical assessment. Hendin (1975) in his study of Columbia University students found few young women who regarded marriage or motherhood as desirable goals.

More in regard to adolescence, it was only a generation ago that the use of psychoactive drugs, beyond, perhaps, an occasional experiment, was regarded as a token of serious pathology. Marijuana was, in those innocent days, found only on the fringes of respectable society among blacks, delinquents, and jazz musicians. Now, of course, we have come to the point at which Jonathan's ultra-middle-class, law-abiding, politically active stepmother has asked him and his brother for a supply of "pot" for a Christmas present. I would even venture to say that there are many professionals who have had some experience with it. Here then, is a classic illustration of the way in which social change affects our values, including professional values and the supposedly objective judgments we base on them.

Hartmann (1960) has said that the only values to which psychoanalysis is committed are "health values." How are we to define health values today? Those that place a premium on adaptation? To what average expected environment? Those values that foster flexibility as opposed to rigidity? Does flexibility encompass opportunism? Bending to the wind? Bisexuality? Trying everything? Is adherence to the work ethic adaptive or maladaptive in a time of growing unemployment, reduced work weeks, and rampant consumption values? Is a commitment to monogamous heterosexuality healthy? Or is it an uptight hangup? Ticho (1968) talks of her difficulty in assessing the conduct of a respectable, upper class male patient she saw after her arrival in South America following her emigration from Vienna. This man was a regular and guiltless patron of the thriving bordellos in his cosmopolitan city. In Vienna such conduct in a man of his class would have been regarded as distinctly pathological; in Rio de Janeiro it was conventional behavior. Are we all in a position similar to Ticho's today? It is certain, at any rate, that genitality will no longer serve as the index of psychic maturity. The aim and object of the libido are less likely to serve us as such indices than is the affective quality of the relationship to objects.

For many of my generation, at least, work with adolescents and young adults approaches in its complexity cross-cultural investigation, where the therapist is obliged to learn a new language and a new and often strange value system. Though the relentless now-ism fostered by the combination of war and affluence seems to have been replaced by an equally dogged and rather desperate careerism born of economic crisis and disillusion, a pervasive mistrust of adult values and attitudes remains. It is embodied in the rock music and drug cultures which, in the silliest rhetoric of the last decade, Reich (1970) suggested would lead to the "greening of America." They have instead remained in reality underground subcultures with which we must, anthropologically, make contact. In their extremity, however, they reflect the pervasive value shifts that have direct relevance to the conduct of our clinical work with patients of all ages today.

The difficulty of spelling out some of the broader theoretical implications of recent social change, are, of course, far greater. It needs hardly be said that the fundamental elements of what Rapaport (1960) has called "general theory"—the idea that behavior is integrated, that it is meaningful, that it is part of a genetic series, that the crucial determinants are multiple and unconscious—are no more subject to modification than are the concepts of transference and resistance in the clinical theory. Nonetheless, adaptation of our theoretical model to changing conditions and growing knowledge are essential if we are to maintain it as a vital, scientific instrument.

Psychoanalysis originated as a psychology of conflict. In its early days it developed a special focal interest in the conflicts of the oedipus complex which came to be seen by Freud and his followers as the nuclear and crucial elements in human psychological evolution. Even now, with the growth of ego psychology, there are those who, despite so firm a commitment to structural concepts that they are led to the position that all prestructural ideas should be relegated to the dustbin of history, still maintain this view of the central role of the oedipus complex in psychological development and therefore in analytic work and theory.

For many of us, however, the new breed of patients together with the relatively new data of infant and child study tend to throw at least as much weight on the side of developmental disorder as on that of specific unconscious conflict. More and more we find that as analysts and therapists we are concerned with the repair of developmental failures rather than resolution of discrete pathogenic conflicts. If we agree that, as stated earlier, we deal with a spectrum of vulnerability, we must be at least as concerned with the causes of such vulnerability as we are with the conflicts—generally more or less universal—to which our patients fall prey. Thus our recent concern with the problems of narcissism, of separation-individuation difficulties, of addictions, and borderline states, all lead us to some fundamental reconsideration of what are indeed the central issues in clinical theory.

From the work of Mahler, Greenacre, Winnicott, Escalona, and others we are increasingly impressed by the crucial importance of very early experience and maturation in shaping basic personality configurations. Loewald (1962, 1973) has convincingly explicated the critical role of early interactional processes in the development of those psychic structures which form the stage on which the preoedipal and oedipal conflicts are played out. We have not even begun to understand the influence of television on development—in a world in which by age three young children spend at least as much time with the TV set as they do with their parents. Is it possible that the four to five hour-a-day bombardment by visual imagery and ready-made fantasies—never mind the content—does

29

not have a significant affect on the child's way of seeing the world and of regulating his drives? Cohen (1975), an eminent educational researcher, has said:

> Analysis will show that it is not farfetched to hypothesize a relationship between certain kinds of child behavior now appearing and the technology in children's lives, especially such behavior as resistance to expending effort, even when the goals are child-appropriate goals; inability to tolerate frustration and time delay in the pursuit of gratification, even when these are required for self-chosen tasks; mistaking titillation for genuine learning; decrease in imagination and play; an easy-is-best orientation to life; confusion between image and reality; fear of coping; and a tendency toward shallowness of feeling and superficiality of thinking. Such behavior, taken together, has the look of aborted ego development and the mark of anomie and alienation.

Already, the children she describes are today's adolescents.

On the other hand, our traditional assumption that basic personality patterns are set for all time by age six is very much open to reassessment. Erikson (1950), Blos (1967), and others are making us more aware of the plasticity of early personality and its responsiveness to later developmental influences, particularly in adolescence. As Werman (1974) has discussed the differences between the college students of 1968 to 1969 and 1974 to 1975, "In view of the importance we attach to the early years of life for personality development, how can we explain the apparently massive shifts in (overt) youthful behavior in as short a time span as five years?"

Thus, it seems that psychoanalysis must increasingly become a psychology of development rather than merely a psychology of conflict. As Silverman, Rees, and Neubauer (1975) have put it:

> We are referring to a shift in emphasis from a formulation which depicts the oedipus complex as the cause of the neurosis to one which would consider the oedipus complex as a dynamically central feature of a developmental process which may or may not predispose to neurotic solutions of developmental tasks.

In metapsychological terms, we are forced to consider the primacy of genetic as opposed to dynamic issues.

But further, we are obliged, not by social changes but by increased scientific sophistication, to reconsider whether the economic point of view is of any real value at all in understanding the operations of the mental apparatus. All of us are more or less enmeshed in habitual linguistic patterns in which we find it comfortable to employ such usages as "discharge," "cathexis," and "neutralization" and to reify and anthropomorphize psychic structures, despite our awareness of their limitations as scientific concepts (cf. Grossman and Simon 1969). But in the new world such terminology will prove less useful and tenable and will, I believe, tend increasingly to isolate us from the rest of the scientific community. It is particularly striking, incidentally, that Kohut (1971), the man who has most decisively moved us away from the closed system, fluid level model of viewing self- and object-related interests and motives, is himself most fixed and unswerving in his dedication to the use of economic concepts and pseudoexplanatory "libido economic" jargon. Schafer (1972, 1973a, 1973b) has, I believe, discerned one way in which we can accommodate our theory to new concepts of language and thought in a scientific world that is less and less tolerant of analogic, metaphoric, or anthropomorphic usages. Klein (1970) suggested another approach through which psychoanalysis could, by focusing on clinical, phenomenological data regarding aims, wishes, purposes, and meanings in their developmental context, purge itself of archaic "process" explanations and return to its basic purpose—the exploration and explications of motivations in human psychology.

Conclusions

Let me be perfectly clear. I am not proposing that psychoanalysis seek to accommodate theory to the shifting winds of social change, or, alternatively, that it seek to provide explanations for broad social phenomena. As Heilbroner (1975) stated, there is and will be no psychoanalytic theory of the business cycle as there is not and will never be an adequate socioeconomic theory of dreams. But I do suggest that psychoanalysis must, perhaps more than before, be prepared to reexamine some of its general and clinical theoretical assumptions in the light of changes in the social matrix within which it operates. Just as we must insist on holding to what is sound and timeless in our theoretical structures, we must as well be willing to modify or abandon what time and experience have proved perishable.

Forty-five years ago, Freud (1930) said:

Men have gained control over the forces of nature to such an extent that with their help they would have no difficulty in exterminating one

31

another to the last man. They know this, and hence comes a large part of their current unrest, their unhappiness and their mood of anxiety.

Today we can see this mood magnified by a sense of loss of control—not over nature, but over those very technological resources of which Freud spoke. If psychoanalysis is to speak to our time, it must, through what Freud called the "small voice of reason," make some contribution to allaying this sense of helplessness—or, at the least, to understanding it.

REFERENCES

Blos, P. (1967). The second individuation process of adolescence. *Psychoanalytic Study of the Child* 22: 162-186.

Brierley, M. (1947). Notes on psychoanalytic and integrative living. *International Journal of Psycho-Analysis* 28: 57-105.

Cohen, D. (1975). The technological distortion of the child's world: The loss of interaction. Presented at American Association for the Advancement of Science Annual Meeting, January 1975.

Comfort, A. (1972). *The Joy of Sex*. New York: Simon and Schuster.

Deutsch, A. and Ellenberg J. (1973). Transience vs. continuance of disturbances in college freshmen. *Archives of General Psychiatry* 28: 412-424.

Erikson, E. (1950). Growth and crises of the healthy personality. In *Identity and The Life Cycle*. New York: International Universities Press, 1959.

Esman, A. (1972). Review of Toffler, A., "Future Shock." *Psychoanalytic Quarterly* 41: 143-145.

Freud, A. (1965). *Normality and Pathology in Childhood*. New York: International Universities Press.

Freud, S. (1905). On psychotherapy. *Standard Edition* 7: 267 (quoting F. T. Vischer). London: Hogarth.

———(1930). Civilization and Its Discontents. *Standard Edition* 21: 64-145. London: Hogarth.

Gagnon, J. (1974). Quoted in New York Society for Adolescent Psychiatry Newsletter, January 1975.

Gardner, G. (1957). Present day society and the adolescent. *American Journal of Orthopsychiatry* 27: 508-517.

Ginsberg, G., Frosch, W. and Shapiro, T. (1972). The new impotence. *Archives of General Psychiatry* 26: 218-220.

Grossman, W. and Simon, B. (1969). Anthropomorphism: motive, meaning and causality in psychoanalytic theory. *Psychoanalytic Study of the Child* 24: 78-111.

Hartmann, H. (1960). *Psychoanalytic and Moral Values.* New York: International Universities Press.

Heilbroner, R. (1975). Personal communication.

Hendin, H. (1975). *Youth in Crisis.* New York: W. W. Norton.

Kernberg, O. (1970). Factors in the psychoanalytic treatment of narcissistic personalities. *Journal of the American Psychoanalytic Association* 188: 51-85.

———(1974). Contrasting views regarding the nature and psychoanalytic treatment of narcissistic personalities: A preliminary communication. *Journal of the American Psychoanalytic Association* 22: 255-267.

Klein, G. S. (1970). The ego in psychoanalysis: A concept in search of identity. *Psychoanalytic Review* 56: 511-525.

Kohut, H. (1971). *The Analysis of the Self.* New York: International Universities Press.

Loewald, H. (1962). Internalization, separation, mourning and the superego. *Psychoanalytic Quarterly* 31: 483-504.

———(1973). On internalization. *International Journal of Psycho-Analysis* 54: 9-18.

Nietzsche, F. (1882). Die Frohliche Wissenschaft, quoted in Kaufman, W. (1968), *Nietzsche: Philosopher, Psychologist, Antichrist* (3rd edition). Princeton, New Jersey: Princeton University Press.

Offer, D. (1969). *The Psychological World of the Teenager.* New York: Basic Books.

Rapaport, D. (1960). The structure of psychoanalytic theory. In *Psychological Issues* 2. New York: International Universities Press.

Reich, C. (1970). *The Greening of America.* New York: Random House.

Schaefer, R. (1972). Internalization: process or fantasy. *Psychoanalytic Study of the Child* 27: 411-436.

———(1973a). The idea of resistance. *International Journal of Psycho-Analysis* 54: 259-286.

———(1973b). The concepts of self and identity and the experience of separation-individuation in adolescence. *Psychoanalytic Quarterly* 42: 42-59.

Sherfey, M. (1966). The evolution and nature of female sexuality in relation to psychoanalytic theory. *Journal of the American Psychoanalytic Association* 14: 28-128.

Silverman, M., Rees, K. and Neubauer, P. (1975). On a central psychic constellation. *Psychoanalytic Study of the Child* 30: 127-157.

Ticho, G. (1968). Cited in Jackson, S., Panel report: aspects of culture in psychoanalytic theory and practice. *Journal of the American Psychoanalytic Association* 16: 660.

Toffler, A. (1971). *Future Shock*. New York: Random House.

Trilling, L. (1972). *Sincerity and Authenticity*. Cambridge: Harvard University Press.

Werman, D. (1974). Personal communication.

3] DISCUSSION OF
AARON H. ESMAN'S CHAPTER

RICHARD C. MAROHN

Dr. Esman's thesis is that psychoanalysis has its own value system which "significantly influences both its theory and its practice." Characterizing this value system as "the primacy of reason, the acceptance of delayed gratification in the service of future goals, the idea of stable monogamous heterosexual bonds, and a commitment to a life-long career (love and work)," he notes that these values are under considerable assault today, and wonders what effects sociocultural changes have had on the adolescent process and on psychoanalytic theory. The changes to which he refers can be partially characterized in the observations of Trilling who has noted the decline of sincerity in relations with other people and the ascendancy of authenticity which reflects a self-oriented system of self-expression. I would not agree that this is paralleled by a shift from superego to instinctual primacy, for indeed sincerity and authenticity can be closely related, though the former involves an interpersonal focus and the latter, an individualistic or intrapsychic. It may well be, as Dr. Esman comments, that there is a parallel between this value shift and increasing interest in psychoanalysis in problems of narcissism and the self.

The increased interest in adolescent psychiatry, like the increased interest in problems of narcissism, need not suggest increases in pathology in either of these realms. These shifts may be the result of new discoveries, new conceptualizations, and newly described configurations to which we had heretofore been blinded. The case of Jonathan is suggestive of a new kind of pathology, though we must keep in mind the possibility that the Jonathans emerge because of our new found abilities to see narcissistic problems. Jonathan's search for self-objects in girlfriends and boyfriends and our young peoples' fervent devotion to new religious and mystical ideals is, indeed, part of the focal adolescent process of divergence from internalized and archaic parental representations to newly created identifications of one's own which ultimately become consolidated into some sort of internal self-regulating system. In the meantime, bereft of parental self-support systems, the adolescent binds himself slavishly to a myriad of narcissistic relationships. The fact that young people are turning "increasingly" outside the family for their new identifications does not seem a significant change; it has always been that way, and such is the nature of adolescence.

Prolonged adolescence has frequently been attributed to the increasing complexity of our culture and the long-term demands of higher education. Higher education, though, may actually facilitate the separation-individuation process insofar as it provides the late adolescent with a variety of new peer experiences and throws him more decidedly on his own internal regulating devices. The work of higher education, however, is primarily in the conflict–free area, and I believe we must be careful not to equate the completion of one's training and the assumption of meaningful career work with the closure of the adolescent period. Adolescence is an internal process characterized by shifts of internal value object ties, as well as by the integration and mastery of genital sexuality and increased aggressive urges. Career pursuit need not be the outstanding herald of the close of adolescence except to the judges of a work ethic society. And one could say that certain youths who are able to work at these adolescent tasks in a slower, less hurried way (this may be one reason Offer (1969) finds less turmoil in his sample) are able to work through the separation and integration issues without the peremptory displacements and reversals that Anna Freud (1958) described.

However, I do agree with Dr. Esman that contemporary pathology seems different. Boredom, depression, alienation, and the search for stimulation signify values and internal regulators that, not idealized, provide the self with little gratification, and result in a chronic sense of depletion. As Kohut (1975) has suggested, the somewhat explosive, seductive, incestuous, dramatic, and multiple object relationships of the families of yesterday required defenses for such dangerous and stimulated drives. The vitality of the seductive young mother, the rage of the punitive father, the envy associated with sibling rivals, the stimulation inherent in extended families who live together, the expanding and open frontiers where motherhood, childbearing, and child-survival were all important, probably produced different kinds of problems best characterized as conflicts, internal and neurotic. Today, the older, less vibrant mother, the more controlled father, the fewer, if any, siblings, the distant aunts and uncles and grandparents, the closed bedroom doors, may produce different pathology, subtle chronic deficits, perhaps not because of the "intense and potentially explosive object ties" that Dr. Esman suggests, but perhaps because of the very lack of intensity of current family life in which we are now too sophisticated to idealize, admire, respect, fear, love, struggle with, or dream.

It is certainly true, then, that the adolescent process is experienced by many as diffuse and ill-defined as one gropes to separate from representations that are themselves diffuse and ill-defined. Yet the diffusion and poor definition exists also for the psychoanalyst, the therapist, and the researcher. Whether Jonathan today turns to homosexuality and years ago turned to football, booze, or heterosexuality may simply reflect cultural variations on a long-existent theme of problems in tension regulation and lack of adequate structuralization. It would appear that the sexual revolution has not eliminated neurosis, but only served to confuse some of us who work in this field. Oedipal guilt may now appear as sexual hyperactivity whereas before it took the form of sexual inhibition. Yet we must also consider the possibility that the problem may, in part, be due to issues of self-esteem regulation, self-cohesion, and tension modulation. Yes, it is true that one can now compulsively and perfectionistically search for an orgasm everytime, just as before one was scrupulously chaste. However, I am not sure that the new liberation movements have added "additional stresses to the developmenal process." Are they really additional, or are they simply different?

One way of viewing the issue of our society providing less support for young people to regulate these value shifts as the traditional institutions of society crumble, is to paraphrase questions raised by Klumpner (1972) about the role in adolescence of the secret academic societies described by Wolf, Gedo, and Terman (1972). Just as Klumpner wondered whether these societies really facilitated the separation process, or whether they should be more accurately described as manifestations of the internal shifts that were occurring, we might ask ourselves if it is necessary for a society to provide supporting institutions for its children or whether, indeed, the children, themselves, will create institutions and other manifestations by means of their own intrapsychic activity. Perhaps more significant is the issue of whether or not the representations from which they are shifting are well-defined and available, rather than whether or not the society provides other well-defined and available supports to facilitate the shift.

In addition to our newfound vision, we are also dealing with more numerous developmental failures. But I am not sure that the values of psychoanalysis have changed; our theory still tells us that behavior is meaningful, has genetic roots, and is unconsciously determined. Therapeutically transference and resistance still occur, but perhaps in new forms. The use of marijuana can be judged similarly as the use of alcohol. As therapy has always been devoted to the patient experiencing and realizing his potential it does not necessarily include judgments about monogamy, divorce, and career.

But some things are different today. Our adolescents are given the rights of adults; they commit suicide, they are bored, and they grope as they attempt to separate from something with which they were never united. Dr. Esman's chapter reflects and integrates much of what our colleagues have begun to understand about this process.

REFERENCES

Freud, A. (1958). Adolescence. *Psychoanalytic Study of the Child* 13: 255-277.

Klumpner, G. H. (1972). Discussion of E. Wolf, J. E. Gedo, D. M. Terman (1972), "On the Adolescent Process as a Transformation of the Self." Presented before the Chicago Psychoanalytic Society.

Kohut, H. (1975). Personal communication.

Offer, D. (1969). *The Psychological World of the Teenager.* New York: Basic Books.

Wolf, E. S., Gedo, J. E., and Terman, D. M. (1972). On the adolescent process as a transformation of the self. *Journal of Youth and Adolescence* 1: 257-272.

4] ON CHILDREN'S RIGHTS AND
THERAPEUTIC INSTITUTIONS

DEREK MILLER AND ROBERT A. BURT

Legal rules regulating access for adolescents to residential facilities offering psychiatric care are currently being reexamined by both courts and legislatures. In the past, the law has provided two paths into such institutions: placement by an adolescent's parent or by the juvenile court. Both routes provided the adolescent no legally sanctioned voice in the matter. Regardless of whether he or she wanted such a placement or protested it, adult authority made the legally recognized decision. New rules, however, are being offered which replace parental authority by stipulating that hospitalized adolescents may protest their placement, thereby obtaining court review with representation by appointed attorneys. To liberalize juvenile court authority, a new ethos is being proclaimed that courts may take custody of an adolescent only to protect society, never solely to protect the adolescent from self or environment.

Critiques of the old law begin by revealing the manifest inadequacies of residential facilities for children and adolescents, particularly those under the aegis of the juvenile court. But in their effect, these critiques sweep beyond these well documented targets to include all psychiatric hospitals for children. They reject any therapeutic possibility for any psychiatric facility without the explicit consent of the adolescent. These critiques rest on a fundamental misconception of adolescent psychology. If they are accepted by courts and legislatures, the results will disadvantage those adolescents who need psychiatric services, their families, and the rest of society that might also benefit from the successful provision of such services.

The purpose of this chapter is to sketch those critical aspects of adolescent psychological development which must be considered in any

39

decision for psychiatric residential placement. The issue of adolescent consent will be reviewed in the context of developmental psychology. A role for court supervision of adolescent psychiatric placements that achieves a fundamental sympathy with the psychological needs of adolescents will be identified.

Techniques of Intervention in Adolescent Maladjustment

Whenever adolescents are involved with social systems designed to control their antisocial behavior or personality maladjustment, certain principles should apply. Interventions with any adolescent may be nonspecific and nonindividualized, or specific and individualized (Knesper and Miller 1976). The former includes social, educational, psychological, and biological interventions designed to offer maturationally appropriate protection and reinforcement of developmental strivings; physical, educational, and psychosocial. Specific interventions involving the same subgroups are individualized to deal with the unique problems of each child. Before either intervention is invoked, however, adequate diagnosis is essential. The etiology of the presenting problems, the effect of these problems on society, their influence on the attitude of others, and the effect on the personality development of the adolescent, require clarification.

If interventions are to be optimal, adolescent techniques of communication, which differ from those of adults, require illumination. Depending upon maturational age (a concept which involves an awareness of physical and psychological maturation), adolescents may be significantly concrete in their thinking (Piaget 1963) and have little or no affective awareness that the future is influenced by actions in the present. Adolescents are both self-referent and altruistic, impulsive and omnipotent, easily depressed, and very sensitive in perceiving themselves as persecuted.

Regarding communication, words may be considerably less significant than action. Least meaningful in infancy, words obtain optimum communicative meaning by adulthood. Autonomous middle-class adolescents may be able to give words abstract significance, while lower socioeconomic groups usually retain concrete thinking for some considerable time. Abstract thought carries a maximum capacity for future orientation. Yet, the nearer an adolescent from any social class is to physiological puberty (usually early adolescence), the more likely is adolescent verbalization concrete.

The most significant communication techniques of adolescents are behavioral; these include a number of devices:

1. Acting Out: Impulsive relief of internal tension or externalizing internal conflict by the conscious or unconscious manipulation of external reality.
2. Acting Up: Socially unacceptable behavior apparently designed to test the adult capacity for care and control. Some types of delinquent behavior may fall into this group.
3. Play Acting: Experimental behavior designed to gain personal experience of the world and the environment, to test oneself. Sexual activity may initially involve this.

All these techniques of communication may become developmental stumbling blocks when so much gratification is gained from them that growth becomes impossible, or when emotional immaturity makes movement from that developmental level impossible. Words themselves may be an action communication. Adolescents struggling for autonomy may defy authority and, for example, deny any need for adult assistance: thus, acting out independent wishes; acting up to test the strength of the external world; play acting, the experience of defiance. The denial may also occur because verbal agreement is perceived as an inappropriate surrender.

Although it is clear that society provides an inadequate range of facilities for disturbed and disturbing adolescents, it is questionable whether psychiatric adolescent treatment facilities are a special problem. General inadequacies in this area are, however, blatant. There are insufficient medical and psychiatric outpatient facilities for the young; training in understanding the physiology and psychology of the age group is inadequate; society lacks adequate educational resources for disturbed children; good community group homes are few and far between. Long stay residential care, whether in or out of hospitals for adolescents who need it is almost nonexistent.

Legislatures and courts have not significantly attempted to redress these inadequacies. But, for reasons which are not yet clear, these bodies have recently chosen most dramatically to intervene in parent-child relationships in the provision of psychiatric treatment (Ellis 1974). The Supreme Court has considered a case in which a lower court required an appointed attorney to represent every child placed by his parents in a residential psychiatric institution.[1] One state court has recently provided that adolescents may themselves decide to leave treatment at age sixteen unless they are committable under adult standards.[2] One state legislature provides that adolescents of thirteen may invoke court hearings to protest their parents' placement decision, and that treatment personnel must initiate "therapeutic" contact with the adolescents by "warning" them of these rights.[3]

These rules disregard central issues of adolescent psychology. Inevitably in adolescence there is a covert and often overt conflict between parents and child, if only because the latter is struggling for autonomy. The legal rules which automatically gave unexamined authority to parents to make significant decisions on behalf of their children previously supported the stable urban, rural middle-class, and artisan nuclear family: historically, units of a stable network of human relationships. To some extent, the law reinforced a preexisting sense of worth, which adolescents gave to parents even though conflicts might exist. Paradoxically, the more adolescents are able to make meaningful stable relationships with peers and extraparental adults, the more are they able to deal successfully with autonomy issues in their families and to retain a positive relationship with their parents (Miller 1974).

However, the more children are isolated from stable social networks, the greater the stress on the relationship with their parents. A need exists for such parents to be invested with the support of society at large. The legal system should represent the positive mores of the society, but recent changes ironically reinforce the weakening of the nuclear family—a weakening produced by societal instability and an increasing isolation due to horizontal and social mobility. Legal changes have reinforced the likelihood of nuclear family disintegration, particularly with those adolescents whose relationship with their parents is, in any case, difficult.

In many states, adolescents may have treatment for venereal diseases or drug abuse without the knowledge or consent of parents (Riatt 1975). There are, as yet, no figures to indicate whether this type of intervention is successful. Clinical psychiatric evidence reveals that when authority figures act with children against their parents, even implicitly, the results of treatment are not generally satisfactory. If the law reinforces the pseudo-autonomy of adolescents rather than a real autonomy, by implying that parental intervention will be unsatisfactory, it is likely that results will be equally disappointing.

Parents tend to be blamed by society for the misbehavior of their children, but it has been impossible to find any current evidence in the technical literature, or anywhere else, indicating that parents of recent decades have been able to use the psychiatric system to place psychologically disturbed children in residential facilities without proper cause. The subtleties of family dynamics have rarely been understood by the legal system, which appears to believe that truth can be arrived at by adversary techniques that strives, albeit without success, to deal with absolutes. Such an approach to human behavior occludes the ambiguous issues of unconscious parental collusion and provocation of disturbed behavior (Miller 1974), the need of some parents to maintain family homeostasis by maintaining the maladjustment of their children, and the reinforcement of disturbed behavior by the vicarious satisfaction it may give parents. The problem in the psychological treatment of disturbed adolescents appears to be the reluctance of parents to support therapeutic endeavors, not their anxiety to place their youngsters.

The law is now making a substantial intervention in the area of residental treatment of adolescents recognized as psychologically disturbed, though there seems to be no rational reason for focusing reformist zeal on psychiatric inpatient facilities where they exist. The legal concept approves the right of juveniles to decide on actions affecting their lives and freedom, unless found incapable of making reasoned decisions. Adolescent's rights will be protected by offering individual court hearings for those patients who verbally protest against the initiation or continuation of treatment. At times, adolescents attempt to use this type of legal intervention to bargain about the amount of responsibility they feel they should have within psychiatric hospital settings, thus invoking legal authority, which by definition requires submission, against medical authority, which should be based on an alliance with expertise (Miller 1976).

The attitude that adolescent's rights will be protected by court hearings mirrors the traditional legal attitude toward the rights of the mentally ill; if the need is verbally denied, treatment should not be insisted upon unless the individual is dangerous to himself or others. Ironically, this approach makes it more difficult to provide helpful services for the young, because such youths tend to deny in words their need for help.

Now the result of this legal change is that those adolescents who can currently be treated in inpatient psychiatric facilities may not get it there or anywhere else. It is almost inevitable that psychologically disturbed adolescents, who are still able to struggle for autonomy, must defy authority by denying in words that they need help. The more immature the adolescent, the more intense is the struggle, along with a primitive, self-referent stance, which implies that everyone and everything should be subordinate to the adolescent's wishes. These are the youngsters who most vociferously deny the need for help. Unfortunately they often have parents who are least able to withstand this type of pressure.

A fifteen-year-old boy was referred to a psychiatrist because his parents had heard him on the telephone discussing drug abuse. When interviewed, he revealed that he was using street drugs moderately,

43

but also that he was a very active dealer, although only a middle man. He talked of his dealing with much affective coldness and indicated that his goal was to make as much money as possible. He said that if his father attempted to interfere with him, he would have to use physical force to stop him. When an inquiry was made about this, he said that he kept a knife and gun at home. He would carry either one to school every day in order to protect himself against possible attack by other students, but he had never yet been in a situation to need to do this. He said that if he was attacked, he would use his weapon.

This young man was a candidate for admission to a hospital in a state whose law invited judicial review of adolescent admissions. He seemed to have some minimal capacity to make meaningful emotional relationships with others, and thus might be potentially treatable. However, he refused to be admitted without a court order. His parents were quite unable to stand up to this possibility; they felt they could not risk having the judge refuse to have their son admitted and they indicated that they would then be fearful for their lives. Nothing was done. In the days when parental wishes and medical judgment was sufficient, such adolescents could have been hospitalized and successfully treated.

Many residential settings now refuse to consider admitting young people who are likely to be involved with the court; they feel that the treatment of disturbed adolescents is sufficiently difficult without the complication of attorneys who are easily seduced by adolescents, and who appear competitive with physicians, often because of the automatic application of an adversary relationship. Physicians may recognize their own defensiveness with attorneys and prefer not to be involved.

When adolescents are told that they have recourse to the court if they do not want treatment, they are likely to feel rejected. One boy said to his therapist:

> I know what you and Dr. T. and all of the ward staff mean when you tell me over and over again about my rights, and that I can go to court if I don't want to stay, and all that. What you really mean is that you don't want me.

Since most adolescents must deny their need for assistance by verbal protest, most adolescent admissions appear involuntary, particularly as parental assistance does not produce overt agreement.

Adolescents demonstrate willingness in action. Hospitals are entered with only token resistance or with no trouble. When young people run away from hospital settings, it is rare for them to arrange not to be caught, or not to return voluntarily. Running away appears to be a test as to whether or not parents want their adolescent children to be treated, or whether the hospital staff care enough about the well-being of the individual.

Most adolescents need to feel that they have some choice, even if this is not so. A legal commitment is likely to incite an adolescent to rebellion in order to assert independence, either by overt action or by emotional withdrawal. Legal insistence on adolescents going to a hospital is likely, even in good treatment settings, to lead to overcompliance, emotional withdrawal, institutional paranoia, and, occasionally, planned absconding. Furthermore, when an adolescent who is in the residential setting invokes the court in an attempt to leave, and the psychiatrist who treats the adolescent expresses the opinion that treatment should continue, the patient may feel that the therapist is being intolerably seductive.

A sixteen-year-old boy in treatment in a psychiatric hospital demanded a hearing, insisting that he should be released. A strong case was made by his psychiatrist for his retention in a hospital because of suicidal wishes. The court agreed that he should stay. The immediate response on the boy's part was that now he was in the hospital because the psychiatrist wanted him. However, in addition he began to lie by omission to his therapist; previously he had been quite honest and direct. He planned to abscond, and within a week did this most skillfully. On his return, he told his therapist that he had been planning to do this for a week before he left, and he said that he was not going to talk to his psychiatrist or to the staff again. Eventually his passive withdrawal convinced his parents that the boy ought not to be in the hospital. His attitude toward the psychiatrist was, "You forced me to be here, now do what you want with me," and treatment floundered.

•

Finally, if the court does not agree that the youngster should stay in residential care and recommends outpatient treatment, the psychiatrist who previously looked after the youngster is no longer able to do so. The psychiatrist's opinion has been so devalued by the court that it is highly unlikely that he will be of any benefit to the boy or girl in the future.

The request to invoke legal assistance may be looked upon therapeutically as an expected, initial communication from some adolescents who are either newly admitted to a psychiatric hospital or who are resisting internal characterological change. Prior to the present legal involvement with adolescent care it was not uncommon for individual adolescents who were admitted to psychiatric hospitals to challenge the worth of the individuals within the therapeutic system, by testing behavioral limits in a variety of ways including absconding. More recently, the legal system has been used in the same way.

The communication should be handled both in terms of external reality and for its therapeutic significance.

A fifteen-year-old boy was admitted to an adolescent psychiatric unit in a teaching hospital in a state wherein non-committed patients could give five days notice to leave the hospital. Unless legal intervention to force a continued stay was successfully invoked discharge was obligatory. The boy's admission had been precipitated by his attacking his father and a policeman with a knife when he was toxic on diazepam. He had a two year history of chronic drug use including alcohol, marijuana, hallucinogens, and hypnotics. He was also a drug dealer. Some three weeks after hospital admission he called the American Civil Liberties Union to establish his "rights" and he wrote out a formal request to leave the hospital. The therapist told him that he was in the hospital at the parents' request and that if they wished to go to court to seek his commitment the therapist would support this choice. If the therapist was required to give evidence about his clinical condition he would of course do this as he was of the opinion that the parents were right to want their son in the hospital.

In the event that the court found that the boy could be discharged he would have to have another physician because he knew that it was important to him that his psychiatrist be seen as a worthwhile person. If the law contradicted his doctor's opinion this meant the opposite of this. On the other hand if the law agreed with his doctor's view the therapist felt sure that he would feel as if all his freedom of choice had been taken away by his doctor which would be intolerable. All this meant that either way he would have to get another psychiatrist. The boy's immediate response was to tell his doctor to go to hell. Four hours later he said that he had torn up his "five day notice." The young man was discharged from inpatient care two months later, continued in outpatient treatment and four months after the above episode was living at home, making A's at school, dealing competently with his distended family, and avoiding both drugs and alcohol. He complained that some of his old friends did not know of the many exciting aspects of the city in which he lived. His expressed wish at this stage of therapy is to be a policeman who has studied "psychology and criminology."

The episode described might legally be termed "coercive." Without question the clarification of the reality that would occur was helpful and the boy's expressed vocational wish is a striking identification with the attitude that is often thought necessary to treat individuals suffering from antisocial disorders of personality.

Legal preoccupation with the psychiatric treatment of adolescents may be based on a proper concern that young people receive adequate therapy, particularly in institutions. However, currently proposed legal reforms seem to be based on three inaccurate assumptions.

1. The parents of the disturbed children have no mixed feelings about wanting their offspring helped, and incline readily towards institutionalization. Clinical evidence proves this incorrect. It is inordinately difficult for parents to maintain their children in residential care.
2. Psychiatrists may keep children in hospitals for an unnecessarily long period of time. There is no evidence for this. The disappearance of a problem in a protective setting does not mean that the adolescent is now ready to live in the larger community. The issue is whether the problem is a typical response to stress of the individual concerned.
3. Adolescents mean what they say. There is evidence that this is inaccurate.

Direct and explicit confrontation and the legal imprimatur of an adversary relationship between the adolescent and helping agents at the time of admission, or at times of stress during hospitalization on the issue of whether the individual should remain, is therapeutically harmful. It dramatically interferes with the possibility of a successful resolution of issues concerning autonomy, which are at the heart of typical adolescent disturbances. The ultimate goal of psychiatric hospitalization is to provide adolescents with opportunities for unlocking their potential for successful and constructive confrontation with the adult world. This is the goal of therapeutic endeavors, it cannot be their precursor.

The law apparently is interested in guaranteeing legally defined patient rights. To psychiatrists, this seems to ensure that an individual's needs will not be met. Individual court hearings to review adolescents placed in psychiatric facilities by their parents are not the best way to accomplish the goal of ensuring that abuse does not take place.

A Proper Role for the Courts

There is, however, a useful role for courts to prohibit abuses regarding adolescents in residential placement. That role cannot be played in individualized court hearings, but is possible in litigation enforcing "rights to treatment" generally for children in all residential facilities with an explicit therapeutic goal. The Supreme Court has recently endorsed the proposition that involuntarily committed adults have a constitutional "right to treatment" in psychiatric facilities.[4] Lower courts have established wide-ranging standards to define and guarantee the content of treatment rights for involuntarily confined adults. More recently, this litigation has been extended to facilities for adolescents and younger children who are considered psychologically disturbed or mentally retarded (Burt 1976).[5]

Because these treatment rights, in the adult facilities, were linked to an involuntary commitment, courts have been reluctant to confer similar rights on all hospitalized children, and thus far have restricted their remedies to those children explicitly committed in court proceedings: an artificial limitation at best. It is clear that most children in psychiatric facilities, because of their parents' decisions, are placed without effective regard to their stated wishes and are thus involuntarily placed. It is further clear that, insofar as this parental placement power is sanctioned by law, the child's involuntary placement is achieved under state authority. Current legal reformers argue from these two propositions that a court hearing must precede every such placement as a matter of constitutional law. But this reasoning is not compelling. There are, in fact, competing constitutional norms at stake in parental placement of children. The constitutionally sanctioned logic that personal liberty cannot be deprived without due process of law requires mandating court hearings in each individual case. But the constitutional norm that parents have authority to make important child-rearing decisions without state interference points in a different direction (Burt 1975).[6]

The competing values expressed in these constitutional propositions can be accommodated, but not through the psychologically false notions that children are always victimized by their parents' placement decisions (and thus should have ready access to court protection), or that children are never victimized by such decisions (and thus always should be viewed as volunteering patients). Courts can accommodate both of the competing values at stake in parental placement decisions by viewing children placed in psychiatric facilities as voluntary patients, for one purpose—so that individualized hearings need not precede placement—but as involuntary patients for a different purpose—to permit courts to guarantee the right to treatment for children in *any* therapeutic residential facility. (Even private facilities are included by this reasoning, because parental placement authority comes from state law and thus children are placed by virtue of those laws.)

In deciding the precise content of the court-guaranteed treatment right, a balance must also be struck between the competing constitutional norms of maximizing personal liberty while deferring to parental child-rearing discretion. For this purpose, courts must scrutinize with special care the degree to which psychiatric residential placement in fact interferes with the child's personal liberty. Courts should be skeptical of all custodial aspects of such hospitalization. The use of locked wards, of isolation cells for individual youngsters, of physical and chemical restraints, and more generally restriction of contact with the extra-hospital community necessarily involved in geographically remote institutional placement—all of these elements should be rigorously disfavored by courts enforcing treatment rights in facilities for children.

If a psychiatric facility is located within a community, has many opportunities for contact by its residents with the extra-hospital community, and does not use more than token confinement within physical facilities, then hospitalized adolescents' right to personal liberty is implicitly safeguarded, while considerable weight is explicitly granted to parents' discretion in placement. The adolescent's liberty is protected in such facilities because of the implicit opportunities for the adolescent to protest his placement by running away.

For most psychiatrically disturbed young people, the implicit opportunity to run away, without pressure for an explicit commitment to stay, provides a reasonably accurate gauge of the patient's essential evaluation of the worth of their placement. And yet, importantly these absconding opportunities avoid the therapeutic trap (set by individualized court hearings) of forcing an explicit acquiescence or protest in response to hospitalization. When an adolescent runs away from an open institution and does not return spontaneously (or with a protest designed to save face) this should be viewed by therapeutic personnel as an indication that that individual's entire treatment needs review. When, in a significant number

49

of cases, such flight occurs this is an appropriate indication for external review agencies—peer review mechanisms perhaps overseen by judicial agencies enforcing treatment rights—to scrutinize both the overall worth of that facility's program and the techniques of treatment used for the individual.

Some psychologically disturbed adolescents should be placed in facilities with a capacity for effective security. Such placement should be reserved, however, for those adolescents who, if free in the community, will act in ways that are seriously dangerous to themselves or others. Placement in facilities with more than token security should be restricted to those for whom social control is found appropriate in a juvenile court hearing.

Individualized hearing as a prerequisite to secure placement would have the same psychological impact on the adolescent as discussed. But the visible security aspects of the placement itself and its confining impact on the adolescent in themselves have critically important (but not necessarily conclusive) antitherapeutic implications. The adolescent is forced, in such a secure facility, to sacrifice many autonomous values. The court hearing and its inevitable adversary posture does not reduce the antitherapeutic impact of the facility, but does give high visibility to the proposition that society has found it appropriate to interfere with the autonomy of the confined adolescent in extraordinary ways. The visibility of this proposition, resulting from court proceedings, can assist skilled therapists to confront the confined adolescent on precisely the reasons for his confinement and the dangerous antisocial or self-destructive implications of his conduct.

Such stark confrontation is appropriate for few psychiatrically hospitalized adolescents, and, for most, unnecessarily complicates therapeutic possibilities. It is thus critically important to invoke court hearings, and their explicitly confrontational modality, only for those cases where confrontation is already necessary due to the patient's problems and personality difficulties. To assume, however, that all residential psychiatric facilities for adolescents are equally prisons, no matter how open, estranges the possibility of therapeutic work for adolescents who are otherwise amenable to treatment. Legal rules regulating access of adolescents to psychiatric residential facilities should thus differ, depending on the critical differences among such facilities reflected by their degree of security. With this differentiation clearly drawn, the proper uses of residential psychiatric care and of differing degrees of security for adolescents can then be assessed.

Conclusions

The decision as to the type of residential placement required for disturbed adolescents must not be based solely on the severity of the adolescent's symptomatic behavior, but rather on the basis of how successfully that behavior can be contained within the context of human relationships— with parents, therapists, extra-parental adults, peers, and general social systems. For an adolescent who is drug dependent, absconding from home or school, or seeking nurture in sexual promiscuity, outpatient interventions are failures unless a very rapid adult attachment is made. Usually no individual can offer the adolescent the instinctual gratification which is obtained from these types of activities. When an adolescent's ability to make one-to-one relationships is inhibited, and thus antisocial behavior cannot be abandoned because of attachment to adults, intervention commonly fails. This failure may, however, be a function of inadequate training and the inability of adults to recognize the significance of their relationships with the young. For this cluster of problems, residential psychiatric care is appropriate, but that care need not be provided in secure facilities. This kind of residential care, however, removes the adolescent from a psychonoxious environment, and permits him to initiate problem solving which could not begin while he remained living in the community.

For more destructive problems—suicidal, homicidal, or seriously antisocial conduct—which cannot be contained within the context of an interpersonal relationship, more secure residential placement is appropriate. Yet, the very seriousness of the problems and the visibility of invoked social controls makes individualized court hearings also appropriate. At such hearings, the bases for predicting such conduct by the adolescent must be made explicit.

Such placements, though, should not be made solely on the ground that the community needs protection from the adolescent. There is an important reality, which should not be obscured, that such confinement can be equally (if not more) in the personal interests of the adolescent. In this country, the inadequate character of juvenile court placement facilities has acutely retarded such favorable results. The hypocritical promises for such benefits made by juvenile courts in the past have led many critics to urge abandonment not only of any rehabilitative rhetoric, but of any rehabilitative intention for any juvenile court placements. This seems to be the underlying premise of recent recommendations announced by the Commission on Juvenile Justice Standards, chaired by Judge Irving

Kaufman (New York Times 1975). In calling for fixed-term (and in some cases mandatory) incarcerations for juvenile offenders, and prescribing that the sentence term be fixed solely with reference to the "seriousness" of the offense, the Kaufman Commission is abandoning any attempt to make individualized dispositions based on the psychological characteristics and treatment needs of the individual offender.

As with currently proposed reforms for adult criminal justice, this kind of proposal has attractions for both conservatives and liberals. The conservative argument maintains that the rehabilitative intentions of the juvenile court only protects bad actors and encourages crime. But the notion that punitively intended incarcerations will deter juvenile crime has no relevance at all to the seriously characterologically disturbed adolescent. To such an individual, deterrence has little meaning. He is gratified by antisocial behavior, has little or no sense that present actions have future consequences, and is pervasively omnipotent (Giovacchini 1973).

For liberals, abandoning rehabilitative promises of the juvenile court appears attractive because most juvenile detention facilities currently provide only punitive incarceration. Society's past unwillingness to commit extensive resources to such facilities suggest the continuing hypocrisy of that promise. Though the task of designing effective treatment institutions for disturbed juvenile offenders is formidable, and though much social hypocrisy has attended previous efforts, nonetheless it is questionable that wholesale effacement of the rehabilitative ideal will serve any useful purpose.

The arguments seem to mirror adolescent delinquent reasoning. Magic answers are sought for complex problems, magic fails to work, and then punitive responses are taken. Punitive incarceration holds no potential as a solution for problems posed by the aggressively disturbed young. It only puts a social imprimatur on the currently unsatisfactory way of treating children in residential care which takes place under the auspices of the juvenile justice system, and would signal the end of any social commitment for improvement.

NOTES

1. Bartley v. Kremens. *Federal Supplement* 402: 1039-1058 (1975).
2. Melville v. Sabbatino. *Connecticut Supplement* 30: 320 (1973).
3. *Michigan Mental Health Code,* Section 330. 1417 (1974).
4. O'Connor v. Donaldson. *Supreme Court Reporter* 95: 2486 (1975).

5. Wyatt v. Stickney. *Federal Supplement* 344: 387 (1972).
6. Wisconsin v. Yoder. *United States Reports* 406: 205 (1972).

REFERENCES

Burt, R. A. (1975). Developing constitutional rights of, in and for children. *Law and Contemporary Problems* 39: 118-143.
———(1976). Beyond the right to habilitation. In M. Kindred, ed., *The Mentally Retarded Citizen and the Law*. New York: The Free Press.
Ellis, J. W. (1974). Volunteering children: parental commitment of minors to mental institutions. *California Law Review* 62: 840-916.
Giovacchini, P. L. (1973). Character disorders. *International Journal of Psycho-Analysis* 54: 2: 153-159.
Knesper, D. J. and Miller, D. (1976). Treatment plans for mental health care. *American Journal of Psychiatry* 131: 1: 45-50.
Miller, D. (1974). *Adolescence: Psychology, Psychopathology and Psychotherapy*. New York: Jason Aronson.
———(1976). The ethics of practice in adolescent psychiatry. *American Journal of Psychiatry*. In press.
New York Times (1975). Radical changes urged in dealing with youth crimes. 1: 1: November 30, 1975.
Piaget, J. (1963). *The Developmental Psychology of Jean Piaget*. Edited by J. Flavell. New York: Von Nostrand Reinhold.
Raitt, G. E. (1975). The minor's right to consent to medical treatment. *Southern California Law Review* 48: 1417-1456.

5] ADOPTION AND THE ADOLESCENT: AN OVERVIEW

ARTHUR D. SOROSKY, ANNETTE BARAN, AND REUBEN PANNOR

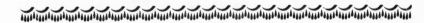

Adoptive family relations are subject to conflicts not found in the typical nuclear family. These conflicts create a particular stress on the adoptive parents with problems similar to those of having a handicapped child (Pringle 1967), or raising a minority child (Lewin 1940). The parental conflict is best epitomized by Seglow, Pringle, and Wedge (1972) who described the adopter as caught in a double bind: implored to "make the child your own but tell him he isn't." Kirk (1964, 1966) has emphasized that if adoptive parents can accept themselves as different than biological parents, rather than denying a difference, they will be better able to communicate openly with the child regarding his adoptive status and to handle any problems that might arise throughout his development with loving support, understanding, and empathy (Lewis, Balla, Lewis, and Gore 1975, Mikawa and Boston 1962, Smith 1963).

In the typical adoptive situation, the couple has accepted a child conceived by others because of their own infertility. It is the inability to accept and work through the stigma of sterility that causes many problems for the adoptive parents and subsequently for their children. Manning (1975) describes the experience of sterility as creating a sense of isolation about being "different," anger at losing control of one's body, and a reaction of guilt over not being able to procreate "genetic children." McCranie (1965) points out the importance of adoptive parents completing their grief over not being able to conceive and to resolve any feelings of bitterness toward the spouse, if only one is found to be sterile.

Many of these issues are raised as the adoptee enters his own

Presented at the International Forum on Adolescence, Jerusalem, July 4-7, 1976.

54

reproductive cycle during puberty. With the adoptive mother there is a revival of envy of women who are capable of having children. This may lead to a sexual rivalry with the father as well, which is further intensifed by the lack of usual sexual taboos (Schechter 1970). For the sterile adoptive father the emerging sexuality of his son may become a threat because of the unconscious association of infertility with a lack of virility (Dawkins 1972). Furthermore, the circumstances of the child's illegitimate birth conflicts with the parents' own moral attitudes and teaching regarding sexuality and reproduction to the youngster, making discussion about the genetic parents extremely difficult for the adoptive parents (Pannor and Klickstein 1968). The resolution of this ambivalence toward the birth parents determines, for the most part, how successfully the parents deal with their teenager's questions about their genealogical forebears (Baran, Pannor, and Sorosky 1974; Sorosky, Pannor, and Baran 1975b).

Communication between the adoptive parents and their children is further complicated by a greater age difference, as adoptive parents tend to be seven to eight years older than their biological counterparts. The widening of the generation gap makes it difficult for parents to empathize with the typical identity conflicts experienced by all adolescents. Furthermore, the adopted adolescent has a special interest in the nature of his or her conception, the reason for the adoption, and the genealogical history. Unfortunately, this healthy curiosity is often construed by the adoptive parents as an indication that they have failed in their role as parents or a sign of their child's lack of love for them. Deutsch (1945) illustrates how the adopted child's insecurity is fed by the mother's insecurity, and a vicious cycle arises, in which the mother's anxious question Does he love me as my own child would? is answered by similar questions on the part of the child: Who are my real parents? Am I loved like a blood child?

Adoptive parents have a particular problem in accepting the developing independence of their adolescent youngster, tending to view any disengagement from themselves and an attachment to others as an abandonment and a return to the lonely, insecure feelings associated with the preadoption childless period. This may result in a tendency to infantilize the adolescent adoptee in a final attempt to prevent an emerging individuation. In order to maintain a sense of integrity, the adolescent is thus pushed into a heightened state of rebellion against his or her parents.

Adoptive parents are also known to be overprotective of their youngsters from infancy on (Humphrey and Ounsted 1963; Pringle 1967). These tendencies unconsciously attempt to prove to the child that they are loved as their own. Adoptive parents have also been described as rigid and pressuring in regards to their child's academic achievement (Hoopes, Sherman, Lauder, Andrews, and Lower 1970, Seglow, Pringle, and Wedge 1972). Their expectation levels are high and may stem from concerns that the child's future may be affected by genetic limitations.

Adoptive parents are often obsessed with fears of hereditary taints coming out during their child's adolescence, and are inclined to see their child's behavior as representing their own unacceptable, repressed sexual and aggressive drives which they readily attribute to constitutional factors derived from promiscuous, impulse-ridden birth parents (McCranie 1965). Often, behavior is mobilized in the child by the suggestive force of the parents' suspicion and he or she is driven by that force into a kind of compulsive acting out through an identification with the birth parents.

Adoptive parents require greater maturity and psychological awareness than biological parents because of the special obstacles they face. They need to know more about themselves and must be capable of empathizing with their child's position. Most significantly, they may require help to realize that they are the true psychological parents and that nothing can happen to alter this role.

The Birth Parents

The National Center for Social Services estimates that in 1971, 60 percent of all children adopted in the United States, about 101,000, were born out of wedlock (Gallagher 1973). The psychodynamics underlying illegitimate pregnancy has been studied in depth. Earlier concepts viewed the phenomenon as a neurotic acting out of underlying conflicts (Clothier 1943, Young 1954). More recent studies (Bernstein 1966, Herzog 1966, Pauker 1969, Pope 1967) have demonstrated, however, that psychopathological features are not always implicated. The unwed father, also studied in depth (Pannor and Evans 1967, Pannor 1971, Pannor, Massarik, and Evans 1971), has demonstrated, contrary to any reputed irresponsibility, concern about the pregnancy, a greater concern about his offspring than heretofore recognized, and in only rare situations took advantage of the unwed mother in getting her pregnant.

Parents who cannot keep their infants have a sense of worthlessness and considerable feelings of guilt (Lewis 1971). Smith (1963) emphasized that the mother who relinquishes her baby is trying to give her child what she knows he needs and what she wants him to have—love, care, and security from two parents in a normal home situation that she cannot provide. It is usually assumed that after the mother has offered her child for adoption that she wants to completely sever her ties with the child and begin life anew. The proof that the unwed mother does not suppress her pregnancy, however, is revealed by the fact that many of them inquire about their child's welfare, from time to time, at the agencies that handled the adoption arrangements. Recent evidence has also demonstrated that for most of these birth mothers the adoption was an indelible, traumatic experience (Pannor, Sorosky, and Baran 1974; Pannor, Baran, and Sorosky 1976).

Once the adoptive proceedings have been completed, the birth parents seem to become the forgotten or "hidden" parents (Rogers 1969) around whom the adoptee and adoptive parents have been able to weave fantasies of a positive or negative nature. This ambivalence is indicated by the wide variety of adjectives used to describe them: first; original; birth; natural; biological; bio; physical; genetic; real; true; other; and blood. Of these names we feel that the terms *birth, genetic,* and *biological* seem the most descriptive and least offensive to each of the parties involved in the adoption triangle.

The Adolescent Adoptee

The psychological problems encountered in adolescent adoptees can be divided into three categories: (a) a continuation of childhood developmental difficulties; (b) an intensification of the typical adolescent conflicts; and (c) unique symptomatology associated with the adoption experience.

CONTINUATION OF CHILDHOOD DEVELOPMENTAL DIFFICULTIES

A number of authors have described a vulnerability of the adopted child to stress and the development of emotional problems requiring psychotherapy (Goodman, Silberstein, and Mandell 1963, Jameson 1967, Reece and Levin 1968, Schechter 1960, Simon and Senturia 1966, Sweeney, Gasbarro, and Gluck 1963). Such problems originate from an outgrowth of early developmental difficulties. Initially, illegitimacy is known to have a higher correlation with poor prenatal care and delivery complications, predisposing the child to various neurological aberrations (Pasamanick and Knoblich 1972, Seglow, Pringle, and Wedge 1972). The unwed mother is also likely to be under greater emotional stress during the gestation period which some feel relates to foetal hyperexcitability and later psychological problems (Dodge 1972, Sontag 1960, Stott 1971). Women giving up children for adoption may have a higher incidence of genetically transmitted mental illness (Horn, Green, Carney, and Erikson 1975).

The severity of emotional problems correlates directly with the age of the child at the time of the adoption placement and the extent of early maternal deprivation (Offord, Aponte, and Cross 1969, McWhinnie 1967, Witmer, Herzog, Weinstein, and Sullivan 1963). The adoptive mother and infant also demonstrate a greater difficulty in establishing secure and stable attachments in the early months of their relationship (Clothier 1942, Humphrey and Ounsted 1963, Lewis 1975, Reeves 1971). These difficulties in early object relationships can lay the foundation for future relationship difficulties in adolescence.

The resolution of the oedipal complex is affected by the absence of the biological incest barrier. Schechter (1960) and Peller (1961, 1963) therefore advised postponing the revelation of the child's adoptive status until after the resolution of the oedipal conflict to avoid complicating this stage of psychosexual development. However, most contemporary adoption experts feel that delaying the revelation of adoption until latency creates a risk that the child will learn of his or her adoptive status from outsiders. Extremely traumatic to the child, learning of the adoption from outsiders frequently leads to mistrust of the adoptive parents and intense retaliatory acting out in adolescence (Lawton and Gross 1964).

Freud (1909) proposed and Conklin (1920) later demonstrated that, as a part of normal child development there were episodes of doubt for the child that he or she was, in fact, the natural child of his or her parents. This "family romance" fantasy is usually a brief state during the latency period and is abandoned once the child accepts that he or she can love and hate the same individual. Adoptees, however, are likely to experience a prolongation of this fantasy with a resulting delay in the development of ambivalence, and a tendency to split both adoptive and birth parents into good and bad (Clothier 1939, 1943b, Eiduson and Livermore 1952, Kohlsaat and Johnson 1954, and Schwartz 1970). Such a capability of keeping good and bad images diffused can lead to problems in ego development with subsequent disturbances in learning and object relationships.

Adopted children seen in psychotherapy are more likely to be referred because of behavior problems and are prone to acting out by aggression, lying, stealing, or running away (Bohman 1970, Goodman, Silberstein, and Mandell 1963, Humphrey and Ounsted 1963, Jackson 1968, Jaffee and Fanshel 1970, Menlove 1965, Offord, Aponte, and Cross 1969, Reece and

Levin 1968, Schechter, Carlson, Simmons, and Work 1964, Simon and Senturia 1966). They also have a higher incidence of school underachievement which may be related to minimal brain dysfunction or a manifestation of passive resistance to parental pressures (Borgatta and Fanshel 1965, Elonen and Schwartz 1969, Taichert and Harvin 1975).

INTENSIFICATION OF
TYPICAL ADOLESCENT CONFLICTS

The internal or intrapsychic conflicts occurring during adolescence include the acceptance, expression, and control of aggressive and sexual impulses, as well as the resolution of the identity crisis. The external or environmental conflicts include dependency-independency issues, peer acceptance and social approval, as well as growing concerns about the future. The resolution of these adolescent conflicts can be adversely affected by the adoption experience (McWhinnie 1969, Tec 1967).

Aggression conflicts. During adolescence there is a great deal of inner turmoil and a need for external firmness, consistency, and establishing limits. Because of their own unresolved feelings about their infertility, adoptive parents seem to have special difficulty in accomplishing these goals, which results in an unconscious fear of losing the child's love or of the child leaving them for the original parents. The youngster thus becomes involved in the classic vicious cycle of testing limits, going beyond the limits without restriction, feeling guilt, and retesting the parents in a futile attempt to find a source of punishment and retribution.

Adopted adolescents are prone to act out their conflicts with impulse ridden outbursts at family members, teachers, and peers (Glatzer 1955, Herskovitz, Levine, and Spivack 1959, Young, Taheri, and Harriman 1975). The acting out can be interpreted as a partial attempt to try out a series of identities developed from fantasies about the birth parents (Simon and Senturia 1966). Certain behaviors, such as running away, seems designed as a test that the adoptive parents love them and won't abandon them as the birth parents did. At the other extreme, we occasionally see overly inhibited adolescent adoptees who fear expressing any anger against the adoptive parents because of the excessive guilt aroused or the fear of being abandoned once again (Toussieng 1962).

Sexual conflicts. Easson (1973) postulated that the adopted adolescent has difficulty in three areas of emotional growth which can affect the development of a stable sexual identity: (1) the process of emancipation from the adoptive parents; (2) the resolution of incestuous strivings in the adoptive relationship; and (3) the final identification with the parent of the same sex and the establishment of a stable growth-productive relationship with the parent of the other sex. Because of these conflicts adopted adolescents have a greater tendency toward sexual acting out. This is particularly prevalent with girls who are attracted to the image of a promiscuous birth mother. By sexually acting out, this image becomes a self-fulfilling prophesy that the hereditary taint is appearing in poor impulse control. Furthermore, Lawrence (1975) cites a high incidence of homosexuality among her sampling of adoptees.

Identity conflicts. Erikson (1968) described the essential task of adolescence as the development of a sense of identity and described how the failure of the process results in identity confusion. The development of identity is partially established through identification with the parents, especially the one of the same sex. In the case of the adopted adolescent the process is complicated because he or she has the knowledge that an essential part of the self has been cut off and remains on the other side of the adoption barrier (Kornitzer 1971), thereby confusing the psychological identity of the adoptee (American Academy of Pediatrics 1971, 1973, Anglim 1965, Barinbaum 1974, Livermore 1961, Mech 1973, Schoenberg 1974). Sorosky, Baran, and Pannor (1975) described these adoption-related conflicts as resulting in "identity lacunae." And these problems can lead to a sense of shame, embarrassment, and lowered self-esteem (Schwartz 1975).

Dependency-independency conflicts. Anna Freud (1958) described the typical adolescent struggle as centering around denying, reversing, loosening, and shedding of ties to the infantile objects. Blos (1962) asserted that the process of detachment from the parents during adolescence is accompanied by a profound sense of loss and isolation equivalent to the experience of mourning. Adolescence becomes a second stage of individuation from the parents. During this phase the youngster vacillates regularly between denying his or her dependency needs and regressing to infantile levels with a desperate search for dependency gratifications.

The adoption experience results in an actual object loss, in contrast to the symbolic loss experienced by the adolescent as he or she emancipates his or herself from the parents. Thus, the adolescent adoptee becomes particularly vulnerable to any experiences of loss, rejection, and abandonment (McWhinnie 1969, Rogers 1970). Threatening to leave home or run away is the youngster's counterphobic attempt at covering up these abandonment fears. Unfortunately, these strivings for individuation are often met with an overreaction on the part of insecure adoptive parents.

Social conflicts. During adolescence the child gradually transfers his interests and emotional attachments from the family to the outside world. Acceptance by peers and sexual attractiveness take precedence among the youngster's priorities. The adopted adolescent who feels ashamed of his or her adoptive status may avoid close relationships for fear of being exposed (Reynolds 1975). Some youngsters will seek company in fundamentally different social groups, on a lower level than the rest of the family. This pursuit seems to be an effort to establish a group identity corresponding to the predestined group to which the child imagined he belonged (Frisk 1964). Other youngsters will compensate for these feelings of inadequacy by wearing their adoption as a badge and telling everyone (Barinbaum 1974).

Dating is another experience affected by adoption. Because of an unconscious fear of being hurt or rejected the teenager may be reluctant to get too close to his or her companion. Some are concerned about a negative reaction from their date's parents when they learn about their adoptive status. The deeper issue, however, is the terrifying fear of establishing an incestual liaison with an unknown biological relative.

Future conflicts. The older adolescent becomes more concerned about his or her academic or vocational future. A sense of fear and uncertainty about the adult world is often more intense for the adoptee, who is likely to be preoccupied with existential concerns and a feeling of isolation and alienation due to the break in genetic continuity that the adoption represents. For some, the existing block to the past may create a feeling that there is a block to the future as well. Furthermore, a fear of an unknown hereditary illness may make the adoptee apprehensive about the prospects of marriage in the future.

UNIQUE SYMPTOMATOLOGY ASSOCIATED WITH THE ADOPTIVE EXPERIENCE

There are certain behavioral patterns and emotional conflicts whose dynamics are somewhat unique to the adoption syndrome, including: (a) genealogical bewilderment; (b) compulsive pregnancy; (c) the roaming phenomenon; and (d) the search for biological relatives.

Genealogical bewilderment. Clothier (1943) stated that the trauma and severing of the individual from his or her racial antecedents typifies what is peculiar to the psychology of the adopted child. Frisk (1964) conceptualized that the lack of family background knowledge in the adoptee prevents the development of a healthy "genetic ego" which is then replaced by a "hereditary ghost." When this genetic ego is obscure one does not know what is inherited. During adolescence, these issues become intensifed when heightened interests in sexuality make the adoptee more aware of how man and his characteristics are transmitted from generation to generation.

Under normal circumstances, special attention is not paid to one's genealogy; it is usually accepted as a matter of fact. Wellisch (1952) pointed out that a lack of knowledge about birth parents and ancestors can be a cause of maladjustment in adopted children. Elaborating further by introducing the term "genealogical bewilderment," Sants (1965) described a state of confusion and uncertainty developing in adolescent adoptees who become obsessed with questions about their biological roots.

Compulsive pregnancy. Adopted youngsters, both male and female, may demonstrate a compulsive urge to procreate, thus providing them with their first contact with a blood relative. Conceived within or outside of marriage, this can lead to a pregnancy at a very young age. For some, the pregnancy may serve as a means of disproving fears about hidden genetic anomalies. The pregnancy can also be seen as a means of identifying with the adoptee's birth mother. Then, if the child is kept, the youngster is provided with an opportunity to undo his or her abandonment neurosis created by the relinquishment for adoption. In still other cases, the pregnancy provides an adopted girl with a chance to get back at her adoptive mother by accomplishing something she failed at—conceiving.

The roaming phenomenon. Toussieng (1962) described a number of cases in which adopted children in adolescence start "roaming" almost aimlessly, though occasionally they claim to be intentionally seeking the fantasied "good real parents." Toussieng later reinterpreted this phenomenon as an acted-out search for stable objects and introjects that were never provided by elusive adoptive parents. Frisk (1964) also described a restless wandering by some adoptees, interpreted as a symbolic search for the biological parents motivated by a desire to discover their true character.

A variant of the roaming phenomenon is a state of turning inward seen in some adopted youngsters (Kornitzer 1971). Lewis (1971) explained that the reason so many adolescent adoptees become dreamy and inaccessible derives from a preoccupation with fantasies about their forebears. Rogers (1969) described the emotional turmoil experienced by adopted adolescents whose biological parents have been "hidden" from them.

The search for biological relatives. There is considerable controversy as to the extent of interest that adoptees have in knowing about or meeting their biological relatives. Some authors feel these concerns are ubiquitous to most adolescent and young adult adoptees (Kirk 1964, Linde 1967, McWhinnie 1967, Pringle 1967, Schechter, Carlson, Simmons, and Work 1964). Others postulate this curiosity is greatest in adoptive homes where

here has been a strained relationship and difficulty in openly communicating about the adoptive situation (Clothier 1942, Eldred et al. 1976,
Hubbard 1947, Jaffee and Fanshel 1970, Lemon 1959, Smith 1963,
Triseliotis 1973). In contrast. Senn and Solnit (1968) maintain that
fantasies about the birth parents are usually built from disguised
impressions and wishes about the adoptive parents and have little to do
with the birth parents per se.

There is a general consensus, however, that certain developmental stages
seem to intensify the adopted person's curiosity and interest in their
genealogical background. Initially, the pubescent youngster becomes
aware of the biological link of the generations and begins to visualize him
or herself as part of a chain that stretches from the present into the remote
past (Rautman 1959). As late adolescence and young adulthood ushers in
accelerated identity concerns, the feelings about adoption become more
pronounced and questions about the past increase. When marriage is
imminent or when the adoptee becomes pregnant, these concerns overtly
intensify. Furthermore, the death of one or both of the adoptive parents
create a feeling of loss or relieve the burden of guilt and concern about
hurting them (Lemon 1959). A separation or divorce may also trigger off
feelings of rejection and abandonment, with an increased interest in past
ties (Triseliotis 1973).

In recent years adult adoptees have insisted that they have a civil right to
their original birth certificate which is presently sealed after the adoption
proceeding has been completed. Some have organized into activist groups
(Fisher 1973, Paton 1968) and are challenging the courts in an attempt to
institute legislative changes affecting adoption. Much publicity has been
given to their plight and it appears that they have a reasonable chance of
altering the law, enabling emancipated adults to gain access to their records
which contain the actual names of their birth parents. It is interesting to
note that birth records are available to adult adoptees in other countries:
Scotland (Triseliotis 1973), Finland (Rautenan 1971), Israel (Ministry of
Justice, State of Israel 1960), and in England and Wales (Dept. of Health
and Social Security 1975).

The authors of this chapter have studied the outcome of reunions
between adult adoptees and their birth parents (Baran, Sorosky, and
Pannor 1975, Sorosky, Baran, and Pannor 1974, Sorosky, Baran, and
Pannor 1976). For the most part, these experiences have been quite
successful in establishing a greater sense of identity and ego integrity in the
adoptees. The encountered birth parents were very cooperative and, for
many, it put to end years of concern about the welfare and outcome of the
child they had relinquished for adoption. Although many of the adoptive

63

parents were initially uncomfortable with the reunion, in almost all cases the relationship between the adoptee and adoptive parents was actually improved. It was also discovered that the need to search for the birth parents was related more to the innate personality characteristics of the adoptee and less to the nature of the adoptive family relationship.

It is important to speculate on what effect a change in the sealed record statutes might have on adolescent adoptees. Some have argued that it might create much anticipatory anxiety, and a disruption in the adoptive parent-child relationship. This should not be the case if the adoptive parents can emotionally dissociate themselves from their adolescent youngster's genealogical concerns and curiosities, make themselves available to assist their child in obtaining his or her records, and searching for the birth parents if this is still a pressing issue when the youngster reaches adulthood.

During the adolescent years, however, and as the adoptee is still too immature to put the entire experience into a healthy perspective, we feel that any attempts at searching for the birth parents should be discouraged. The adolescent process of individuation is complicated enough without the introduction of another set of parent figures. It is important, of course, for adolescents to be provided with every opportunity to express their feelings about their birth parents, and with as much of the non-identifying background information available.

Adoption agencies must revise their traditional approach to the matter of secrecy and confidentiality (Dukette 1975, Smith 1976). In withholding or distorting information the agencies have become watchmen and censors of the truth, and this aura of secrecy has been more of a burden than a protection to adoptive parents. On the other hand, adoption agencies have insisted that adoptees be told early and clearly about their adoption. On the other hand, little help has been provided to adoptive parents in dealing with the complicated feelings arising out of their adoptee's dual identity. For the adoptee, the information offered by the agencies has been recognized as shadowy, unreal and, therefore, unsatisfying. Withheld data does not protect adoptees, but instead initiates a feeling that full information would reveal awful truths. At no time during the adoptee's psychological development is openness and honesty more vital than during adolescence.

Future Trends

There are a number of trends that will have a significant effect on future adoptive practice. Most important, there are fewer babies available for adoption today as a result of improved contraception for unwed teenagers, liberalized abortion laws, and an increasing tendency for unwed mothers to keep and raise their child. Subsequently, more couples will choose to adopt less desirable children: older, handicapped, retarded, and mixed-racial. Others may be willing to accept "open adoption" arrangements in which there is an understanding that the birth mother will be able to visit her child periodically after the relinquishment (Baran, Pannor, and Sorosky 1976). We are also likely to witness an increase in the use of artificial insemination as a means of procreation for infertile couples.

These trends and policy changes will undoubtedly create new pressures and concerns for parents of adolescent adoptees. The child adopted at an older age is more likely to experience an intensification of many of the problems discussed. Raising a handicapped, retarded, or mixed-racial youngster will require a very special psychological awareness on the part of the parents. Ability to handle an open adoption arrangement will necessitate considerable openness of communication on the part of all parties to the adoption triangle: adoptee, adoptive parents, and birth parents. The unique psychological problems created by artificial insemination have yet to be studied. Even though the youngster is not told about the nature of his or her conception there may be a sense of undisclosed information if the parents have not resolved their feelings about the nature of the child's birth.

Conclusions

The turmoil of adolescence creates strains on all families, but particularly reveals vulnerabilities inherent in the adoptive family. The adopted adolescent has a more difficult time integrating experiences and personal introspections into a healthy sense of identity. The adoptive parents are confronted with a reawakening of a painful infertility stigmata and have difficulty accepting their youngster's emerging independence. Furthermore, the birth parents are thrown back into prominence because of the adoptee's genealogical concerns, and the adoptive parents' fears that undesired hereditary traits will appear in their children.

The healthiest adaptation occurs when the adoptive parents have been reasonably successful in resolving their feelings about infertility and are willing to acknowledge that their role is different, in certain respects, than that of biological parents. On the other hand, they must appreciate that they are the true psychological parents and must learn to emotionally detach themselves from their youngsters' curiosity and interest in background information. It would be helpful if the original adoption agency would provide the adoptive parents with ongoing reports on the outcome of the birth parents which can be used to answer their children's inquiries. The more open the communication about all adoption related matters, the less likely the adolescent will have to resort to excessive fantasizing or acting out in an attempt to fill in identity lacunae.

REFERENCES

American Academy of Pediatrics, Committee on Adoptions (1971). Identity development in adopted children. *Pediatrics* 47: 948-949.

American Academy of Pediatrics, Committee on Adoption and Dependent Care (1973). *Adoption of Children.* Evanston: American Academy of Pediatrics.

Anglim, E. (1965). The adopted child's heritage—two natural parents. *Child Welfare* 44: 339-343.

Baran, A., Pannor, R., and Sorosky, A. D. (1974). Adoptive parents and the sealed record controversy. *Social Casework* 55: 531-536.

————(1975). Secret adoption records: the dilemma of our adoptees. *Psychology Today* 9 (7): 38-42, 96-98.

————(1976). Open adoption. *Social Work* 21: 97-100.

Barinbaum, L. (1974). Identity crisis in adolescence: the problem of an adopted girl. *Adolescence* 9: 547-554.

Bernstein, R. (1960). Are we stereotyping the unmarried mother? *Social Worker* 3: 100-110.

Blos, P. (1962). *On Adolescence.* New York: Free Press.

Bohman, M. (1970). *Adopted Children and Their Families.* Stockholm: Proprius.

Borgatta, E. F., and Fanshel, D. (1965). *Behavioral Characteristics of Children Known to Psychiatric Out-Patient Clinics.* New York: Child Welfare League of America.

Clothier, F. (1939). Some aspects of the problem of adoption. *American Journal of Orthopsychiatry* 9: 598-615.

————(1942). Placing the child for adoption. *Mental Hygiene* 26: 257-274. Reprinted in E. Smith, ed. *Readings in Adoption.* New York: Philosophical Library, 1963.

————(1943a). Psychological implications of unmarried parenthood. *American Journal of Orthopsychiatry* 13: 531-549.

————(1943b). The psychology of the adopted child. *Mental Hygiene* 27: 222-230.

Conklin, E. S. (1920). The foster-child fantasy. *American Journal of Psychology* 31: 59-76.

66

Dawkins, S. (1972). The pre-adopter and infertility. *Child Adoption* 67: 24-32.

Dept. of Health and Social Security (1975). Children act: main provisions and arrangements for implementation. *Local Authority Circular* (75): 21: 1-4.

Deutsch, H. (1975). *The Psychology of Women, A Psychoanalytic Interpretation, Vol. II (Motherhood).* New York: Grune and Stratton.

Dodge, J. A. (1972). Psychosomatic aspects of infantile pyloric stenosis. *Journal of Psychosomatic Research* 16: 1-5.

Dukette, R. (1975). Perspectives for agency response to the adoption-record controversy. *Child Welfare* 54: 545-555.

Easson, W. M. (1973). Special sexual problems of the adopted adolescent. *Medical Aspects of Human Sexuality* July: 92-105.

Eiduson, B. T., and Livermore, J. B. (1952). Complications in therapy with adopted children. *American Journal of Orthopsychiatry* 23: 795-802.

Eldred, C. A., Rosenthal, D. Wender, P. H., Kety, S. S., Schulsinger, F., Welner, J., and Jacobsen, B. (1976). Some aspects of adoption in selected samples of adult adoptees. *American Journal of Orthopsychiatry* 46: 279-290.

Elonen, A. S. and Schwartz, E. M. (1969). A longitudinal study of the emotional, social and academic functioning of adopted children. *Child Welfare* 48: 72-78.

Erikson, E. (1968). *Identity, Youth and Crisis.* New York: W. W. Norton.

Fisher, F. (1973). *The Search for Anna Fisher.* New York: Arthur Fields.

Freud, A. (1958). Adolescence. *Psychoanalytic Study of the Child* 13: 255-278.

Freud, S. (1909). Family romances. Reprinted in J. Strachey, ed. (1950), *Collected Papers* 5: 74-78. London: Hogarth Press.

Frisk, M. (1964). Identity problems and confused conceptions of the genetic ego in adopted children during adolescence. *Acta Paedo Psychiatrica* 31: 6-12.

Gallagher, V. M. (1973). Changing focus on services to teenagers. *Children Today* 2: 5: 24-27.

Glatzer, H. T. (1955). Adoption and delinquency. *Nervous Child* 11: 52-56.

Goodman, J., Silberstein, M. R., and Mandell, W. (1963). Adopted children brought to child psychiatric clinics. *Archives of General Psychiatry* 9: 451-456.

Herskovitz, H. H., Levine, M., and Spivack, G. (1959). Anti-social behavior of adolescents from higher socio-economic groups. *Journal of Nervous and Mental Disorders* 129: 467-476.

Herzog, E. (1966). Some notes about unmarried fathers. *Child Welfare* 45: 194-197.

Hoopes, J. L., Sherman, E. A., Lauder, E. A., Andrews, R. G., and Lower, K. D. (1970). *A Follow-up of Adoptions (Vol. II): Post-Placement Functioning of Adopted Children.* New York: Child Welfare League of America.

Horn, J. M., Green, M., Carney, R., and Erikson, M. T. (1975). Bias against genetic hypotheses in adoption studies. *Archives of General Psychiatry* 32: 1365-1367.

Hubbard, G. L. (1947). Who am I? *The Child* 11: 130-133.

Humphrey, M., and Ounsted, C. (1963). Adoptive families referred for psychiatric advice: part I. the children. *British Journal of Psychiatry* 109: 599-608.

Jackson, L. (1968). Unsuccessful adoptions: A study of 40 cases who attended a child guidance clinic. *British Journal of Medical Psychology* 41: 389-398.

Jaffee, B., and Fanshel, D. (1970). *How They Fared in Adoption: A Follow-Up Study.* New York: Columbia University Press.

Jameson, G. K. (1967). Psychiatric disorder in adopted children in Texas. *Texas Medicine* 63: 83-88.

Kirk, H. D. (1964). *Shared Fate.* New York: The Free Press.

———, Jonasson, K., and Fish, A. D. (1966). Are adopted children especially vulnerable to stress? *Archives of General Psychiatry* 14: 291-298.

Kohlsaat, B., and Johnson, A. M. (1954). Some suggestions for practice in infant adoption. *Social Casework* 35: 91-99.

Kornitzer, M. (1971). The adopted adolescent and the sense of identity. *Child Adoption* 66: 4: 43-48.

Lawrence, M. (1975). The adoption study project. Personal communication.

Lawton, J. J., and Gross, S. Z. (1964). Review of psychiatric literature on adopted children. *Archives of General Psychiatry* 11: 635-644.

Lemon, E. M. (1959). Rearview mirror—an experience with completed adoptions. *Social Worker* 27, No. 3: 41-51.

Lewin, K. (1940). Bringing up the Jewish child. *The Menorah Journal* 28: 29-45. Reprinted in: *Resolving Social Conflicts.* New York: Harper and Row, 1948. pp. 539-551.

Lewis, D. O., Balla, D., Lewis, M., and Gore, R. (1975). The treatment of adopted versus neglected delinquent children in the court: a problem of reciprocal attachment? *American Journal of Psychiatry* 132: 142-145.

Lewis, H. (1971). The psychiatric aspects of adoption. In J. G. Howells, ed., *Modern Perspective in Child Psychiatry*. New York: Brunner/Mazel.

Linde, L. (1967). The search for mom and dad. *Minnesota Welfare* Summer: 7-12, 47.

Livermore, J. (1961). Some identification problems in adopted children. Presented at the annual meeting of the American Orthopsychiatric Association, New York.

Mech, E. V. (1973). Adoption: a policy perspective. In B. M. Caldwell and H. N. Ricciuti, eds., *Review of Child Development Research, Vol. 3*. Chicago: University of Chicago Press.

Menlove, F. L. (1965). Aggressive symptoms in emotionally disturbed adopted children. *Child Development* 36: 519-532.

Menning, B. E. (1975). The infertile couple: a plea for advocacy. *Child Welfare* 54: 454-460.

Mikawa, J. K., and Boston, J. A. (1962). Psychological characteristics of adopted children. *Psychiatric Quarterly* 42: 274-281.

Ministry of Justice, State of Israel (1960). *Laws of The State of Israel* 14: 97. Jerusalem. Government Printer.

McCranie, M. (1965). Normal problems in adapting to adoption. *Journal of the Medical Association of Georgia* 54: 247-251.

McWhinnie, A. M. (1967). *Adopted Children and How They Grow Up*. London: Routledge and Kegan Paul.

————(1969). The adopted child in adolescence. In G. Caplan and S. Lebovici, eds., *Adolescence—Psychosocial Perspectives*. New York: Basic Books.

————(1970). Who Am I? *Child Adoption* 62: 36-40.

Offord, D. R., Aponte, J. F., and Cross, L. A. (1969). Presenting symptomatology of adopted children. *Archives of General Psychiatry* 20: 110-116.

Pannor, R. (1971). The teen-age unwed father. *Clinical Obstetrics and Gynecology* 14: 446-472.

————, Baran, A., and Sorosky, A. D. (1976). *Journal of the Ontario Association of Children's Aid Societies* 19: 4: 1-7.

————, and Evans, B. W. (1967). The unmarried father: an integral part of casework services to the unmarried mother. *Child Welfare* 46: 150-155.

————, and Klickstein, M. (1968). An agency looks at attitudes of adoptive parents towards the biological parents. Unpublished manuscript.

————, Massarik, F., and Evans, B. (1971). *The Unmarried Father*. New York: Springer.

————, Sorosky, A. D., and Baran, A. (1974). Opening the sealed record in adoption—the human need for continuity. *Journal of Jewish Communal Service* 51: 188-196.

Pasamanick, B., and Knoblich, H. (1972). Epidemiologic studies on the complication of pregnancy and the birth process. In S. I. Harrison, eds., *Childhood Psychopathology.* New York: International Universities Press.

Paton, J. M. (1968). *Orphan Voyage.* New York: Vantage.

Pauker, J. D. (1969). Girls pregnant out of wedlock. *In Double Jeopardy, The Triple Crisis, Illegitimacy Today.* New York: National Council on Illegitimacy.

Peller, L. E. (1961). About telling the child about his adoption. *Bulletin of The Philadelphia Association for Psychoanalysis* 11: 145-154.

————(1963). Further comments on adoption. *Bulletin of the Philadelphia Association for Psychoanalysis* 13: 1-14.

Pope, H. (1967). Unwed mothers and their sex partners. *Journal of Marriage and the Family* 29: 555-567.

Pringle, M. L. K. (1967). *Adoption—Facts and Fallacies.* London: Longmans, Green.

Rautenan, E. (1971). Work with adopted adolescents and adults—the experience of a Finnish adoption agency. In *The Adopted Person's Need for Information About His Background.* London: Association of British Adoption Agencies.

Rautman, A. (1959). Adoptive parents need help too. *Mental Hygiene* 33: 424-431. Reprinted in E. Smith, ed., *Readings in Adoption.* New York: Philosophical Library, 1963.

Reece, S., and Levin, B. (1968). Psychiatric disturbances in adopted children: a descriptive study. *Social Work* 13: 101-111.

Reeves, A. C. (1971). Children with surrogate parents: cases seen in analytic therapy, an etiological hypothesis. *British Journal of Medical Psychology* 44: 155-171.

Reynolds, W. F., and Chiappise, D. (1975). The search by adopted persons for their natural parents: a research project comparing those who search and those who do not. Presented at the American Psychology-Law Society meeting, Chicago, Ill.

Rogers, R. (1969). The adolescent and the hidden parent. *Comprehensive Psychiatry* 10: 296-301.

————(1970). The relationship between being adopted and feeling abandoned. *Pediatrics Digest* 12: 21-27.

Sants, H. J. (1965). Genealogical bewilderment in children with substitute parents. *Child Adoption* 47: Summer: 32-42.

Schechter, M. D. (1960). Observations on adopted children. *Archives of General Psychiatry* 3: 21-32.

———(1970). About adoptive parents. In E. J. Anthony and T. Benedek, eds., *Parenthood, It's Psychology and Psychopathology.* Boston: Little, Brown.

———, Carlson, P., Simmons, J. Q., and Work, H. (1964). Emotional problems in the adoptee. *Archives of General Psychiatry* 10: 109-118.

Schoenberg, C. (1974). On adoption and identity. *Child Welfare* 53: 549.

Schwartz, E. M. (1970). The family romance fantasy in children adopted in infancy. *Child Welfare* 49: 386-391.

———(1975). Problems after adoption: some guidelines for pediatrician involvement. *Pediatrics* 87: 991-994.

Seglow, J., Pringle, M. L. K., and Wedge, P. (1972). *Growing Up Adopted.* Windsor, Berks: National Foundation for Educational Research.

Senn, M., and Solnit, A. (1968). *Problems in Child Behavior and Development.* Philadelphia: Lea and Febiger.

Simon, N., and Senturia, A. (1966). Adoption and psychiatric illness. *American Journal of Psychiatry* 122: 858-868.

Smith, E., ed. (1963). *Readings in Adoption.* New York: Philosophical Library.

Smith, R. (1976). The sealed adoption record controversy and social agency response. *Child Welfare* 55: 73-74.

Sontag, L. W. (1960). The possible relationship of prenatal environment to schizophrenia. In D. Jackson, ed., *The Etiology of Schizophrenia.* New York: Basic Books.

Sorosky, A. D., Baran, A., and Pannor, R. (1974). The reunion of adoptees and birth relatives. *Journal of Youth and Adolescence* 3: 195-206.

———(1975a). Identity conflicts in adoptees. *American Journal of Orthopsychiatry* 45: 18-27.

———(1975b). The psychological effects of the sealed record on adoptive parents. *World Journal of Psychosynthesis* 7: 13-18.

———(1976). The effects of the sealed record in adoption. To be published in *The American Journal of Psychiatry.*

Stott, D. H. (1971). The child's hazards in utero. In J. G. Howells, ed., *Modern Perspectives in International Psychiatry.* New York: Bruner /Mazel.

Sweeny, D. M., Gasbarro, D. T., and Gluck, M. R. (1963). A descriptive study of adopted children seen in a child guidance center. *Child Welfare* 42: 345-349.

Taichert, L. C., and Harvin, D. D. (1975). Adoption and children with learning and behavior problems. *The Western Journal of Medicine* 122: 464-470.

Tec, L. (1967). The adopted child's adaptation to adolescence. *American Journal of Orthopsychiatry* 37: 402.

Toussieng, P. W. (1962). Thoughts regarding the etiology of psychological difficulties in adopted children. *Child Welfare* 41: 59-71.

Triseliotis, J. (1973). *In Search of Origins—The Experiences of Adopted People*. London: Routledge and Kegan Paul.

Wellisch, E. (1952). Children without genealogy—a problem of adoption. *Mental Health* 13: 41-42.

Witmer, H. L., Herzog, E., Weinstein, E. A., and Sullivan, M. E. (1963). *Independent Adoptions: A Follow-Up Study*. New York: Russell Sage Foundation.

Young, I. L., Taheri, A., and Harriman, M. (1975). Adopted and non-adopted adolescents in residential psychiatric treatment. Presented at the American Association of Psychiatric Services for Children, New Orleans, La.

Young, L., (1954). *Out of Wedlock*. New York: McGraw-Hill.

ANOMIE: ITS INFLUENCE ON
IMPULSE RIDDEN YOUTH AND THEIR
SELF-DESTRUCTIVE BEHAVIOR

EDWARD M. LEVINE AND CHARLES H. SHAIOVA

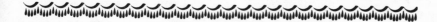

While the effects of urbanization and industrialization were a source of interest to others who preceded him, Durkheim (1897) first sensed the significance of stable social structures and values for the psychopathology termed suicide. Those he categorized as "anomic" suicides were urbanites lacking important values and social attachments.

With crude statistical methods and far from adequate data he was, nonetheless, able to show that anomic suicides were inversely related to close attachments to socially cohesive communities and fundamental values. Durkheim found, for example, that suicide rates for married individuals were less than for single people, and less for Catholics than for Protestants.

Of equal importance, if less empirically conclusive, was Durkheim's explanation that higher rates of suicide during periods of growing prosperity and recessions were both attributable to the inadequacy of personally meaningful standards for coping with such drastic changes in one's living conditions. For example, those whose economic gains or declines were severe were most subject to psychic strain, since they were unusually hard pressed to find new values that would be effective in helping them cope with vastly altered standards of living into which they were suddenly introduced.

From a psychoanalytic perspective, to the extent that a lack of personally meaningful values and social attachments were correlated with suicide, they are its proximate causes; ultimate causes reveal serious emotional disturbances. Yet among the other-directed (those generally lacking internalized basic values), well-educated, urban middle class in contemporary America, such basic values and stable social structures are increasingly lacking. Later, I will show how such conditions are dysfunctional for the development of integrated egos and superegos.

Sociopsychologically, the utility of values in stabilizing individual behavior and for reducing the individual's uncertainty concerning how to respond to others (in both primary and secondary groups) was identified by Mead (1934), who indicated how both children and adults are dependent on "significant others" for support and approval. Later, psychoanalysts examined the interpersonal psychodynamics affecting the needs and dependencies of the child during the course of its emotional development in considerable detail (Diggory 1967, Litman 1967). This work, however, did not entail the social comprehensiveness of those social psychologists who have extended their observations into other phases of life for both children and adults (Becker 1963, Blumer 1969, Goffman 1959, 1967). Still, the emphasis in both psychoanalysis and social-psychology has focused on the functions and character of interpersonal relationships, while tending to assume the general availability of values effective in the socialization of children.

Other social scientists, especially sensitive to urban social problems, have conducted studies which lent support to this same assumption. The leading scholars in the field of social deviance, for example, have concluded from their work that antisocial deviant behavior is the result of: inaccessibility to valued opportunities leading to success (Merton 1958); status frustrations (Cohen 1955), and inadequate socialization (Cloward and Ohlin 1970, Cohen 1955, Sutherland and Cressey 1970); male gender uncertainty (Parsons 1947, Cohen 1955); and the adoption of deviant values from deviant peers (Becker 1963).

Antisocial deviant behavior has not been attributed by these scholars to the ambiguous, or weak values commonly associated with modernity. Instead, the inference is that most, if not all, such deviants could become socially and individually responsible by more thorough exposure to socially appropriate values. Banfield (1974) stands almost alone in contending that inadequate (present-oriented) values are largely responsible for antisocial deviant behavior. However, he attributes these values to a "class-cultural" setting (essentially low-income communities) where they predominate, and has not drawn attention to their growing prevalence among white youth in middle and higher income suburban communities.

Psychoanalysis, while not questioning these conclusions and the conditions on which they were based, has qualified them with its knowledge that much, perhaps most, antisocial deviant behavior is an expression of emotional disturbances whose precipitating causes stem from objective social factors (Aichhorn 1925, Eissler 1949, Friedlander 1949, Glover 1960, Waelder 1960). Furthermore, psychoanalysis has shown that dominating impulses, neuroses, and self-preservative defensiveness may at times render the internalization of values difficult or impossible—that even values which are deeply internalized and greatly prized may, under some conditions, be at least temporarily overwhelmed by impulses and anxieties which motivate deviant behavior. Still, while adding such appropriate qualifications to sociological research, psychoanalysis has not asked whether the values characteristic of the other-directed in urban-industrial society are effective for the emotional development of children.

Impulse-Freeing Values:
The Urban-Industrial Ethos

By identifying the "other-directed" individual as the emergent character of middle class, urban-industrial society, Riesman (1950) drew sociology and psychoanalysis closer toward a common concern with a psychological utility of values. Illuminating their uncertainty about and lack of internalized basic values, and the indecisiveness of such people in their interpersonal relations, he went on to show how numerous people, shorn of their ethno-cultural and religious psychosocial moorings, had become unusually dependent on their peers ("significant others") for social approval and appropriate social values, tastes, and attitudes. Taking for granted the material abundance of this increasingly service-producing, consuming society, other-directed individuals—particularly today's youth—are more than ever concerned with narcissistic gratifications (exemplified in rock and roll dances and music; Blum 1966, Levine 1966) and much less with interests involving self-determined assertion and restraint. In considerable measure, the values of their peers, parents, and society support this trend.

Riesman (1950) also observed that the values that other-directed adults transmit to their offspring stress sensitivity and responsivity to others' interests and wishes. Today, parents rarely encourage their children to internalize impulse-controlling values which emphasize and result in a self "inner-directedness," rather than allowing others to determine basic moral values, desirable behavior, and life style. Furthermore, while parents have continuing, if clearly diminished, responsibility for the emotional development and the socialization of their children, peer groups have none. The former explain, justify, and enforce their moral values. Yet, peer groups do not claim filial responsibilities and can, unlike parents, reject the dissident or misfit from their midst with impunity and by virtually any exclusionary means. Consequently, when children, particularly pre- and post-adolescents, are aware of important differences or conflicts between the values of their parents and those of their peers, the latter will evermore steadily increase their influence and simultaneously weaken parental authority (Bettelheim 1965, Eisenstadt 1956, Levine and Shaiova 1971, Riesman 1950). This, in turn, further diminishes parents' effectiveness to instill in their children those values remaining to them which they deem important for their children's welfare.

The Nature and Functions of Values: Sociological and Psychoanalytical Perspectives

Values are explicit or implicit statements which clearly indicate the kind of behavior preferred, permissible, appropriate, or required, and the conditions under which it is expected—as well as indicating that behavior which is, in varying degrees, disapproved or prohibited and the conditions of its definition. Values (norms defining the appropriate behavior in specific situations) thereby provide human beings with a sense of direction and its limits, informing us of the ways and boundaries within which self-assertion can arise. Further clarifying the meaning values imparted are the rewards and punishments prescribed for their observation and transgression, inclining the individual to examine and understand their meaning and limits more carefully.

By establishing limits, values serve as boundaries against which the individual can test, experience, and come to understand himself both cognitively and affectively. They are as crucial to the ego for reality testing and, thus, its integration, as they are to the development of the superego for assisting the individual to adjust to others. Values, in this sense, are indispensable in helping the ego acquire coherence, for in responding safely in terms of the directions and limits they provide, increments of emotional strength accrue to it. Furthermore, the necessity, need, preference, or desire to understand values, to use them correctly, to modify, object to, or reject them are all acts of self-assertion and, therefore, contribute to the further development of the emotional strength of the ego when undertaken with emotional safety. Such interpersonal actions are the central psychosocial factors in the process of self integration, and in the development of a stable gender-ego identity (Levine and Shaiova 1974).

In contemporary urban-industrial society, rapidly changing values and those which replaced more traditional ones concerned with individual restraint, obligation, and responsibility tend, among other-directed parents, to indulge and encourage impulse gratification, a trend which Aichhorn (1925) noted several decades ago. Among such parents, there is increasingly less concern to inculcate in children a clear sense of self-discipline and of deferring immediate gratification, which is characteristic of an affluent economy with considerable social mobility (Fletcher 1966, Levine and Shaiova 1971, Riesman 1950). The weakness and paucity of self-regulatory values, which are necessary for developing and stabilizing the self and providing it with functional ego-constraints, will result over time in a growing vulnerability to the influence, if not the domination, of the impulses (Freud 1953, Gaylin 1968, Waelder 1960). Increasingly this will precipitate both conscious and unconscious feelings of anger and depression when impulses are denied gratification; the impulse-ridden individual, with an already weak and unrealistic ego, is less able to cope effectively with such impulse frustrations. In these circumstances the pleasure principle will ever more frequently be elevated over the reality principle.

Contemporary evidence attests to the increase in impulse-motivated behavior among a special population heretofore little associated with social problems—white and upper-middle class youth. In 1974, for example, the Illinois State Superintendent of Education publicly stated that the use of marijuana is as common among such youths in the schools of suburban communities as it is among youth in inner city schools. And although peer group influences and curiosity account for some of it, a good deal of the use of marijuana—and of amphetamines, barbiturates, heroin, and alcohol—are the outcome of emotional problems which lack adequate ego controls. It was also reported that the public schools in Chicago suburban communities suffered a million dollars in damage due to vandalism in 1973. Additionally, the use of marijuana and pills in private schools in Chicago and in public high schools serving students from affluent families in the northern suburbs is reputed to be as prevalent as in innercity schools in lower-income neighborhoods.

This points up one of the most unexpected and striking paradoxes of our times—the antisocial values, outlook, and impulse-governed behavior long found almost exclusively among low-income (often nonwhite) youth are now found in growing numbers of white, well-educated youth from middle and upper-middle income families in suburban communities. Banfeld (1974) has described the former as being primarily interested in action- and pleasure-seeking behavior, those whose orientation is bound to a present of immediate gratifications. He described such individuals (youth and adults) as belonging to the "lower class culture" whose values generally legitimatize impulse gratification. That such acting-out behavior is now increasing found among the economically and educationally advantaged white, city and suburban youth attests to the prevalence of impulse-dominated behavior among that stratum which historically has no more than dabbled with vandalism, delinquency, and drugs.

Still other, if limited, evidence confirming this analysis reveal that psychoanalysts and other therapists are discovering growing numbers of young patients with egos so deficient (borderline syndromes) their prospects in therapy are extremely problematical (Freedman 1968, Grinker 1968). And still other analysands are unable to function occupationally because their egos are too weak (narcissistic personalities) to counteract the self-destructive force of their neuroses.

These are disturbing trends which raise questions about present and prospective social policies and programs concerned with behavioral problems of youth. There exists evidence to illustrate the ineffectiveness of publicly funded programs specifically designed to rehabilitate drug users (Epstein 1974, O'Donnell 1969, Wilson 1972). Yet if present trends in drug use continue among the enormously populous post World War II generation, more programs seem sure to be funded simply because the numbers of those needing help will support arguments that something must be done to cope with so widespread and serious a problem. The issue will not be whether the rate of young drug users is increasing—it will be simply a matter of numbers—a segment of the population may become so large that its size alone will suffice to justify efforts to alleviate its problems. The precedent of established drug programs and the influence of bureaucratic and other interests will also add their weight to the drive for more funding.

This grim prognosis rests on evidence familiar to psychoanalysis, for the entire gamut of serious antisocial behavioral problems subsumed under deviance is largely the manifest expression of emotional disturbances. Therefore, future funding of public and private programs attempting to cope with drug and other troubling problems of impulse-ridden youth will, as in the past, concentrate resources on symptoms, not causes. It is consequently imperative that both professionals and the public recognize the immense costs involved in such remedial efforts—those of funding, staffing, and operating the programs; the lost years, lives, and productivity of those who cannot cope without drugs; the taxes which could be used for other purposes; and the professional skills and time which are sorely needed elsewhere.

Conclusions

While emotionally disturbed individuals almost surely have existed in all societies, tightly knit social structures and deeply internalized basic values have been the instrumental socio-cultural bulwarks in constraining or confining within socially approved limits the behavioral expression of their impulse-dominated or conflicted feelings. Today, however, such vital social controls have been eroded by the forces of urbanization and industrialization, leaving modern other-directeds shorn of these critically supportive social moorings. It appears, therefore, that unless substantially greater concern is expressed by both society and parents in effectively instilling in children impulse constraining values emphasizing self and social responsibility, discipline, and obligation, the number of impulse ridden youth, particularly among the middle income more affluent whites (the prototypical contemporary other-directeds), will probably increase considerably. Should this eventuate, as seems likely, it is also quite probable that the problems of drug use and other kinds of self-destructive and antisocial behavior among such youths will expand far beyond present, already worrisome, levels.

REFERENCES

Aichhorn, A. (1925). *Wayward Youth.* New York: Viking Press, 1935.

Alexander, F. (1948). *Fundamentals of Psychoanalysis.* New York: W. W. Norton.

Banfield, E. (1974). *The Unheavenly City Revisited.* Boston: Little Brown.

Bettelheim, B. (1965). The problem of generations. In E. Erikson, ed., *The Challenge of Youth.* Garden City: Doubleday.

Becker, H. (1963). *The Outsiders.* New York: The Free Press.

Blum, L. (1966-1967). The discotheque and the phenomenon of alone-togetherness. *Adolescence* 1: 4: 351-366.

Blumer, H. (1969). *Symbolic Interactionism: Perspective and Method.* Englewood Cliffs, N.J.: Prentice Hall.

Cloward, R. and Ohlin, L. (1960). *Delinquency and Opportunity: A Theory of Delinquent Gangs.* Glencoe: Free Press.

Cohen, A. (1955). *Delinquent Boys.* Glencoe: The Free Press.

Diggory, J. (1967). Components of personal despair. In E. S. Shneidman, ed., *Essays in Self Destruction.* New York: Science House.

Durkheim, E. (1897). *Suicide.* New York: The Free Press, 1961.

Eisenstadt, S. (1956). *From Generation to Generation.* New York: Free Press.

Eissler, I. R. (1949). *Searchlights on Delinquency.* New York: International Universities Press.

Epstein, E. (1974). Methadone: the forlorn hope. *The Public Interest* 29: 36: 3-24.

Fletcher, J. (1966). *Situation Ethics.* Philadelphia: Westminster Press.

Freedman, L. (1968). Psychoanalysis, delinquency, and the law. In J. Marmor, ed., *Modern Psychoanalysis.* New York: Basic Books.

Freud, A. (1953). The bearing of the psychoanalytic theory of instinctual drives on certain aspects of human behavior. In R. Loewenstein, ed., *Drives, Affects, Behavior: Contributions to the Theory and Practice of Psychoanalysis and its Applications.* New York: International Universities Press, 1960.

Friedlander, K. (1947). *The Psychoanalytic Approach to Juvenile Delinquency.* New York: International Universities Press.

Gaylin, W. (1968). Epilogue: the meaning of depair. In W. Gaylin, ed., *The Meaning of Despair.* New York: Jason Aronson.

Glover, E. (1960). *The Roots of Crime.* New York: International Universities Press.

Goffman, E. (1959). *The Presentation of Self in Everyday Life.* New York: Doubleday Anchor Books.

———(1967). *Interaction Ritual.* Garden City, N.Y.: Anchor Books.

Grinker, R., Sr., Werble, B., and Drye, R. (1968). *The Borderline Syndrome.* New York: Basic Books.

Levine, E. (1966). The twist: a symptom of identity problems as social pathology. *Israel Annals of Psychiatry* 4: 198-210.

———, and Shaiova, C. (1971). Equality and rationality v. child socialization: a conflict of interests. *Israel Annals of Psychiatry* 9: 107-116.

———(1974). Biology, personality, and culture: A theoretical comment on the etiology of character disorders in industrial society. *Israel Annals of Psychiatry* 12: 10-28.

Litman, R. (1967). Sigmund Freud on suicide. *Essays in Self Destruction.* New York: Jason Aronson.

Mead, G. (1934). *Mind, Self, and Society.* Chicago: University of Chicago Press.

Merton, R. (1938). *Social Theory and Social Structure.* Glencoe: The Free Press.

O'Donnell, J. (1969). *Narcotic Addicts in Kentucky.* U.S. Government Printing Office.

Parsons, T. (1947). Certain primary sources and patterns of aggression in the social structure of the Western world. *Psychiatry* 10: 167-181.

———(1951). *The Social System.* New York: The Free Press.

Riesman, D., Glazer, N., and Denny, R. (1950). *The Lonely Crowd.* New Haven: Yale University Press.

Sutherland, E. and Cressey, D. (1970). *Principles of Criminology.* Philadelphia: Lippincott.

Tonnies, F. (1887). *Gemeinschaft und Gessellschaft.* C. P. Loomis, translator and editor. New York: Harper and Row, 1963.

Waelder, R. (1960). *Basic Theory of Psychoanalysis.* New York: International Universities Press.

Wilson, J. (1972). The problem of heroin. *The Public Interest* 29: 3-28.

Wirth, L. (1938). Urbanism as a way of life. *American Journal of Sociology* 1-24.

7] COLLEGE STUDENTS IN THE FIFTIES:
THE SILENT GENERATION REVISITED

ROBERT P. WOLENSKY

For American youth, the decade 1960 through 1970 was one of the most turbulent periods of social unrest. Among college students, a leftward shift in political ideology was a dominant trait influencing views toward civil rights, ecological reform, global peace, wealth redistribution, and institutional redefinition.[1] With these and other issues, youth often espoused ideas and values which were antithetical to those of the older generation.

Despite recent social unrest, the United States has been characterized by relative harmony between generations. Feuer (1969) referred to this as "generational equilibrium" noting that basic values of younger generations have generally harmonized with those of their parents and the larger society. A cogent example of generational equilibrium can be seen in the "silent generation" of the 1950s. Regarding their general image, silent generation members were said to be noninvolved, acquiescent, security minded, and disinterested. Their essential value system was said to harmonize with that of their parents and this facilitated an anxious integration into adult life.

The "silent generation" developed from the popular literature of the period and, although it often applied to youth in general, the term was directed mainly at the college student cohort.[2] In discussing the silent generation Holmes (1952) stated, "Contemporary historians express mild surprise at the lack of organized movements, political, religious or otherwise among the young." Goldsen, Rosenberg, Williams, and Suchman (1960) found "the present generation of college students . . . politically disinterested, apathetic, and conservative." And Jacob (1957) observed students to be "rubber stamps" of conformity.

Interest in the silent generation had reemerged in the early 1970s and the impression was much the same. Adler (1970), a self-proclaimed member of the silent generation, authored *Radicalism and the Skipped Generation* and reinforced the silent image: "In college under Eisenhower, we were known for nothing, or for our apathy." *The Silent Generation Meets the Class of 1970,* written by Gartner (1970), another self-proclaimed member, described his college days and concluded that, "we were the last, and quietest, of the silent generation." A *Time* essay (1970) additionally said that, while this generation may eventually have taken a different identity, the image in the fifties was one of apathy and remoteness.

By focusing on the college student cohort of youth in the fifties, this chapter revisits the silent generation with two objectives in mind. The first is to address the term, *silent generation.* The second is to develop a theoretical framework for understanding this category. The foundation of the latter objective is generational theory which, among other things, deals with continuities and conflicts between generations. The point argued is that the silent generation failed to establish a distinct generational character (defined as distinct values, beliefs, and attitudes) because of a socialization process which encouraged continuity of life with the previous generation. Two elements in this socialization process are scrutinized: (1) students' adaptation to the social and cultural environment of the era and (2) the educational institution.[3]

Defining the Silent Generation

The silent image began with mass circulation publications of the 1950s and was then furthered by social science research. Content analysis of mass circulation publications revealed two dimensions of silence. One related to the nonvocal stance of students in regard to social, political, economic, and other matters; it stated that they were literally silent about contemporary issues. The other related to their complacency with and virtual unquestioned acceptance of the world around them and an impatient ambition to gain a mooring in that world as an adult.

The first dimension is self-explanatory; students simply had little to say about most issues and events. "They are a generation with no responses— apathetic, laconic, no great loves, no profound hates and pitiful few enthusiasms. They are a wordless generation. If they have ideas they don't seem to like to rub them against other people's ideas" *(Life* 1951). In describing these characteristics, Trilling (1957) said, "the undergraduate of today is not very much committed to anything; if he is they are secret commitments."

The second dimension, however, is more complex since it deals with a rather complete socialization of students into the mainstream of American life. Conformity, security, apathy, and acceptance of the status quo were the blatant results. This was clearly illustrated in a *Life* editorial (1957) entitled, "Arise, Ye Silent Class of '57!" The editorial contained excerpts from the addresses of various commencement speakers. Brandeis President Sachar, speaking at the University of Massachusetts, deplored "a growing cult of yesmanship [in which] security becomes a craven disguise for servility. . . ." At Depauw University, IBM President Thomas Watson said, "We hear of a 'silent generation,' more concerned with security than integrity, with conforming than performing, with imitating than creating." And philosopher-theologian Paul Tillich, speaking at the New School for Social Research, criticized those who displayed "an intensive desire for security both internal and external, the will to be accepted by the group at any price and an unwillingness to show individual traits, acceptance of a limited happiness without serious risk." Tillich made a plea for nonconformity: "We hope for nonconformists amongst you, for the sake of the nation and for the sake of humanity."

While the silent image was firmly implanted in the popular literature of the period, social science research also documented these traits. The Cornell Values Study began research in 1950 on a panel of students and later studied larger samples at eleven colleges and universities, leading to the book *What College Students Think* (1960). Again the study found students to be models of the status quo. They had few real commitments and valued a happy family life above everything else, with the security of employment (preferably in a large corporation) running a close second. Education was viewed pragmatically, as a means to these goals. In regard to politics and government, the dominant traits were apathy and conservatism.

Similarly, Jacob (1957) reviewed five major studies on students and conducted his own research on thirty campuses only to conclude that homogeneity was the dominant characteristic. In a critical mode he wrote:

American college students today tend to think alike, feel alike, and believe alike. To an extraordinary degree, their values are the same wherever they may be studying and whatever the stage of their college careers. The great majority seem to be turned out of a common mold, so far as outlook on life and standards of conduct are concerned.

Silent, therefore, encompassed much more than taciturnity. It touched upon a philosophy of life and provided an entire approach to society and one's place in it. Most students were not only unwilling to speak up, but unquestionably accepted the ongoing institutional framework and its accompanying value system.

The Silent Generation in Theoretical Perspective

While the identification of the silent generation was clear in both popular and social science literature, theories alluding to why it existed present another problem. The task here is to relate the silent generation to generational theory and provide at least one possible explanation for its existence.

GENERATIONAL THEORY

Ortega y Gasset (1961) noted that inherent in each generation is a distinct character, a unique style. For a generation to make a new mark on history, it must liberate this character from the mode of life passed on to it by the previous generation. Accordingly, life for each generation has two aspects: the reception of ideas, values, and institutional patterns of the previous generation, and the liberation of the creative genius inherent in the generation concerned. The character of a generation will depend on which of these two aspects predominates:

> There have been generations which felt that there was perfect similarity between their inheritance and their own private possessions. The consequence, then, is that ages of accumulation arise. Other times have felt profound dissimilarity between the two factors and there ensue ages of elimination and dispute, generations in conflict.

Mannheim (1952) also noted that a distinct character (or entelechy) is inherent in every generation. Like Ortega y Gasset, he said that a generation is often blocked from liberating its uniqueness:

> Such generations, frustrated in the production of an individual entelechy, tend to attach themselves where possible to an earlier generation which may have achieved a satisfactory form or to a

85

younger generation which is capable of evolving a new form. . . . In this way the impulses and trends peculiar to a generation may remain concealed because of the existence of the clear-cut form of another generation to which they have become attached.

Whether or not a generation can liberate a distinct character could be greatly influenced by socialization, the basic process through which an individual becomes part of the society through cultural assimilation. Yet, while socialization is first an individually unique process, it also has a societal dimension. As Eisenstadt (1956) pointed out, age groups such as the silent generation can be part of a smooth generational transition when, in the society at large, the family supports the prevailing value orientations so that, "the preparatory socialization effected in age groups is compatible with the main institutional patterns of symbols, norms, and values of the social structure."

The data from mass circulation and social science publications indicated that students had indeed been socialized into the values, norms, and symbols of the larger society as reflected to them by their parents. While there may have been some peripheral differences in dress, language, and music, there was an essential congruity in value orientations toward major institutions resulting in great value continuity and harmony between generations.

It could be argued, then, that the socialization of the silent generation prevented a distinct character from emerging. By becoming attached to the orientations of an earlier generation the establishment of a unique character failed to take place. Assuming this theoretical approach to be workable, the next question becomes; what factors influenced the smooth socialization process and, hence, prevented a unique generational character from emerging? There are several possibilities that can be considered.

EXISTENTIAL ADAPTATION: INTEGRATION AS A RESPONSE TO CONFUSION[4]

CONFUSION THEME—WITHDRAWAL THEME—INTEGRATION THEME

(Helplessness)   (Resignation)   (Security)

ADAPTATION MODEL

The confusion theme suggests that the silence of students was a response to their place in a confusing and paradoxical world. It was illustrated in the view that many of life's situations—including social, political, international, and domestic matters—have direction, but the greater shape of things is controlled by circumstances and people over which the individual has no influence. The confusion theme shows that at least part of students' silence was due to their being convinced that, as individuals, they were helpless and and could do little to influence many of life's events.

Being convinced that the shape of things was beyond control brought about the withdrawal theme where individuals began turning inward so as to withdraw from a resulting confusion. The withdrawal was not from the mainstream of American institutions and values, as occurred with the Beat Generation (Holmes 1952, Cook 1971), but from situations perceived as or actually uncontrollable.

Students moved away from the uncontrollable to the controllable, to life situations where a definite amount of assuredness was available. The integration theme shows that they became preoccupied with security, with success in educational, occupational, and familial goals, pursuing a course of integration into the mainstream of American middle class life. As a result, an age of accumulation arose, characterized by continuity of values between generations.

Thus a distinct generational character did not emerge within the silent generation because its members adapted to the confusing social and cultural environment by integrating into the mainstream of life. The socialization process which this implies becomes clearer as each of the three themes is examined in the literature.

THE CONFUSION THEME

This confused attitude among college students was discussed in numerous magazine articles. Consider the Johns Hopkins University student who described his peers by saying, "we are resigned to a position of grayness and indecision. If my generation seems inert, it is not because we do not care, it is because we feel helpless" *(Newsweek* 1960). It was evident in the Ohio State University student who felt that he couldn't vote in the 1956 presidential election because he was inadequately informed on most political issues and because "no one really knows the facts except the few at the top." This student was one of many who possessed such attitudes in a Gilbert Youth Research survey for *Look* (October 2, 1956: 100ff). Published under the title, "Tragic Fact: Our Young Voters Don't Care," it concluded that, regardless of where the students went to college, they didn't care about the election or "are so confused that it amounts to the same thing."

A respondent to a Gallup Poll *(Saturday Evening Post,* December 23, 1961: 63-80) echoed the helpless feeling when he said, "Look . . . we neither have the naivete nor the urgency of our parents. They felt that they mattered; that they could do something about conditions. We feel that nothing we do will make any difference."

Time (February 9, 1953: 66ff) reviewed a book about youth *(Seventy Five: A Study of a Generation in Transition,* 1952) written by "a distinguished group of greying Yalemen and professors." It provided one explanation for student apathy, namely, helplessness in the face of a swiftly changing world. The authors stated that youth lacked "the conviction that they ought or that they can significantly affect their world." This attitude was primarily a result of life in a mass society where people find themselves as individuals among billions and eventually become confused about their ability to "make a difference."

Goldsen, Rosenberg, Williams, and Suchman (1960) also found evidence of the confusion theme in their research on student political attitudes. The apathy they discovered was not only related to an unquestioned acceptance of the status quo, but went deeper, into a genuine disenchantment with issues, causes, and the efficacy of individual involvement. Students were convinced of the complex nature of political issues and chose to keep their distance. They were aware of paradoxes in the political process, but were more cognizant of their inability to significantly influence that process.

This sampling of items indicates that the literal silence of students was due to more than disenchantment or simple disinterest. It was also a manifestation of a socialization process in which students internalized feelings of helplessness, powerlessness, and confusion in regard to their ability to effectively shape their environment.

THE WITHDRAWAL THEME

Goldsen, Rosenberg, Williams, and Suchman (1960) noted the withdrawal of students and found it to reside in their psychological device of "playing it cool":

If they are conservative and apathetic, they are so in part by default. There are no clearly defined answers to the problems their generation confronts. In social psychological terms we would say that they react to baffling complexity by withdrawing. In the slogan of their own campus culture, they "play it cool."

In more recent observation about students in the fifties, Lipset and Schaflander (1971) found the trait of "turning inward" to be an important part of students' adaptation to their environment. They stated, "The students under these circumstances turned inwards. They became concerned with their psyches, their personalities, and their feelings. The fact that *The Catcher in the Rye* was a collegiate best seller in the 1950s should occasion no surprise."

Erikson in *Childhood and Society* (1950) observed that American youths often defend themselves against rejection and anxiety by not getting too "worked up" and involved, elevating ego restriction to a dominant defense mechanism. In their research on youth, Gallup and Hill (1961) uncovered significant evidence of this lack of willingness for personal involvement. More than half their respondents expressed interest in making this a better world, but in keeping distance from concerted action. "They plan to improve it by improving themselves. They tell us that reform can come if 'I reform myself' or 'understand others.' " Perhaps, in keeping with the withdrawal theme, students found it well within their power to bring changes in themselves, whereas possible changes in the political, social, and economic structures seemed impossible.

The personal and individual emphasis of the withdrawal theme not only resulted in a great concern for occupational, marital, and educational success and security, but brought other dimensions of life, especially social life, into a personalized egotistical framework. Personal social acceptance, the desire to belong was paramount, exemplified by the popularity of fraternities, sororities, and other social organizations as well as the various proms, cotillions, dances, parties, and outings which flourished on the campus.

That the withdrawal maneuvered students toward immediate life situations over which they could exert an amount of control was indicated by Hofstadter (1957) who said that students "feel . . . there is nothing much they can do about many things like radioactive fallout. So today, college students are serious about their careers, and that's about all they can do." Birney (1957) agreed when he said that students "try to be able to cope with what they can control. They don't worry about what they can't."

The withdrawal theme, therefore, emphasized the personal dimension and was characterized by a blocking out by means of an uncontrollable, preoccupation with the controllable, thereby facilitating the social integration of students as they turned away from confusion toward personal success and advancement.

THE INTEGRATION THEME

This theme shows students' acceptance of the values and institutional definitions passed on by the previous generation and the resulting integration into the dominant culture. Characteristic of the integration was pursuit of security, one which, at least partially, was a reaction against the insecurity of the confusion theme and the resignation of the withdrawal theme.

The expanding postwar economy, the demand for college trained personnel, and the growing higher education system provided the context for integration. These conditions gave students the opportunity for educational and occupational advancement and security. As a result, they became more concerned with success, being established, and joining the adult world, than with beliefs or values that could have led to alternative principles of life.

Assuming that students adjusted to their environment by withdrawing from confusing and paradoxical situations and integrating into the mainstream of society, the next task is to explore specific factors which played important socializing roles.

THE EDUCATIONAL SYSTEM: INSTITUTIONAL MECHANISM AS A VEHICLE OF INTEGRATION

One reason for the great impact of Jacob's (1957) study of changing values in college was his convincing argument on the "leveling effect" of the college experience. Contrary to many popular beliefs, Jacob reported that higher education produced only a slight change in the values of some students and had no fundamental effect on the values of the overwhelming majority. Indeed, the changes which did occur were such as to "bring greater consistency into the value patterns of students and fit these patterns into a well-established standard of what a college graduate in American society is expected to believe and do." The college experience, therefore, acted as a great leveler of values, producing "cultural rubber stamps" rather than innovators of new patterns of thought and behavior.[5] It reinforced the predominantly middle class values a student brought from the home, the community, and the high school:

College has a socializing rather than a liberalizing impact on values. It softens an individual's extremist views and persuades him to reconsider aberrant values. It increases the tolerance potential of students toward differing beliefs, social groups, and standards of conduct so that they can move about with a minimum of friction in a heterogeneous culture. It strengthens respect for the prevailing social order.

Riesman (1963) noted the manner in which the university as a bureaucratic institution fostered an acceptance of the prevailing social order and, simultaneously, reinforced feelings of helplessness in the student. Through its authoritarian workings, the university convinced students that it was immutable, infallible, and monolithic, dictating policies and regulations as though it were commissioned by an absolute power. Furthermore, university professors, whether as a matter of policy or an indirect result of it, often created a feeling of passivity and helplessness within their students. As a consequence, "students feel even less qualified than heretofore to influence their fate as students; and so they tend to leave matters in the hands of the constituted authorities. . . ."

Further data on the integrating influences of the educational system emanated from Friedenberg (1963) who, in the late 1950s, researched the leveling effects of the American high school, the institution which, of course, students must pass before entering college. His extensive study revealed the conclusion that secondary education has the main objective of fostering a middle class value system which includes traits such as initiative, competition, respect for authority, and the demand to "get ahead and be somebody." In return for accepting these values, students could count on a rising standard of living, higher social status, and occupational advancement. In fact, "the youngsters by and large agreed with the high school that they were being given an unprecedented opportunity." Goldsen's (1960) finding that students had a very favorable attitude toward the educational institution reflected this appreciation at the college level.

Friedenberg discerned that students were not judged by their personal worth, but by their ability to conform to the prescribed standard of values. He concluded that the educational system fulfilled two primary functions: it operated to reinforce the values of the larger, middle class Protestant society and served as a Darwinian function—the latter referring to its providing those who accepted the value system the necessary credentials for success and security, while instilling in others who could not accept it, "a sense of inferiority and [a] warning [to] the rest of society against them as troublesome and untrustworthy."

This Darwinian analysis suggests that by the time young people were in college they had learned to accept the value system and were therefore on the way to success. It is here that we see the linkage between the socializing influences of this institutional factor and the failure of the silent generation's unique generational character. Through the educational system, students were socialized with the value system of the larger society; the acceptance of this value system was necessary in order to acquire the credentials paramount to success, security, and advancement. In the process of accepting this value system, however, an "age of accumulation" resulted, characterized by continuity of values and acceptance of the prevailing institutional definitions.[6]

Conclusions

The purpose of this chapter has been to define and theoretically investigate students in the fifties, part of the silent generation. Definitionally, silence was found to consist of two traits: literal silence regarding social, political, economic, and other contemporary matters, and an unquestioning acceptance of the institutional status quo and its accompanying values.

Utilizing generational theory, an attempt was made to explain the existence of the silent generation phenomenon. It was concluded that students internalized the value system of the previous generation and were thus unable to exhibit a distinct generational character. Two elements in this socialization process were explored: adaptation to the social and cultural environment of the period, and the socializing influences of the educational institution.

NOTES

1. For a review of attitude polls concerning student cohorts in the late 1960s to early 1970s see Lipset and Schaflander (1971: Chapter 2). As Lipset, who authored Chapter 2 said, "the majority of students have been politicized in a left direction by the events of the 1960s. . . ." See also Flacks (1967, 1971).

2. A cohort is defined as "an aggregate of individuals each of which experienced a significant event in its life history during the same chronological interval." See Ryder (1965, 1968).

3. Content analysis was the methodological tool utilized in this research.

Special attention was given to qualitative content analysis as discussed by Bereleson (1952) and Holsti (1969). Through this method, both mass circulation and social science publications were examined: the former because it was crucial in determining the etiology of the term "silent generation" and because of its enduring discussion of this social category throughout the fifties; the latter because it had systematically approached the study of college students.

Information from mass circulation magazines was obtained in the following manner. Articles were selected from the *Reader's Guide to Periodical Literature* from the years 1950 to 1960 under the topics "Colleges and Universities," "College Students," and "College Graduates." Because of the volume of articles, each could not be read and, furthermore, many were clearly irrelevant. The method of sorting was to note whether the title of an article displayed relevance to a description or analysis of college students as a silent generation or to a specific aspect of student culture or values. To further limit selection, titles in only five magazines were used *(Time, Life, Look, Newsweek,* and *Saturday Evening Post),* since these were the most popular mass circulation magazines of the period. Any title giving even the slightest hint of dealing with the topic was read and analyzed. Out of a total of 254 articles under the three headings, fifty-six dealt directly with the silent generation or an aspect of student values or culture and thus became the basis of research.

The books by Goldsen, Rosenberg, Williams, and Suchman (1960), and Jacob (1957) served as the main sources of social science data. Although other sources were used, these books were among the most comprehensive studies found.

Specifically, the mass circulation and social science sources were content analyzed with particular attention given to student values orientations toward religion, work, marriage and family, education, and government.

4. The analysis which follows is an example of "grounded theory" (Glaser and Strauss 1967). After extensive research in the mass circulation and social science literature it was noted that three interrelated characterizations were present: confusion accompanied by helplessness, withdrawal accompanied by resignation, and yet acceptance of the ongoing value system accompanied by smooth-social integration. In an attempt to unify these apparently disjunct themes, the following theory was generated. It describes a process which had the net effect of socializing students into the mainstream of American middle class life.

5. In this regard Goldsen, Rosenberg, Williams, and Suchman said, "if young people are exposed for four years to institutional norms and values

in the very milieu in which they are explicit and authoritative, they will become socialized to the predominant values of that milieu and will come to acknowledge their legitimacy."

6. An obvious question at this point is: did the educational system change in the 1960s so as to promote conflict between the generations? Of course, this is an issue beyond the scope of the present research and, while the author believes the influences of the educational institution were considerable in this regard, this complex question has not been systematically examined and, therefore, no definite conclusions can be made. Those seeking more information may want to begin with Flacks (1970, 1971).

REFERENCES

Adler, R. (1970). Radicalism and the skipped generation. *Atlantic* 225 (February): 53-57.

Arise ye silent class of '57! (1957). *Life* 42 (June 17): 94.

Bereleson, B. (1952). *Content Analysis in Communication Research.* Glencoe, Ill: The Fress Press.

Birney, R. (1957). Quoted in *Time* (November 18): 52.

Cook, B. (1971). *The Beat Generation.* New York: Charles Scribner's Sons.

Eisenstadt, S. N. (1956). *From Generation to Generation.* New York: The Free Press.

Erikson, E. H. (1950). *Childhood and Society.* New York: Norton.

Feuer, L. (1969). *Conflict of Generations.* New York: Basic Books.

Flacks, R. (1967). The liberated generation. *Journal of Social Issues* 23: 52-75.

———(1970). Social and cultural meanings of student revolt. *Social Problems* 7: 340-357.

———(1971). *Youth and Social Change.* Chicago: Markham.

Friedenberg, E. Z. (1959). *The Vanishing Adolescent.* New York: Dell.

———(1963). *Coming of Age in America.* New York: Vantage.

Gallup, G., and Hill, E. (1961). Youth, the cool generation. *Saturday Evening Post* 223 (December): 63-80.

Gartner, M. (1970). The silent generation meets the class of 1970. *Saturday Review* 53 (August): 52ff.

Generation in transition (1953). *Time* 63 (February 9): 66ff.

A generation of esthetes? (1951). *Life* 31 (November 26): 96.

Gilberg, E. (1956). Tragic fact: our young voters don't care. *Look* 20 (October 2): 100ff.

Glaser, B. and Strauss, A. (1967). *The Discovery of Grounded Theory.* Chicago: Aldine.

Goldsen, R., Rosenberg, M., Williams, R., and Suchman, I. (1960). *What College Students Think.* Princeton: Van Nostrand.

Hofstadter, R. (1957). Quoted in *Time* 70 (November 18): 52.

Holmes, C. (1952). This is the beat generation. *New York Times Magazine* 95 (November): 10ff.

Holsti, O. R. (1969). *Content Analysis in the Social Sciences and Humanities.* Reading, Mass: Addison Wesley.

Jacob, P. (1957). *Changing Values in College.* New York: Harper and Brothers.

Lipset, S. M. and Schaflander, J. (1971). *Passion and Politics: Student Activism in America.* Boston: Little, Brown.

Mannheim, K. (1952). The problems of generations. In P. Kecskemeti, ed., *Essays on the Sociology of Knowledge.* London: Routledge and Kegan Paul.

———(1957). No nonsense kids. *Time* 70 (November 18): 51-52.

Ortega y Gasset, J. (1961). *The Modern Theme.* New York: Norton.

Riesman, D. (1958). Review of the Jacob report. *American Sociological Review* 23: 732-739.

———(1963). The college student in an age of organization. In H. M. Ruitenbeck, ed., *The Dilemma of Organizational Society.* New York: Dutton.

Rootless class of '60 (1960). *Newsweek* 55 (June 13): 60-61.

Ryder, N. (1965). The cohort as a concept in the study of social change. *American Sociological Review* 30: 843-861.

———(1968). Cohort analysis. *International Encyclopedia of the Social Sciences* 2: 546, New York: MacMillan and The Free Press.

The silent generation revisited (1970). *Time* 95 (June 29): 38-39.

Trilling, L. (1957). Quoted in *Time* 70 (November 18): 52.

The younger generation (1951). *Time* 56 (November 5): 46ff.

8] SEXUALITY IN ADOLESCENT MALES

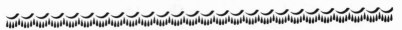

JUDITH BASKIN OFFER AND DANIEL OFFER

The psychoanalytic theory of adolescent sexual development classically describes a strengthening of libido, reawakening of oedipal strivings, and consequent need for the adolescent to separate from parents. The process of adolescence is defined as a search for new object relationships (Blos 1961). With the reawakening of oedipal fantasies, the home situation becomes more tumultuous for the teenager whose ambivalence toward parents will now forcefully express itself.

Most psychoanalytic theoreticians believe that the healthy young adolescent experiencing this upsurge of aggressive and sexual feelings will not immediately turn to heterosexual activities to relieve tensions, but will sublimate sexual impulses through intellectualization, asceticism, and idealism (A. Freud 1936). Sexuality will also be channeled through masturbation, fantasies, and homosexual strivings before the adolescent enters into heterosexual activities. During this period of early adolescence, the teenagers are described as needing time to consolidate their identities (Erikson 1968), to consolidate their narcissistic selves (Kohut 1972), and to disengage themselves from parents (Deutsch 1967) before attempting heterosexual experimentation. Early adolescent heterosexuality is regarded as being primarily motivated by defensive counter-oedipal maneuvers and defensiveness again against homosexual strivings (Blos 1961, Deutsch 1967).

In this chapter, sexual behavior and attitudes of adolescents are discussed as they relate to overall personality development. We diverge from the traditional psychoanalytic position not because the theory is inconsistent, but because it lacks proof as a general statement explaining adolescent development. Our questions regarding the theory of sexuality start long before discussing sexual behavior for adolescents. Returning to the developmental process, there is, of course, the question as to whether adolescence is preceded by a period of latency, when sexual feelings are thought to be muted, following the intensity of the oedipal period. The whole idea of "sexual reawakening" has come under question, and with it the question of the extent to which adolescence needs to be a period of storm and stress (Offer and Offer 1975a, b).

Following psychoanalytic theory further, we have tried to evaluate its applicability to the data which we have gathered on adolescence. This chapter will concentrate on our results when correlating sexual behavior with general patterns of development. Empirical findings can then be viewed within current theories.

The Offer Self-Image Questionnaire (O.S.I.Q.)

The Self-Image Questionnaire is a self-descriptive personality test that can be used for measuring the self-system of teenage boys and girls between the ages of 13 and 18. The self-system is directly correlated with the mental health and adjustment of adolescents (Offer and Howard 1972, Offer, Marohn, and Ostrov 1975), measuring adjustment in eleven content areas which are considered important in the psychological world of the teenager. The questionnaire was originally developed to provide a reliable means for the selection of a representative group of modal or "normal" adolescents from a larger group of high school students (Offer and Sabshin 1963, Offer 1969), and has since been used in many studies, administered to over 20,000 teenagers in the United States, Australia, Ireland, Israel, and Brazil. The populations sampled include males and females; younger and older teenagers; normal, disturbed, and delinquent adolescents; rural, urban, and suburban representatives in about thirty different metropolitan centers. The samples cover the range of the middle class, but has recently been given to rural, ghetto, and lower class teenagers.

Normal Adolescent Project

Gagnon and Simon (1973) have emphasized the need for regarding sexual behavior within its more general role appropriateness. Our smaller but long-term intensive study portrays sexual behavior and attitudes within the context of total psychological functioning. Within the longitudinal study of normal, healthy, or typical adolescent males, seventy-three adolescents were interviewed during the four-year period of their high school years, sixty-one of whom were followed further for the four years post high school (Offer and Offer 1975a, b). The latter were interviewed during an eight-year period (1962-1970), when they grew from the ages of fourteen to twenty-two. In addition, psychological testing was given twice (at ages sixteen and twenty-one), parents were interviewed, questionnaire forms were compiled, and grades and teachers' ratings were utilized to help provide an understanding of the subjects' functioning. The subjects came from two suburban, Midwestern, predominantly white Protestant communities. The range of the middle-class were represented, although most came from middle-middle class and upper-middle class backgrounds. Using the Offer Self-Image Questionnaire (O.S.I.Q.), we chose as subjects for the longitudinal research study those male freshman high school students whose answers were within one standard deviation of the mean in nine out of ten scales. The sexual attitudes and behavior scale was not used for the selection process.

Within the relatively psychologically and sociologically homogeneous group which we chose for the eight-year study, three groups could be distinguished: (1) *Continuous Growth Group;* (2) *Surgent Growth Group,* (3) *Tumultuous Growth Group.*[1] A group of mixed scores were also obtained but not included in this analysis and description. The group with mixed scores comprised less than twenty percent of the total sample.

No factors such as age of first date, frequency of dating, or age of first sexual intercourse are useful in differentiating between the three groups. A general positive correlation was found between a conservative attitude toward sexuality and good academic performance. A closer examination shows that the differentiation comes not by counts of "scoring," a behavior which Gagnon and Simon (1973) describe as typical for adolescence, but by examining the nature of the relationships formed by the members of the three groups.

In previous reports of our research (Offer and Offer 1975a, b), case examples statistically most typical for each route through adolescence were used to illustrate the functioning of members of that group. Here we shall utilize one case example from the Continuous Growth Group with attention focused upon developing heterosexual attitudes and behavior.

CASE EXAMPLE

Tony, as a fifteen year-old freshman in high school in the spring of 1963, told the psychiatric interviewer that he had a girlfriend. He said that he did not generally place much importance on social activities and did not go around in a gang.

During his interview the following fall, the subject of heterosexual relationships was hardly discussed. When asked about three problems for adolescents and three wishes for himself, Tony did not mention social relationships. When asked whom he would like to have on a desert island with him, Tony selected his brother. Tony said that the idea of dating makes him nervous.

In the spring of 1964, shortly before his seventeenth birthday, Tony was asked to give examples of times when he had felt anxiety, depression, shame, and guilt. Again, his examples came from home and school situations which did not relate to heterosexual experiences. We can obtain some idea of Tony's feelings about gender roles from his descriptions of an ideal father and mother. The ideal father, according to Tony, is someone whom you can respect. He should be strict, but not too strict. What about the ideal mother? Tony responded, "She gives you love and shelters you."

In his junior year of high school the interview focused on heterosexual behavior. Tony was then going out in groups with "girls and fellows." He said that it was nice to have a girlfriend, but not important to have a steady one. He himself had had a "steady" for about three months. He expressed more confidence about himself in saying that the most difficult thing about a first date was in choosing the girl.

Did Tony think that teenagers should participate in sexual relationships? "The wisest thing for teenagers is to double date and not to stay alone. If one stayed alone, then temptation is always present. It is not all right for high school age teenagers to have sexual intercourse." Why? "You could get into trouble and get a bad reputation. Everything else but intercourse is O.K."

When Tony was twenty-two, his sexual and dating experiences had broadened but without dramatic changes, as was true for his behavior in general, He was going steady with a different girl. He was discussing the pros and cons of getting married at his age as well as the pros and cons of having sexual intercourse. He had not yet had sexual intercourse and asked whether he "should feel his wild oats or not" with his steady or with any girl. When the interviewer was noncomittal, Tony said that he did not like it when his father tells him to play around before he settles down. He said that the reason he does not have sexual intercourse has nothing to do with morals. Tony told the interviewer that he was afraid that sleeping with a girl might ruin his career, if the girl became pregnant.

In the spring of 1970, before graduating from college, Tony had decided to marry his girlfriend, but not before they could be financially independent from his parents. He was continuing his reasoned, meditating approach toward a rational solution to the tasks which he set for himself.

Results of the Offer Self-Image Questionnaire

As can be seen in Tables 1-8, the O.S.I.Q. differentiated significantly between a random sample of normal adolescents; male and female; young and old; and a contrasted sample of delinquents and emotionally disturbed adolescents. This was true for all scales and the total score, with the exceptions of Scale 6 (Sexual Attitudes and Behavior). In the other cultures (Irish and Israeli) there were more polarities between the sexes, i.e. males are more liberal than females in their description of their sexual attitudes and behavior (Scale 6).

For the older adolescents (ages sixteen to eighteen), the differences between the sexes in the United States is not as great as in the other three cultures. Is this finding a result of the impact of the woman's liberation movement? The data are not conclusive, but it will be of interest to follow up on this speculation with further studies over the next decade in order to obtain more solid results.

We are aware that there are many methodological limitations in a cross-culture study such as ours. The instrument was constructed and validated in the United States on a middle class teenage population. How valid these same items and scales are in another culture (even if they speak English) is open to question. The nuances that the meaning of words carry, and the meaning of taking such a questionnaire altogether might differ considerably in different cultures.

Discussion

Most of the juniors in high school, in our intensive study, disapproved of sexual intercourse for teenagers. There was clearly a fear of engaging in coital behavior. The expression of the fear was seen through comments about impregnating a girl, getting a bad reputation, contacting a disease, or, frequently, the worry of an inability to manage the experience of sexual intercourse. The phrase, "we are not mature enough" was heard repeatedly. The subjects were unwilling to reveal even a great deal in the way of fantasizing heterosexual acts. Their expressed fantasies were more often about great personal success in the areas of studies or sports than as being the Don Juan of the school. The blush and the daydream about women were there, but did not preoccupy these youth who as yet felt unsure of themselves as individuals apart from their parents. Thus, there was a delay between biological genital maturity and the heterosexual expression of this maturity. Psychosocial variables intervened, leading neither necessarily to better or worse overall functioning, but creating the internal time schedule which bound these middle-class youth.

Both the young adult (eighteen or twenty-two) and the adolescent counterpart (fourteen to eighteen) have the biological maturity to be able to have sexual intercourse. But, while the adolescent often has avoided the experience, the young adults will have begun to engage in more intensive heterosexual relations and will more openly admit to fantasizing about heterosexuality. One half of our study group population had by the third year out of high school experienced sexual intercourse. Different patterns of sexual practices are exemplified in the cases presented above. For Tony, the Continuous Growth Group example, sexual intercourse was linked to commitments to a career, marriage, and family.

The reason that we found no significant difference between the sexual attitudes and behavior on the O.S.I.Q. among psychologically different subgroups shows the complexities of sexual development during adolescence. There is no one variable which can be tied to sexuality. We need to do more research in this area before we can clearly point to single or multiple factors which make a person behave sexually in one way as contrasted to another.

Engaging in heterosexual activities for our subjects can be related to psychological maturity or immaturity. This is true within a given frame of reference of societal expectations. However, when journalists and professionals describe sexual revolutions and rampant promiscuity, in an area of the birth-control pill, the adolescents do not necessarily follow the societal license to change their behaviors (Davis 1971, Simon, Berger, and Gagnon 1972, and Offer 1972). Not only are the societal pressures more subtle and complex, but so too are the psychological variables less flexible. Because the individual is biologically able and sociologically thought to be enjoying sexual freedom does not mean that he or she is able to handle the emotional implications of an intimate bedroom scene (Ginsburg 1972). Conversely, engaging in sexual intercourse does in no way imply the expression of sexual freedom; it may or may not. For our research subject population, psychoanalytic theory offers a rationale for the internally timed progression toward heterosexual behavior. The theory is useful if it can be seen as one rationale among other possibilities.

Conclusions

To spin psychological theories implies a knowledge of the expectable for the wider range of individuals of any given cultural grouping. Within our large scale questionnaire data, sexual behavior and attitudes could not be meaningfully related to other psychological variables, except for the two large total groups; that of males versus females and younger adolescents versus older youth. Thus, we went from the major quantitative analyses data to the study of seventy-three adolescents for whom sexual behavior and attitudes could be seen as typical of overall patterns of functioning.

This chapter has described the heterosexual behavior and attitudes of a group of nonpatient adolescent males. The particular timing of a sexual act as related to age of the adolescent appears to reveal little about personality development within this group of subjects. Heterosexual behavior was motivated by chance, by biological urges, by a desire for acceptance, and by societal pressures, just as it was inhibited by a lack of opportunities, by a fear of close interpersonal involvement, by a fear of rejection, and by the restraining cultural mores.

A discrepancy of several years between biological maturity and emotional readiness for heterosexual involvements is psychologically neither mentally healthy nor harmful to the individual's total development. It may, however, allow the adolescent to bide for time when developing in other ways, but it is just as likely to decrease adolescent self-confidence as he or she remains untested in this important area of adult achievement. Thus, our psychological evaluations ought to be based on total behavioral patterns rather than on sexual activities alone. Our efforts to relate "scoring" to any cluster of personality variables were unsuccessful. The channeling of the sexual drive by adolescents is indicative of how young people control, define, and express themselves.

APPENDIX I.

Sexual Attitudes and Behavior Scale

1. The opposite sex finds me a bore.
2. It is very hard for a teenager to know how to handle sex in a right way.
3. Dirty jokes are fun at times.
4. I think that girls/boys find me attractive.
5. I do not attend sexy shows.
6. Sexually I am way behind.
7. Thinking or talking about sex frightens me.
8. Sexual experiences give me pleasure.
9. Having a girl/boy-friend is important to me.
10. I often think about sex.

APPENDIX II: TABLES

TABLE ONE:

Comparison of Offer Self-Image Questionnaire Sexual Attitudes Scale and Total Score Means: Normals vs. (Delinquent and Disturbed)—Americans Only

Offer Self-Image Questionnaire Scale[2]	Normals	Delinquent and Disturbed	Probability Levels		
			Analysis #1	Analysis #2	Analysis #3
Scale Six—Sexual Attitudes	2.71	2.68	.58	.66	.38
Total Score	2.27	2.73	.0001	.0001	.0001

1. 240 subjects were used in each of three analyses; the 240 subjects were drawn in each analysis from a grand pool of 965 Normals, 199 Disturbed, and 362 Delinquents; in each analysis there were 80 Normals, 80 Disturbed, and 80 Delinquents.

2. The higher the score, the less well-adjusted.

TABLE TWO:

Comparison of Offer Self-Image Questionnaire, Sexual Attitudes Scale and Total Score Means: Delinquent vs. Disturbed Subjects—Americans Only

Offer Self-Image Questionnaire Scale[2]	Delinquent[1]	Disturbed[1]	Probability Levels		
			Analysis #1	Analysis #2	Analysis #3
Scale Six: Sexual Attitudes	2.54	2.83	.12	.001	.01
Total Score	2.59	2.87	.01	.001	.01

1. 160 subjects were used in each of three analyses; the 160 subjects were drawn in each analysis from a grand pool of 199 Disturbed and 362 Delinquents; in each analysis there were 80 Disturbed and 80 Delinquents

2. The higher the score, the less well-adjusted.

TABLE THREE:

Cross-Cultural Comparison of Offer Self-Image Questionnaire Sexual Attitudes Scale and Total Score Means: Male vs. Female Subjects from America, Australia, and Ireland—Young (13-15-year-old) Normal Adolescents Only

Offer Self-Image Questionnaire Scale[2]	Male[1]	Female[2]	Probability Levels		
			Analysis #1	Analysis #2	Analysis #3
Scale Six: Sexual Attitudes	2.54	2.99	.0001	.0001	.0001
Total Score	2.45	2.47	.38	.73	.05

1. 1056 subjects were used in each of three analyses; the 1056 subjects were drawn in each analysis from a grand pool of 1193 Men and 1432 Women; in each analysis there were 528 Males and 528 Females.

2. The higher the score, the less well-adjusted.

TABLE FOUR:

Cross-Cultural Comparison of Offer Self-Image Questionnaire Sexual Attitudes Scale and Total Score Means: Male vs. Female Subjects from America, Ireland, and Israel—Older (16-18-year-old) Normal Adolescents Only

Offer Self-Image Questionnaire Scale[2]	Male[1]	Female[1]	Probability Levels		
			Analysis #1	Analysis #2	Analysis #3
Scale Six: Sexual Attitudes	2.51	2.86	.0001	.0001	.0001
Total Score	2.37	2.39	.98	.64	.61

1. 366 subjects were used in each of three analyses; the 366 subjects were drawn in each analysis from a grand pool of 322 American, Irish and Israeli Males and 346 American, Irish and Israeli Females; in each analysis there were 183 Males and 183 Females.

2. The higher the score, the less well-adjusted.

TABLE FIVE:

Cross-Cultural Comparison of Offer Self-Image Questionnaire Sexual Attitudes Scale and Total Score Means: American vs. Australian vs. Irish Subjects—Young (13-15-year-old) Normal Adolescents Only

Offer Self-Image Questionnaire Scale[2]	Americans[1]	Australians[1]	Irish[1]	Probability Levels: Americans vs. Others		
				Analysis #1	Analysis #2	Analysis #3
Scale Sx: Sexual Attitudes	2.67	2.75	2.88	.05	.001	.01
Total Score	2.35	2.48	2.52	.0001	.0001	.0001

1. 1056 subjects were used in each of three analyses; the 1056 subjects were drawn in each analysis from a grand pool of 611 Americans, 1352 Australians, and 662 Irish Men and Women; in each analysis there were 352 Americans, 352 Australians, and 352 Irish subjects.

2. The higher the score, the less well-adjusted.

TABLE SIX:

Cross-Cultural Comparison of Offer Self-Image Questionnaire Sexual Attitudes Scale and Total Score Means: Irish vs. Israeli vs. American Subjects—Older (16-18-year-old) Normal Adolescents Only

Offer Self-Image Questionnaire Scale[2]	Americans[1]	Irish[1]	Israeli[1]	Probability Levels: Americans vs. Others		
				Analysis #1	Analysis #2	Analysis #3
Scale Six: Sexual Attitudes	2.80	2.52	2.73	.01	.05	.01
Total Score	2.18	2.49	2.48	.0001	.0001	.001

1. 366 subjects were used in each of three analyses; the 366 subjects were drawn in each analysis from a pool of 354 Americans, 162 Irish, and 142 Israelis, in each analysis there were 122 Americans, 122 Irish, and 122 Israelis.

2. The higher the score, the less well-adjusted.

105

TABLE SEVEN:

Cross-Cultural Comparison of Offer Self-Image Questionnaire Sexual Attitudes Scale and Total Score Means: American vs. Australian vs. Irish Males and Females—Young (13-15-year-old) Normal Adolescents Only

Offer Self-Image Questionnaire[2]	Americans[1]		Australians[1]		Irish[1]		Probability Levels:		
	Male	Female	Male	Female	Male	Female	Analysis #1	Analysis #2	Analysis #3
Scale Six: Sexual Attitudes	2.41	2.93	2.50	3.00	2.72	3.03	.05	.32	.12
Total Score	2.36	2.33	2.41	2.55	2.57	2.53	.001	.23	.01

1. 1056 subjects were used in each of three analyses; the 1056 subjects were drawn in each analysis from a grand pool of 330 American Males, 281 Females, 687 Australian Males, 665 Australian Females, 176 Irish Males, 486 Irish Females; in each analysis there were 176 subjects per cell.

2. The higher the score, the less well-adjusted.

TABLE EIGHT:

Cross-Cultural Comparison of Offer Self-Image Questionnaire Sexual Attitudes Scale and Total Score Means: American vs. Irish vs. Israeli Males and Females—Older (16-18-year-old) Normal Adolescents Only

Offer Self-Image Questionnaire Scale[2]	American[1]		Irish[1]		Israeli[1]		Probability Levels: 2 Degrees of Freedom		
	Male	Female	Male	Female	Male	Female	Analysis #1	Analysis #2	Analysis #3
Scale Six: Sexual Attitudes	2.75	2.86	2.33	2.71	2.45	3.01	.01	.05	.05
Total Score	2.19	2.17	2.52	2.46	2.41	2.54	.19	.44	.07

1. 366 subjects were used in each of three analyses; the 366 subjects were drawn in each analysis from a grand pool of 169 American Males, 185 American Females; 72 Irish Males, 100 Irish Females; 81 Israeli Males, 61 Israeli Females; in each analysis there were 61 subjects per cell.

2. The higher the score, the less well-adjusted.

NOTE

1. A description of the developmental psychology of each of these groups can be found in Offer and Offer (1975a, b).

REFERENCES

Blos, P. (1961). *On Adolescence.* New York: The Free Press of Glencoe.

Davis, K. E. (1971). Sex on campus: is there a revolution? *Medical Aspects of Human Sexuality* 5: 128-142.

Deutsch, H. (1967). *Selected Problems of Adolescence.* New York: International Universities Press.

Erikson, E. H. (1968). *Identity: Youth and Crisis.* New York: W. W. Norton.

Freud, A. (1936). *The Ego and The Mechanisms of Defense.* New York: International Universities Press.

Gagnon, J. H., and Simon, W. (1973). *Sexual Conduct: The Social Sources of Human Sexuality.* Chicago: Aldine-Atherton.

Ginsberg, G. L., Frosch, W. A., and Shapiro, T. (1972). The new impotence. *Archives of General Psychiatry* 26: 218-220.

Kohut, H. (1972). Thoughts on narcissism and narcissistic rage. *Psychoanalytic Study of the Child* 97: 360-401.

Offer, D. (1969). *The Psychological World of the Teen-ager.* New York: Basic Books.

————(1972). Attitudes towards sexuality among 1500 middle class adolescents. *Journal of Youth and Adolescence* 1: 81-90.

Offer, D., and Howard, K. I. (1972). An empirical analysis of the Offer Self-Image Questionnaire for adolescents. *Archives of General Psychiatry* 27: 529-537.

Offer, D., Marohn, R. C., and Ostrov, E. (1975). *Psychiatric Studies of Juvenile Delinquents.* New York: Basic Books.

Offer, D., and Offer, J. B. (1975a). *From Teenage to Young Manhood: A Psychological Study.* New York: Basic Books.

————(1975b). Three developmental routes through normal male adolescence. *This Annual* 4: 121-141.

Offer, D., and Sabshin, M. (1963). The psychiatrist and the normal adolescent. *Archives of General Psychiatry* 9: 427-432.

Simon, W., Berger, A. S., and Gagnon, J. H. (1972). Beyond anxiety and fantasy: the coital experiences of college youth. *Journal of Youth and Adolescence* 1: 203-222.

PART II

DEVELOPMENTAL ISSUES: NARCISSISM, PSYCHIC DEVELOPMENT AND THE ADOLESCENT PROCESS

EDITORS' INTRODUCTION

Adolescence as a developmental phase is a topic of almost universal interest. As childhood has proved to be crucial for the organization of drives, adolescence or rather the adolescent process results in the consolidation of the structure of personality. Of course, when mentioning the adolescent process, we are aware of referring to something significantly open-ended, a series of psychic processes that demand considerable exploration.

Throughout these volumes, the formation of psychic structure during the adolescent period has been constantly stressed. We are now in a position to observe the crystallization of specific trends.

Narcissism, as an aspect of psychopathology, has throughout the years received considerable attention, but only recently, within the last several years, has it been emphasized as an aspect of psychic development. Freud considered both the psychopathological and developmental aspects of narcissism and placed it in an hierarchy of structuralization. Today, there is great enthusiasm about understanding patients suffering from structural pathology in terms of narcissistic defects. Inasmuch as adolescents are struggling with structural problems, narcissism is a particularly apt topic. Here, some of the latest ideas on the subject are presented, as well as an evaluation and critique that attempts to place them in a proper perspective.

Narcissism focuses upon early phases of development, recapitulated during adolescence. Later stages gain prominence as the teenager struggles toward adulthood; the interplay of all infantile steps toward psychic structuralization constitutes the panorama of adolescence. The dominance of sexual feelings, for example, is in phase with biological maturation. As a sexual identity evolves, the adolescent is faced with the task of integrating it with many other facets of the self-representation while he seeks his place in the world through the establishment of meaningful object relationships.

Peter Giovacchini discusses the change in psychoanalytic focus from the hydrodynamic model of Freud to an ego psychological perspective with characterological problems of the adolescent becoming especially important. Reviewing theories of early ego development, the author presents his own synthesis, with specific interest in narcissism, as well as a treatment experience which allowed verification of these theories in a structuralizing setting provided by psychoanalytic therapy.

Warren J. Gadpaille discusses the interplay between puberty as a spurt in biological maturation and adolescence as the psychosocial response to puberty. He believes that there exists a sequence, a primacy, and a qualitative difference in the operations upon one another of human psychobiology and culture, concluding that the entire style of a culture may come to bear on how it responds to adolescent sexuality.

Maurice J. Rosenthal is concerned with tracing the effects on development of the universal, filial obligation toward parents. He views the feeling of filial obligation as an autonomous system providing its own motivation, attitudes, behavior, and distinctive conflicts. Dr. Rosenthal, tracing development through the progression of self and object relationship growth, concludes that expressions of filial obligation persist throughout the entire life span, enriching the social well-being.

Andre P. Derdeyn and David B. Waters discuss therapeutic tasks involved in treating the adolescent as a member of his family. Beyond the psychotherapy of the adolescent, they define goals in the reestablishment of empathic communications. With sufficient attention to the developmental problems of parents, the therapist can support them, help them to achieve a better sense of self, and enlist their aid in freeing their child from an ambivalent attachment to them. This, the authors state, can result in a unique opportunity for parental growth.

Richard C. Marohn discusses the normal transformations of primitive narcissistic structures during adolescence and proposes that delinquency as a defense involves significant pathology in this developmental area. He describes the treatment of narcissistically fixated adolescents and emphasizes the importance of recognizing and dealing with self structures rather than distortions of object relationships. Peter Giovacchini discusses Dr. Marohn's chapter and raises significant questions concerning the use of Kohut's metapsychological ideas on narcissism as a separate developmental line.

9] PSYCHOANALYTIC PERSPECTIVES ON ADOLESCENCE, PSYCHIC DEVELOPMENT, AND NARCISSISM

PETER L. GIOVACCHINI

While there has been an increase of interest in the study of the mental processes of the adolescent, I believe it noteworthy that numerous clinicians are focusing upon an ego psychological, theoretical perspective, emphasizing characterological attributes, rather than the usual id-ego hydrodynamic model which Freud found so useful and productive.

Insofar as the adolescent demonstrates characterological pathology, an ego psychological viewpoint is particularly apt since it chiefly involves psychic structure. Thus, it becomes perfectly understandable that our changing theoretical frame should stimulate a study of adolescent patients. Of course, there are many other reasons why such studies would be undertaken, social-cultural factors and clinical necessity being especially compelling forces. However, even without these, the natural progress of psychoanalysis would, most likely, have led us to concentrate on characterological problems and, with this focus, direct attention to the adolescent patient.

Psychopathology and Character Structure

Other than being a specific chronological period, is there anything typical of adolescence which distinguishes it from other periods of life? Adolescence is a stage of development and, as such, the adolescent has particular tasks to fulfill and problems to overcome that differ from other stages. Adolescence differs from childhood insofar as it concentrates upon socialization and preparation for and integration into the adult world. Whereas the preoccupation of the infant is primarily with the satisfaction of bodily needs (instinctual gratification), the adolescent is concerned with the acquisition of techniques that will help him cope with, that is, adapt to the outer world. The adolescent consolidates his character, and when one encounters psychopathology in this group, characterological defects are invariably present.

Identity problems and existential crises, are commonly found in the adolescent. The self-representation is incompletely formed, and manifestations of insecurity frequently highlight the fluidity of his identity. The adolescent patient is therefore preoccupied with such questions as to who and what he is, the fundamental purpose of life, and the role he will fulfill in a world that he can not yet understand, nor fully accept or reject.

The adolescent patient feels insecure, helpless, and vulnerable because he does not possess the adaptive techniques to cope with an external world that he finds inordinately complex and confusing. Being unable to function only accentuates his identity problems, which, if sufficiently intense, can lead to existential crises and psychoses. Schizophrenia commonly becomes manifest during adolescence.

Perhaps what distinguishes adolescence are the defenses utilized, rather than any particularly unique intrapsychic problems. The latter, as discussed, may be unique insofar as the adolescent has special tasks to fulfill, but for the most part these endeavors will persist throughout life and retain their potential to create psychic problems. The adolescent, being in a transitional phase of development, may nevertheless seek solutions that are different than those seen in what is considered the psychopathology of the adult.

Still, are such defenses particularly different, that is, qualitatively distinct from those encountered later in life? Apart from rebellious acting out, which has been labelled as typically adolescent, can one discern specific reactions and patterns that seem to be more consistent with the adolescent orientation? Here the surrounding culture exerts its significance. *The combination of the adolescent's need to effect psychic equilibrium and those elements of the environment which can be seized upon to oppose or support this need may characterize the manifestations of adolescent psychopathology.*

Furthermore, character traits that have only been recently acquired and only loosely incorporated must have some bearing on symptoms and behavior. Once more one can refer to a combination, this time with an intrapsychic focus. *Character traits that have not achieved stability but which nevertheless determine how executive ego systems function and a relatively amorphous self-representation augment each other in a negative feedback sequence and may eventually lead to psychic collapse.* These factors lie behind much adolescent confusion.

114

Can one define some features that might be considered typical of adolescent psychopathology, or typical of the characterological pathology so often encountered during these years? Certainly, confusion is commonly seen. Feelings of helplessness and vulnerability are often part of the teenager's misery. The adolescent's need to change the external world represents a need to simplify matters, to diminish the complexities they face, and to make their ambience congruent with their lack of adjustive techniques. One of my patients often spoke of living in a world of calculus complexity, while he could only function at an arithmetic level (Giovacchini 1965).

Thus, adolescents and others suffering from similar characterological problems cannot cope with the exigencies of their environment. To some extent, this inability threatens their psychic survival and in extreme instances their survival in general. Adaptive attempts range from such appeals as seen in anaclitic dependent states to defensive denial of inadequacies and rebellious acting out. The psychoneurotic is not invariably quiet and the characterological defect does not necessarily manifest itself in a stormy fashion; still, there is a tendency to develop in these directions. Presumably one is dealing with different levels of development.

Developmental Stages and Narcissism

It has become fashionable to emphasize narcissism as if this were a newly discovered, clinically applicable concept. Freud (1911, 1914), however, defined narcissism and used it in an explanatory psychodynamic fashion as well as including it in a developmental timetable.

The adolescent revives our interest in such matters because the psychopathology he manifests can be thought of as a narcissistic deficit, similar to the way Freud formulated such deficits. From a clinical viewpoint, Freud's basic ideas about this type of emotional disturbance seem little improved upon. Many clinicians do not share Freud's pessimism regarding psychoanalytic treatment of patients suffering from what he called the narcissistic neuroses, but still believe in his fundamental structural and technical principles. It is odd that disagreement chiefly centers around the therapeutic application of Freud's principles insofar as some of us believe they are far more applicable than their innovator believed. Eventually one has to clarify technical issues; such an attempt involves theoretical concepts related to character structure and psychic development.

Curiously, although Freud's tenets about treatment have been frequently challenged, the sequence of developmental phases upon which they are based seldom has. Many analysts who have challenged the energic hypothesis, particularly Colby (1955), Kardiner (1959), Fairbairn (1941, 1954) and Klein (1935), have introduced variations in developmental theory. I believe, however, that the latter modifications represent similar themes with only some variation. They did not make any fundamental changes insofar as they retained numerous adultomorphic elements, introducing products of later development into early neonatal periods.

Klein has been vehemently criticized for having attributed complex mental operations and fantasies to very young infants (Glover 1945, Zetzel 1956). Her formulations, at times, seem ludicrous insofar as she grants the child both perceptual and cognitive qualities that would not be compatible with the immature state of the central nervous system. Fairbairn (1941), not so fanciful, retains many of Freud's ideas regarding psychosexual development. However, he discards the anal stage since it does not preserve biological continuity. Clinical phenomena, he believes, can be better explained as defensive adaptations to basic oral disturbances, and he postulates a schizoid core as being fundamental to psychopathology.

I do not intend making a comparative analysis of these three developmental approaches. Rather, I wish to emphasize their similarity and then introduce variations which will be useful for the understanding and treatment of patients suffering from ego defects.

I will concentrate upon Freud since I hope to demonstrate that his system shares some of the disadvantages that have been considered specific to Klein's theory. I will not consider Fairbairn specifically because he shared, for the most part, Freud's ideas about the earliest developmental phases and questioned ideas concerning only later development (the anal phase).

Freud (1914) postulated a developmental sequence from autoerotism (a stage where the ego is not yet differentiated) to primary narcissism, to secondary narcissism, and finally from part object to whole object relationships. Earlier, Freud (1911) linked such narcissistic phases to megalomania and referred to narcissism as a stage of omnipotent wish fulfillment. These represent very early ego states characterized by feelings of megalomania: "his majesty, the baby," with the capacity for omnipotent manipulation. When inevitable frustration tends to upset this magical balance, the outer world is defended against by projection, and here we might have a paranoid picture. All of this occurs very early with such primitive fixations revived by the regressions of later psychopathology.

Yet many of the arguments leveled against Klein about her attributing sophisticated psychic operations to an unstructured mental apparatus apply to the above formulations as well. Magical manipulation, omnipotence, megalomania, and grandiose feelings are very complicated states which seem to supercede what must be the limited mentational capacity of the neonate. To feel persecuted or to ascribe all evil to something or someone outside oneself requires the capacity to evoke very subtle and sensitive feelings which appear incongruous when one notes that the infant, as yet, cannot smile and whose expression of feeling seems restricted to reactions of comfort or discomfort.

Furthermore, the formulations that the expulsion of something which is perceived as bad as a beginning aspect of development (Freud 1915) is strikingly similar, although more subtle, to Klein's (1946) construction of the paranoid-schizoid position as being part of normal development rather than a psychopathological vicissitude.

Freud did not include the same type of elaborate fantasies that Klein (1935, 1946) believed accompanied paranoid-schizoid and depressive positions, but he considered grandiose and paranoid orientations as the manifestations of narcissistic stages, which are the initial phases of his scheme of psychosexual development. So even though Freud did not elaborate on content, he still described complicated mechanisms which could evoke fantasies that would have a certain degree of complexity—certainly, with far more structure than is possible in a preverbal ego state.

Thus, certain modifications seem appropriate to maintain a hierarchy and be consistent with biological data. At the very beginning of extrauterine life, the neonate does not have much in the way of mental activity. From a psychological viewpoint he is amorphous, and feelings and perceptions are vague and indefinite. A nervous system which is to some extent unmyelinated and which responds in a global fashion (as demonstrated by positive Babinski and Moro reflexes) is not yet capable of fine discrimination or mentation. I realize this viewpoint is at variance with one revived by some South American colleagues who postulate mental activity and fantasy production in the fetus. Still, experiments and observations (Reisen 1947) indicate that perception requires interaction with the environment. To be able to see, for example, requires some maturation of the optic system which will not develop if the child is not visually stimulated. If the ability to form images requires a certain amount of contact with the external world, it seems feasible to assume that the formation of mental representations, memory, and fantasy, would require correspondingly more complex relations and stimuli with and from the environment. Spitz's observations (1965) on institutionalized children raised with an absolute minimum of psychic stimuli poignantly bear this point out.

One can refer to this stage as *prementational.* Its orientation is predominantly physiological. How long it lasts, that is, how long before some mentational activity develops is difficult to ascertain. As some experimental evidence suggests, it is probably of very short duration—perhaps a matter of days.

One can assume, however, that the child swiftly begins to recognize states of comfort and discomfort and that some type of activity can alleviate the latter. He does not yet have distinct perceptions relative to what emanates from within himself or from the environment. The environment is only dimly structured, if at all. To some extent, the infant believes that he is the source of what is happening. This sentence is, of course, blatantly untrue since it is almost as adultomorphic as what I am criticizing; the infant does not believe anything nor does he have any notion about something as complicated as etiological connections. For our purposes, it is important to realize that while he has no concept yet of an external object being relevant to his comfort or discomfort, he recognizes that there are forces and activities which have some bearing on the establishment or disruption of homeostasis. This phase, which we can call a *preobject stage,* may be comparable to what Freud referred to as primary narcissism insofar as there is some awareness of a self that can be both needful and gratified, but very little awareness of anything else separate from one's feeling state. Still, this requires a rudimentary ego organization.

The earlier freudian stage of autoerotism cannot be easily integrated into this developmental sequence. It could perhaps be placed in the first prementational phase where ego has not yet developed, but autoerotic behavior assumes the recognition of parts of the body for the production of pleasure. This achievement would be more consonant with the second stage I have outlined, since the discovery of what Freud (1905) called erogenous zones presupposes the existence of, at least, a primitive body ego.

The next phase of development is characterized by a dawning awareness of a nurturing object, but one that is not separate from the self. Here we have the symbiotic phase which can be considered a transition between a preobject phase and beginning object relations (Giovacchini 1972). This stage has in recent years received considerable emphasis since it is prominently recapitulated in the regressions of patients suffering from ego defects.

From here the psyche progresses to the acquisition of the ability to have part object relations and finally to whole object relations. This sequence may sound familiar and self-evident, but the various qualities attributed to these phases and their relevance to later psychopathology justify some recapitulation and clarification. The latter refers to modifications of Freud's model as well as a comparison with Klein's. The following outline should facilitate this task:

	Freud	Klein
Prementational (primarily physiological)	Possibly autoerotism	No comparable phase
Pre-object	Possibly autoerotism Primary narcissism (Omnipotence)	No comparable phase
Symbiotic	Secondary narcissism (Megalomania)	Omnipotent fusion state
Part object	Oral, anal, phallic	Paranoid-schizoid position
Whole object	Genital	Depressive position

The qualities of omnipotence and megalomania that Freud viewed as the essence of his beginning phases, are, in my scheme, defensive adaptations which develop later, and, then, become part of the regression to early traumatic fixations. When Freud moved up to part-object relations, he distinguished conflict and defense from the properties of the particular psychosexual state. Incorporation, projection, isolation, displacement, etc. are unique defenses associated with conflicts that are characteristic of a specific stage. They represent techniques designed to deal with disturbances in the developmental sequence. This refers to the nature of the trauma as well as its temporal occurrence. Some adaptive techniques are more appropriate than others to ego states of certain developmental phases, and Freud referred to some defenses in terms of the stage they are associated with, such as oral or anal defenses.

I do not wish to distinguish between an ego adaptation and a defensive technique designed to handle intrapsychic disturbance. Perhaps the distinction is simply one of degree. I merely want to emphasize that when Freud described early stages as omnipotent and megalomanic he was, in actuality, discussing defensive techniques that could not possibly have been constructed by an ego associated with an immature central nervous system.

Melanie Klein has been criticized for the same reasons when she speaks of the paranoid-schizoid position as a stage of normal development occurring around the age of two months. She attributes the concepts of good and bad, destroy and being destroyed, and the affects of rage and fear to projective mechanisms that are the essence of this phase. Rescuing, reparation, and ambivalence are assigned to the depressive position, one which occurs at approximately six months and deals with whole objects.

By making some revisions, most of Freud's developmental scheme and much of Klein's can be of value for our study of psychopathology and have important implications regarding treatment. Again, if the qualities of omnipotence and grandiosity are eliminated, then Freud's stages of primary and secondary narcissism are not too different from what I have outlined, which places particular emphasis on object relationships. Klein also concentrated on both internal and external objects, but her confusion of psychopathological reactions with developmental process is immense.

For example, Klein referred to good and bad objects from the very beginning whereas Freud (1900, 1915, 1920, 1923) viewed the psychic apparatus as having an amorphous beginning which acquires structure through the impingements of the outer world. Simultaneously, there is some object differentiation, the good object being incorporated and the bad object extruded, indicating a similarity between Freud's and Klein's paranoid-schizoid positions. Yet, Klein more or less ignores Freud's undifferentiated id and begins with his extruded bad object. The good remains internal and the bad is projected. Both are part objects.

Freud and Klein agree that the bad object is an intrinsic part of development. Freud believed that some frustration was required for growth, and Klein implied the same by assuming that the bad object, the outcome of innate destructive feelings emanating from the death instinct, is an inherent aspect of psychic structure.

By contrast, I believe that the bad object is the outcome of forces that are detrimental to development, implying that frustration is not a necessary condition for development. Theoretically, according to this thesis, optimal development would occur without frustration, clearly a hypothetical situation. Rather than remaining fixated, the ego, because it has experienced satisfaction and because of innate maturational forces, is impelled to structuralize further and explore other areas and modalities to obtain satisfaction and pleasure. Once a person's basic survival needs are met, not frustrated, one can explore the external world and pursue other goals, such as sexual, or higher goals such as creative and asthetic. Gratification does not lead to fixation. There are forces within the psyche which seek greater structure—a developmental drive, so to speak, which is hindered rather than released by frustration.

I do not wish to develop this theme further. However, if it is accepted, the concept of the bad object as a basic given for psychic development becomes superfluous. The production of the bad object and its vicissitudes would be the outcome of frustration which would lead to psychopathology rather than emotional development.

Klein indicates that the progression from part object to whole object relations is achieved through an ambivalent stage, a depressive position where love and hatred are currently directly toward the same object rather than split between good and bad objects. This confluence of love and hate, however, does not lead to the formation of a whole object. It is, as Klein states, an integrative experience insofar as there is some unity, at least more so than when splitting is the predominant mechanism. But, even though love and hate are directed toward the same object, the object, nevertheless, is still a part object. One can view the breast, for example, as the source of goodness or badness; a breast, however, is only part of a person and considerable maturation is required before one can relate to an external object from a unified variety of perspectives.

Viewing development in the terms just described has clinical and technical implications about narcissism and those entities considered narcissistic character disorders. Obviously, Kohut's (1971) concept of narcissism as a developmental stage with an independent progression is inconsistent with this viewpoint (Kernberg 1974, Giovacchini 1976). In fact, narcissism, insofar as it involves self-love, grandiosity, or omnipotence, has no place in early development.

Later, because of trauma or healthy integration, ego states emerge that can be conceptualized as narcissistic. With psychopathology, narcissism is a defensive overcompensatory defense and character trait designed to protect an ego which feels vulnerable, has low self-esteem, and finds itself unable to cope with the exigencies of the outer world. As an outcome of normal development, healthy narcissism, as Federn (1952) long ago described, is characteristic of an ego that is confident of its abilities and enjoys its capacity to function and relate to reality, an ego that is attaining the attributes of the ego-ideal. I believe this regularity occurs with creativity (Giovacchini 1965).

Turning our attention to adolescence and narcissistic character disorders, we observe an ego traumatized during early developmental periods. The difference in clinical outcome between a trauma that is principally experienced (or whose disruptive effects are experienced) during the prementational phase and one that occurs later is enormous.

Our concepts as to what constitutes a psychoanalytic relationship with patients who have suffered very early traumas, and these seem to be more numerous than previously suspected, require close attention and reexamination. This is particularly germane as we focus upon the increasing number of hospitalized patients, especially adolescents. The place of psychoanalytic treatment in an in-patient setting is an extremely fluid question.

The holocausts of wars and ghetto poverty already face us with persons displaying characterological problems of such dimensions that they have effects upon society in general. Violence and crime are rampant and workers are seized with feelings of hopeless misery and impotence when they attempt to rehabilitate certain criminal segments of the adolescent population. These are sad and frightening situations and there may be many good reasons for increasing concern. Maria Piers was quoted recently as saying that many of the South Vietnam war orphans recently brought into this country are going to add to our woes. Because of violence and lack of consistent maternal nurture, she conjectures that severe character problems will develop later and manifest themselves in crime and other forms of antisocial behavior.

It behooves us to see where psychoanalytic treatment fits. Perhaps, in certain cases, it would be ludicrous to even consider it. However, to locate hopelessness will help define the dimensions of hope.

Dimensions of Psychoanalytic Treatment

Interpretation is the essence of psychoanalytic treatment, and Freud placed great emphasis on its verbal form. Secondary process is characterized by the cathexis of word representation (Freud 1915). The transference and nonjudgmental aspects of interpretation have been stressed by many analysts (Boyer and Giovacchini 1967).

If some patients were traumatized during prementational or preverbal phases, how can words have any effect? The word is a secondary process construct, one which patients as sick as I have been describing would presumably be unable to incorporate to achieve further integration. Some adolescents seem particularly inarticulate.

I understand that many hospitalized patients are primitively fixated at such preverbal levels and their accessibility to analysis has been seriously questioned. I wish to discuss this group from a psychoanalytic perspective, that is, in terms of interpretative interaction, but I realize at the outset that I will only be able to raise more questions than to provide answers. Still, I believe it important to be able to structure questions and locate the various positions of our dilemmas and problems.

If the patient does not have enough secondary process to be able to understand, that is, to integrate a verbal interpretation, is there any other kind of activity that may have a structuralizing effect? Can one interpret nonverbally? Can the analyst introduce some secondary process, not as much as in a verbal presentation but sufficient for the patient to be able to grasp what is being offered? The differential between what the analyst offers and the developmental condition of the patient's psychic state could very well determine the amount of structure the patient may be able to achieve.

Before proceeding with a description of a nonverbal interpretation, the question of management requires attention. Many therapists, indeed some of the most skillful and respected (for example, Bettelheim 1967, Ekstein 1966, Winnicott 1947, 1952, 1955) believe that some response to the patient's needs is necessary. Gratifications that have never been or have only been imperfectly experienced should be offered to make analytic contact with the patient. I mention the factor of management because I have found it very difficult to justify analytically on theoretical grounds. Yet when I read about such interactions I am deeply moved by the therapist's humanity and sensitivity, and often impressed by the results.

Interpretation by giving form to inchoate and unconscious constricting elements supposedly releases the ego so it can incorporate potentially adaptive and helpful experiences. Insofar as intellectual insight is supplied within the context of the transference regression, the patient relives the early traumas and is then able to release a developmental drive previously submerged by psychopathology. Admittedly this is a gross oversimplification of what Strachey (1934) referred to as the mutative effects of interpretation, a subject which in itself is inexhaustible. Management, or the attempt to gratify infantile needs, supposedly belongs to another frame of reference and even though it is designed to be helpful, the analyst does not consider such activities as structure promoting. The analyst tries to maintain the patient so that now or later he will be able to become analytically involved.

Superficially, interpretation and management seem at opposite poles. The former presumably occurs in an atmosphere of abstinence whereas the latter is aimed at gratification. These distinctions seem clear and simple. However, when dealing with patients with such embryonic egos, one wonders whether such distinctions are possible. Perhaps an experience aimed at understanding is in some way relevant to the gratification of infantile needs. Perhaps support and management have transference implications which might also have interpretative significance, and thereby promote psychic development.

Consequently, something more specific should be said about the qualities of the early fixations of these severely disturbed patients and how their character pathology is reflected in the transference relation. Whatever transpires between patient and therapist, which is to a large measure determined by the patient's infantile experiences, can be considered from the point of view of transference. Patients with amorphous and poorly equipped egos have some common denominators in their backgrounds characteristically affecting the forms of psychopathology, and leading to various complications in a psychotherapeutic relationship. Let us direct our attention to the patients emphasized here, those who have not progressed much beyond the prementational phase of development.

Fixation on Prementational Phase

As therapists are so used to dealing with others by feelings and words, the situation of dealing with rudimentary or even absent affects is particularly challenging. A patient who is incapable of expressing his needs and emotions can be disconcerting and puzzling. How can one deal with him on a one to one basis? Although therapeutic technique may be challenged, our psychoanalytic orientation may come to our aid in, understanding at least, something about the nature of the patient's traumatic orientation.

This is where the object relationship perspective becomes indispensable. No matter how confusing these patients may be, their inability to relate to people, or to verbally sustain object relationships, becomes strikingly and painfully apparent. This incapability to structure an affect is reflected in their lack of object relations which often manifests itself by an autistic pose.

The treatment, although therapists are sometimes reluctant to term it so, is often characterized by the patient's refusal or inability to acknowledge the analyst's presence. Although this seems to be an impossible situation, it is the way things should be. The patient is reflecting a basic ego defect.

Insofar as the patient was never acknowledged as an individual, he has never been able to distinguish others as distinct from himself. This becomes especially traumatic during adolescence, when the demands to structure an identity vis-à-vis the external world becomes particularly forceful. The outbreak of schizophrenia during adolescence is common enough.

These patients have achieved very little in the way of mentational capacities. Experiences and feelings about the self have only a minimum of mental representation since their egos do not have the structure to perceive beyond the somatic and to support such complex psychological entities as affects, fantasies, and adaptive mechanisms.

What I have just described is, of course, a fiction. No one could have grown and developed to adolescence or adulthood with such lack of structure or differentiation. At best, one would have a living vegetable.

Unfortunately, living vegetables do exist. These are not patients who feel and act as if they were dead. On the contrary, to feel dead means that some part of the self, no matter how poorly conceived, must know something about being alive. And insofar as there is some feeling of aliveness, there is some hope. I am referring to people where it is difficult if not impossible to sustain hope. I remember seeing a nine-year-old girl who had been raised shackled in a dark closet her entire life. It was hard to think of her as a person. She was no larger than a two year old and looked like a monkey rather than a human being as she crawled around blindly and grunted incoherently.

Hopefully, these are extremes, although one wonders whether cataclysmic world conditions may not create more extreme situations. Still most patients have managed to survive in a fashion where they are able to relate in some way to the external world. Even this group, conceptualized as being fixated at prementational levels, have some elements of organization that permit them to make adjustments or grant them the potential to make adjustments in the future.

This minimally hopeful attitude is based upon the fact that fixations are usually partial. If they were total, by definition no development could occur because a completely fixated emotional development would be asynchronous with a biologically innate maturational drive. For most of these patients, then, it is the degree of fixation which determines the severity of the manifestation of psychopathology and the difficulties that will be encountered in a psychotherapeutic relationship.

Again, a few of these patients seem to relate to others and to recognize the fact of an external world apart from themselves. Others seem completely withdrawn as in autism and catatonia; this group is commonly found in hospitals. However, in both groups, the chief ego defect makes it difficult if not impossible to establish distinctions between the self and the outer world. Although the former group seems to relate, in actuality, it is only a superficial relationship devoid of any real affect. Many of these patients go through the motions of relating and have many of the attributes Deutsch (1942) assigned to "as-if" characters.

As there are problems in acknowledging the presence of an external object, this is reflected in the treatment. Indeed, many feel that this deficit is responsible for the patient's inaccessibility to psychoanalytic treatment. Still, it must be remembered that the patient's failure in treatment is also a recapitulation of a situation in childhood that he had never been able to master. He could never form a picture of his mother, one that he could retain as constant and separate from himself. Her presence was never really felt and now there will be problems in feeling the analyst's presence. Furthermore, such an amorphous orientation makes it difficult for the patient to keep past, present, and future separate, making the perception of the outer world even more difficult since reality, to a large measure, is ordered around time sequences.

Although the awareness of the self and outer world is dim and indistinct, the patient still has some ability to feel needs. He may not precisely know their source, since the concept of source is also basically beyond his comprehension; but he does feel something. Also, he must have some capacity to communicate his needful feelings.

The conflict these patients suffer from can be stated simply, even though their condition is far from simple. We have a psyche that can minimally experience and communicate needs, but insofar as the external world has been poorly integrated, the patient does not have the adaptive techniques to take care of himself. Furthermore, he has no security whatsoever that outside forces can be helpful, because he cannot maintain the idea of outside. Needs consequently become dangerous.

There are several possible reactions available. Most likely, the patient will use such primitive defenses as massive denial, and here one notes extreme schizoid or autistic withdrawal. Both inner needs and the outside world are disavowed. Everything is perceived as dangerous because there are few memories of gratifying experiences to draw from. Some extreme cases of anorexia nervosa that end in death are examples of this type of patient. Most patients, however, are not so totally withdrawn and have developed a minimal capacity for hope. Although expecting failure, they may turn to whatever perception of the outer world they can form and mysteriously—that is, mysteriously to us—ask for help.

Other patients act out and may become involved in criminal and destructive behavior. The latter are usually self-destructive and should be distinguished from better organized acting out, where patients externalize rebellious rage. These patients are not particularly angry; in fact, they have not achieved the capacity to structure such an affect as anger (Winnicott 1947). Consequently, their behavior is clumsy and purposeless instead of tendentious and intense. By way of illustration, I recall a patient who would steal from a fruit stand, call up people in order to complain at all hours of the day and night, and send threatening notes demanding ransom to prevent him from kidnapping someone's child. Usually no one paid any attention to him although he succeeded in frightening an intended kidnap victim and landed in jail for a short period of time. The police brought him to the psychiatric ward of a private hospital.

Acting out for these patients represents pathetic attempts at self-assertion. They are pushing themselves onto the external world in order to feel themselves and to master both the inner and outer worlds. To the degree that both worlds are not separated and that they feel themselves only in terms of vaguely perceived biological urges, these attempts at assertion and mastery are very difficult indeed.

If the situation is as problematical as I have described, then how can any rational person believe that such patients can become engaged in a one to one psychotherapeutic relationship and least of all a psychoanalytic one? I believe that there is, in some cases, a possibility of establishing a psychoanalytic relationship in spite of what seems to be insurmountable obstacles. True, the analyst will have to make some adaptations and the form of his relationship will be modified from the traditional one, but the analytic setting can be preserved. In fact, it will be preserved stronger than ever.

Interpretation within the transference context is still what the analyst strives for, although what constitutes both an interpretation and transference requires further scrutiny. These patients cannot sustain the presence of an external object and *one of the analyst's tasks is to make his presence felt*.

This is not usually a problem with many patients who seek analysis on their own and are aware of the analyst from varying perspectives. Thus, the analyst can immediately direct himself to intrapsychic conflict, automatically assuming that the patient can form and retain an introject of the analyst and the analytic relationship.

I am directing myself to inherent limitations that require some type of response that will help the patient link certain inner needs with events in the outer world—in this case, the analyst's presence. Because the patient has structural defects which make it difficult to maintain a mental representation of an external object, the presence of the analyst is either not acknowledged or defended against. Not being acknowledged can be explained as the result of incapacity. A blind person does not see an external object simply because he cannot see. But why defend oneself from seeing by withdrawal, denial, and sometimes protest?

Perhaps the external object is perceived as dangerous, a threatening, destructive, devouring force. This is often true for patients, but not for these patients. Destructive forces are evaluated by feelings and feelings here mean anger and anxiety. Again, this group of patients is nowhere so complex; they have very little capacity for object and goal directed anger and their appraisal of external danger is correspondingly limited.

Rather than dangerous, the external object, when capable of being acknowledged, is perceived as hovering. The patient finds this threatening and sufficiently disruptive to desire withdrawal from the situation. He cannot comprehend it and feels disturbed and confused. If external demands persist he may become further disorganized and panicky—a primitive type of existential terror rather than well organized anxiety that can lead to adaptive defenses.

I have described patients incapable of dealing with certain tasks as lacking the functional introjects that would lead to the acquisition of adaptive techniques by the ego's executive system (Giovacchini 1963). Here, it is not a question of task oriented techniques. Rather, the ego defects of patients fixated on the prementational developmental phase hamper the capacity of the ego to incorporate any experience, even one designed to be helpful. This incapacity makes such an experience uncomfortable and this discomfort can be reflected in the treatment relationship. Besides withdrawing, the patient may indicate to the analyst that he wishes him to leave. In the hospital, this may be the first real communication that the patient is capable of—it is an achievement when he can signal to the analyst and the analyst understands that the patient wishes him to leave.

CLINICAL EXAMPLE

To be able to communicate a wish is an advance from a defensive withdrawal. Let me illustrate this point and then discuss some technical factors. An eighteen year old young man was brought to treatment by his parents because he was "vegetating." They described their son in terms of simple schizophrenia. He showed no interests whatsoever; social, academic, or vocational. He seemed to be totally inept, gauche, and at times appeared retarded although he did well on psychometric tests. The parents were particularly disturbed at his lack of feeling.

He entered treatment with what seemed to be complete indifference. He saw no purpose in anything and kept his appointments only because his parents insisted. His apathy and lack of motivation were so great that I was, to some extent, intrigued. The situation for psychoanalysis seemed so absolutely hopeless that I decided to see what could happen and, identifying with the patient, I had no particular expectations.

Still, the patient was not altogether unappealing. He asked for nothing, but I had the feeling that some part of him was glad to be there, that is as glad as he was capable of feeling.

He kept his appointments regularly and punctually, and lay on the couch without difficulty. For the first three months, he said practically nothing. In many of these early sessions, he simply curled up in a fetal position and lay completely still. His absolute silence did not compel me to intercede. I felt no need to pursue him, to get him to open up or talk. I have had this feeling with other patients, which I have had to control, but not with him. He also seemed comfortable.

Gradually, he began making comments which seemed off-hand but which, since he said so little, achieved great importance and significance for me. To exemplify the flavor of his remarks and our interchange, he once told me about a slight change in the schedule of the train he used for transportation to my office. The change made practically no difference in his convenience in keeping our appointments. In fact, as I later ascertained, it was even more convenient. Instead of finding this material circumstantial and tedious, a reaction which, in retrospect, could have been appropriate, I found myself intensely interested in every little detail of the changed schedule. I asked him further questions about it, and if there had been an outsider present he could easily have concluded that we were engaged in a momentous and fascinating conversation. As I look back at the intensity of my involvement, I still feel surprised. I wish to emphasize that my reactions were spontaneous and not related to management or therapeutic intent. Later, I will discuss reasons for my behavior, reasons which I was totally unaware of at the time.

Gradually, the patient's material developed a theme. Although he seemed to be jumping from one topic to another, he was referring to his inability to understand what was happening to him in the external world or to know how to react to various situations. He was asking to be told how to relate to situations that would have been simple and pedestrian to his contemporaries. He had cast me in the role of an educator and sought my advice, for example, as to what type of shoe would be appropriate for a particular occasion. With him, my natural tendency was to give, whenever possible, the information he sought, again in contrast to the way I reacted to other patients who, on occasion, might ask similar questions. However, I did not expect him to profit from what I told him. He was able to retain some of it, as evidenced by the fact that he took my advice, but I became increasingly convinced that the content of our interaction was secondary. I was forming the impression that the patient was beginning to acknowledge my presence, not necessarily as a person, but simply my presence. In the meantime, I was able to feel his presence although he still seemed to have little in the way of human qualities except for needfulness and confusion.

Now I did something that complicated the treatment and highlighted the importance of being able to communicate in contrast to defensive withdrawal. The first few months of treatment illustrate this point and have important technical implications. In any case, just as the patient was beginning to have a dim awareness of my presence, I took an extended vacation. Considering where we were in treatment, I do not imagine that my departure could have been worse timed. I had announced my intentions well ahead, but what I had not understood was the patient's failure to grasp what I had said.

I do not wish to belabor my poor timing, nor blame myself. True, it was bad for the treatment but then I did not understand this patient as I do now, and, to a large measure, it is the complication I am about to describe that enabled me to understand. Furthermore, I do not know whether I would have postponed my vacation, even if I had understood the kind of importance I had achieved for him. I believe I might have resented the control he would have had over me and this might have been deleterious to treatment. I grant this is an open question where one is caught between the Scylla of guilt and the Charybdis of feeling imposed upon.

Upon returning from my vacation, I received a message that my patient had been hospitalized. According to the attending psychiatrist, the patient underwent a profound regression after I left. Diagnosed as a catatonic schizophrenic, the patient was mute and seemed oblivious to anyone who tried to approach him. He was given phenothiazines and the staff attempted to involve him in programs. He was led to groups but initially remained silent. Curiously, in spite of his withdrawal, the staff remained friendly and found him pleasant and somewhat attractive. He did not stir up the anxiety that the catatonic who seems to be sitting on a volcano does. He was nonthreatening and although the length of stay on this ward was predetermined, the staff seemed to be lax in following their self imposed rules.

Gradually, the patient began speaking and was able to carry on superficial conversations. At this point, the staff had a meeting and decided that since he could now verbalize it might be judicious to continue his psychotherapy with me. Though I am not a member of the hospital staff, I was invited to see him with the aim of determining whether it would be possible to reestablish an outpatient relationship. When the patient was informed of this plan he seemed unconcerned.

He was informed of when I would be there. I was told before seeing him that the patient acted as if he did not even hear the nurse when she told him the day and time of my arrival. On the day of our appointment, he was reminded of it and again he did not seem to hear.

He was in bed when I arrived even though it was afternoon. He was affable enough, although reserved. I asked a few questions, the usual amenities, and then relaxed into silence. Since the patient was lying down, I unconsciously drifted into an analytic frame of mind and the patient began talking. He talked about daily events and some of his experiences in the hospital. He finally reached back into the days shortly after I had departed. There was no visible emotion, but suddenly in the middle of a sentence he shut his eyes. I was startled. Then without particularly thinking about it, I quietly stood up and left.

Naturally, I gave this event considerable thought. I concluded that the patient by closing his eyes was telling me that he wished I leave. For some reason, my presence had become burdensome to him, perhaps it evoked painful associations linked with my abandoning him. Although he did not care to, or was not able to put his wish into words, his method of communicating nevertheless represented an advance from the total withdrawal that one might have expected as his extremely sensitive reaction to a traumatic situation. I definitely felt that my presence had assumed the proportions of such a trauma for him, and the fact that he could limit his reactions to the somatic expression of a wish rather than resorting to massive psychotic denial seemed hopeful.

The patient was eventually discharged from the hospital and on his parents' insistence returned to my office. He occasionally continued as before and presented situations where he wanted to be told how to behave. He seemed tense. His expression often betrayed confusion and there was an embarrassed quality to our relationship.

I felt he was still disappointed in me, that I had betrayed his shaky trust by deserting him. The patient's main affect, however, was confusion. This became increasingly clear, and there were none of the incriminations or anger usually associated with distrust or disappointment.

In a way, many of his hours reminded me of the incident in the hospital. I felt that he was telling me to leave. On the other hand, he did not feel free to leave and did not have the need to withdraw by curling up in the fetal position, as he did at the beginning of our relationship.

I noted, however, that during certain sessions he acted as if I did not exist. He would literally not acknowledge me. He acted as if he did not see me and his associations had all the features of a monologue. He was never silent during these sessions for *to be silent often means not to be talking to someone.* There can be an object relationship quality to silence. Instead the patient was talking to himself. When he seemed to recognize me, he looked confused.

Finally I confronted him with his confusion and added that apparently he found it difficult to accept my presence. Most likely, he perceived me as hovering around him and must have my presence threatening since he did not quite know what to do with me; nor was he certain how to use me or whether he could use me at all.

This interpretation had profound effects. Instead of withdrawing, he now became more conventionally psychotic. He began having visual and auditory hallucinations which consisted simply of my person or voice. There were no longer any boundaries between my office and the outside world; they were blended both spatially and temporally.

This was not a fusion state, at least not yet. Nor was he paranoid in the conventional sense. My hallucinated image was not persecuting him and, in turn, he felt no anger. I was simply hovering and when I talked to him it was of inconsequential and impersonal items.

He continued to feel threatened and confused. The only difference was that instead of these feelings remaining confined to my office, they spread out and encompassed his total environment. Even though I was being carried around with him I was, in a sense, still being kept outside of himself, and, although he felt anxious, it was not disruptive.

Up to this point in the analysis, the patient had never reported a dream. Dreams seemed superfluous since there seemed to be little distinction between sleeping and waking life, between inside and outside. Now he began to dream, but he began to dream while sleeping in my office. Yet, this patient's sleeping did not represent withdrawal. When actually withdrawing, though he seemed to be ignoring everything around him, he had to stay awake to maintain vigilance against a complicated and confusing, dimly perceived outer world—maintaining as much focus as possible upon that

132

which can be perceived or comprehended only with difficulty. It seemed that he could now relax.

Dreaming is also an indication that he was beginning to separate his unconscious from reality, that he was distinguishing the inner from the outer world. The content of his dreams also pointed to this differentiation. He dreamed of being fed and eating. Sometimes, as simply as that, somebody (only vaguely outlined) was feeding him, usually apples. He was very grateful that he was able to enjoy the apples. As a curious aside, he told me that he could never eat apples and, although he liked their flavor very much, he was never able to digest them. He would vomit whenever he tried to eat them. Now, he was able to eat half an apple without throwing up.

There were many other dreams of incorporation as he continued sleeping during most of his sessions, and their manifest content became increasingly complicated. He also reported similar dreams occurring outside of his sessions and at this time he stopped hallucinating me.

I had commented that he was able to put himself in a position where he felt he was receiving something from me, that he was now capable of taking in some parts of me which he experienced as nourishing. He seemed comfortably dependent and recalled many of our conversations during the beginning of treatment. He was also able to put into action some of the answers that I had given to his questions of how to cope with certain situations.

This blissful state was short-lived. It became apparent that he no longer hallucinated me because he had now incorporated me. This became clear in his dreams and associations, and he sometimes directly talked about his feelings that he had swallowed me. But, he found me hard to digest.

The patient kept using the same expression over and over again about having "bitten more than I can chew." Now he was visibly distressed and for the first time during four years of analysis he was able to feel angry—at the moment toward me.

He believed that I was forcing myself upon him and this caused him to feel frightened and angry, but he was not confused.

Once more the patient became psychotic but, in my opinion, his psychosis represented an advance in structure rather than a regressive breakdown of a defensive organization. On the contrary, the psychosis represented a defensive attempt against a state of inner disruption. Freud (1911) spoke of the defensive aspects of psychosis, but this patient's psychosis involved more organization and structure than previously, whereas Freud was describing regression.

The patient was now more typically paranoid. He hallucinated me once again, but this time he felt I was persecuting him. He believed that I had plotted with his parents to have him "put away" and "locked up for the rest of his life." He also was very angry and sent me letters that threatened to expose me to my colleagues.

Remarkably, in spite of all of this, the patient never missed a session. Although it may seem paradoxical, I felt pleased rather than annoyed about his paranoia. As stated, I saw it as a progression; now he could structure the affects of anxiety and anger, and he was able to use the mechanism of projection rather than denial and global withdrawal. Furthermore, it became clear that he was defending himself against a state of symbiotic fusion, a developmental stage that he had not been able to achieve or had done so only to an insignificant degree.

I was able to deal with this material interpretatively and I suppose my rather positive acceptance of his delusions and my concentrating on their adaptive potential must have been reassuring because his gradual discomfort diminished. His delusions also left him as he became increasingly able to talk about rather than experience them.

This is as far as I wish to go in my discussion of this patient. In order not to leave it hanging I will briefly summarize. The patient continued for two more years with me and then felt that he had to resolve his dependence upon me and his parents. He was seeking autonomy and believed that treatment could not go any further unless he paid for it himself and was free of his parents' influence. He emphasized that the analysis had to be truly his own. He left to join the Peace Corps stating that he fully intended to return to treatment.

He never did. After several years he left the Peace Corps, married, had two children, and took over his father's business. He came back to see me once, ostensibly to discuss some problems his older child had. I gained the impression that he was trying to tell me he did not need me any longer.

Technical Principles and Developmental Fixation

The treatment of this patient helps formulate some general principles which may be applicable to all patients suffering from severe psychopathology. His basic characterological defects seemed to preclude the development of a transference that could be analytically useful.

During the first months of treatment when he attempted to use me for educational purposes, I believe he was trying to repair lacunae in the ego's executive systems. However, insofar as he was not able to incorporate any experience with the outer world, even potentially helpful ones, he could receive only minimal help. Still, he was able to tolerate my presence to the extent that when I left on vacation, he reacted catastrophically. Being there and leaving must have been a recapitulation of a very early trauma which occurred when internal controls to maintain homeostasis had not yet developed.

One could say that the patient regressed after I left and that he resorted to even more primitive defenses than those he initially presented. He totally withdrew, not out of anger, because he was incapable of feeling angry, but out of desperation. He was no longer able to recognize the external world and totally ceased communicating.

While in the hospital, the staff tried vigorously to draw him out of his shell, but their success was minimal. With me, however, he was able to communicate a wish; even though he did so nonverbally he somehow managed to convey to me that he wanted me to leave. I believe this was an extremely important and crucial moment in the treatment, one that determined its whole future course.

My response to the patient's psychic state by a definite action, in this case leaving, elevated a vague feeling of discomfort to a definite and circumscribed communication. I believe this interchange evolved into a structural accretion, which led him to some recognition of the external world and helped him achieve some ability to communicate with it. To some extent the dyadic quality of analysis was established. Recognizing the existence of the analyst by being able to send him away indicated that there was another person present, one who would react to his wishes. This also meant that there was another person present into whom he could project or perhaps in the future be able to incorporate.

Both projection and introjection occurred, and the use of such psychic mechanisms represented an advance in emotional development. He was able to structure an affect, and for the first time in his life he was able to feel anger, as evidenced by his transitory paranoid psychosis. He became increasingly able to feel my presence and, even to some degree, incorporate and retain some aspects of myself instead of immediately dismissing them by projection. As a result of progress in treatment we had achieved symbiotic fusion. From this point on he struggled with this symbiosis, feeling both comfortable with it as well as struggling against it, as he became concerned about autonomy.

Discussion

What are the therapeutic implications of responding directly, or at least, of trying to respond directly to the patient's wishes? Here again one is faced with the technical question of management versus transference interpretation.

If my assertion is correct, that my leaving when I believed the patient wished me to leave was the most crucial moment of the treatment, then how can it be explained within a psychoanalytic context? How is a response to a communication related to transference and interpretation? These are decisive questions which confront clinicians who wish to work psychoanalytically with patients similar to the one presented. Our responses have to be understood in a psychoanalytic framework. Can they be integrated into such a framework or are they deviations or parameters?

Fields (1975) and Flarsheim (1975) report a similar situation to the one just described. Their patient turned his back in order to signal his wish that the therapist leave. They suggested acceding to the patient's request, but then to return a little later, perhaps in ten minutes.

By the therapist's leaving, the patient learns that he has wishes of his own and they have effects on the external world. The latter also implies that there is an external world separate from the self and it can be influenced. However, it also means that the external object has disappeared and insofar as the patient is not able to retain a mental representation of an external object, then from this viewpoint, there is no external world. The return of the therapist once more introduces the external world, one which the patient can now link to particular needs. This may be felt as an intrusion, in which case the patient may send the analyst away again or he may withdraw. This latter global defense follows the successful manipulation of a partial acknowledgment of the external world.

Primitively fixated patients have an imperfectly developed time sense and this lack causes difficulties in dealing with transference. The therapeutic handling of transference projections requires some distinction between past and present, some continuity in the flow of time. The patient's withdrawal following the successful manipulation of the analyst helps establish a fixed point in time because the return of the therapist can be linked with the patient's successful communication that he leave. Here one gains the beginning of the recognition of a temporal sequence. Influencing the outer world and a defensive withdrawal are classes of experiences that can be distinguished from one another without requiring any well-developed capacity to retain mental representations. The patient experiences tension; he feels threatened by the presence of the therapist. Having been successful in removing the therapist reestablishes some homeostasis. The patient's tension and his relief achieved by changing the world around him helps establish that internal states can be relieved and that there is an outer world somehow connected with that relief. This aggregate of experiences, since it is closer to physiological needs insofar as survival is involved, can be integrated much more easily into the ego than a mental representation.

The therapist by returning is once again imposing himself upon the patient. Perhaps this evokes the memory of the communication which was able to send the therapist away. So one can distinguish between an outer world which impinges and one that was denied.

This distinction involves a temporal separation which will now enable the patient to relate in a transference context, that is in a psychoanalytic context.

Thus, responding to the patient's wish that the therapist leave helps establish not only a transference relationship but the possibility of utilizing such a relationship for therapeutic purposes since the temporal element is introduced.

In the office, the limits of time are clearly established as an elaboration and further development of the temporal sequence just described. Winnicott (1955) wrote of the constant reliability of the analytic setting as having a structuralizing potential.

The office can be treated by some of these patients in the same way as has been described for the hospital setting. The analyst offers a fixed segment of time on a regular basis. Within that segment, the patient determines whether he stays or removes the hovering analyst by leaving when he feels the need. However, he will return the next day, and the sequence of the removal and the reappearance of the analyst as a representation of the external world is repeated and becomes increasingly fixed within the patient's psyche.

In addition to fixing a temporal sequence, the patient gauges how much he differentiates between the self and the external world and how much of that differentiation he can bear. The analyst by creating a setting which is reminiscent of the one described in the hospital provides the patient with an experience that helps distinguish inside from outside, and hopefully to make the outside tolerable.

The question initially posed referred to the therapeutic efficacy of management, in this instance, trying to gratify infantile needs versus interpretation within the transference context. This discussion has focused upon only one need, the wish to have the therapist leave.

This is a primitive wish and characteristic of patients fixated at early preverbal stages. It can be considered a restorative attempt. The patient feels the external world as imposing and perhaps oppressive, one that he cannot integrate. Consequently, he needs to establish once again a nonintrusive external world. He has to put matters back on a simple uncomplicated basis. To elevate such a primitive need to a wish fulfilling communication through the analytic interaction is an advance.

Does the analyst gratify other needs or wishes, and are such maneuvers compatible with analysis? I doubt it, although I must admit that the examples of such therapeutic interactions given by Bettelheim (1967) and Winnicott (1955) are most impressive. In some instances, these clinicians were directing themselves to such circumscribed needs as oral needs, and sometimes would literally feed the patient.

In view of the primitive psychic structures of the patients they described, especially Bettelheim, one might wonder whether they were dealing with patients similar to those that are being concentrated upon here. It is quite possible that these therapists and others like them may be relating to the patient's inability to accept and acknowledge their presence. Whether the patient is held or fed may simply be the vehicle that will enable him to acknowledge the analyst, and feeding, for example, may come to represent the treatment modality. Insofar as this is true the analyst is not reacting to the patient's infantile oral wishes per se; rather, he is helping to construct a setting in which the patient can establish a temporal sequence and survive the existence of an external world which had, because of early trauma, become impossible to accept.

To consider just one simple need may seem like an oversimplification, but in my opinion it is not. Granted that a human being is a very complex organism with many subtle facets and complicated needs, there are still certain basic fundamental orientations that are reflected in all aspects of the patient's organization and behavior. The single need to send the analyst away reflects both the patient's lack of separation of himself and the external world and his inability to structure an external world which can be integrated within his psyche and can help contribute to its regulation. Thus, rejecting the external world, which in therapy is represented by the analyst, represents the most basic aspect of the psychopathology of persons fixated at the prementational phase. Such a need must somehow be expressed. *Perhaps in one way or another it is being constantly expressed, but only in therapy does it acquire sufficient organization so that it can be communicated.*

From this viewpoint, therapy has a structuralizing potential. This has always been thought to be true, but it is never so true as it is with these patients.

138

My patient after more or less successfully trying to incorporate me was finally able to construct an affect such as goal-directed anger. This occurred when he was moving upwards on the developmental scale from inability to acknowledge my existence toward symbiotic fusion.

I believe this situation, the structuring of anger, distinguishes analysis from other forms of treatment which focus on behavior and symptomatic improvement. From the viewpoint of behavior the patient was incomparably worse. He became phenomenologically psychotic, a typical paranoid schizophrenic. However, from a developmental perspective he was now struggling with problems derived from the traumatic symbiotic phase of infancy, a period when objects are perceived as part objects and split into good and bad objects. The symbiotic phase the patient achieved in treatment was traumatic because the ego defect derived from the prementational phase made him unable to structure and incorporate the external world. The patient had now acquired the ability to be paranoid, and as such, the patient's psychosis represented progress and was treated as a welcome turn of events.

From such a psychosis the patient was able to move forward to the point where he was able to incorporate aspects of the outer world. He still had difficulties, but now his problems focused upon his concern for a circumscribed autonomy.

Can one learn anything about special techniques from the treatment of this patient? I believe the most fundamental impression one gains from this clinical presentation is that even very disturbed patients whose difficulties date back to preverbal periods can be treated psychoanalytically without altering any basic technical principles. True, one has to have a special focus and may have to resort to particular maneuvers, but this is true of any case. Responding to the patient's wish allowed a temporal focus to develop which was essential for the establishment of a transference context. From that point the treatment was concerned with making the analyst's presence felt, but this was done in a transference-interpretative context. Of course, many other factors of general treatment of all patients were also involved, but these have been dealt with elsewhere.

Perhaps it seems wasteful to expend effort concentrating on persons with one particular fixation to the exclusion of so many others whose developmental difficulties belong at other levels. Still, studying patients fixated at the prementational phase forces one to clarify aspects of developmental theory which will shed light on all forms of psychopathology. Furthermore, these patients are quite numerous as one learns from the investigation of hospital populations and the increasing number of adolescents who seek, sometimes desperately, treatment.

Conclusions

The psychopathology of many hospitalized patients and adolescents dates back to preverbal levels of development. By presenting a clinical example, I examine some elements involved in the treatment of such characterologically disturbed patients.

First, one needs a developmental timetable which is consistent with both biology and psychology. Freud and Klein have made momentous and significant contributions, but their formulations are adultomorphically constructed and can become confusing when applied to egos suffering from very primitive fixations. Consequently, I propose a model incorporating most of Freud's and some of Klein's conceptualizations: those without qualities such as grandiosity, omnipotence, and paranoid and depressive positions which are the outcome of later development and subsequent regression when associated with early ego states.

Next, our technical concepts have to be integrated with the special needs one finds among this group of patients. Various structuralizing experiences are emphasized such as the patient elevating a need to a communication, and this achievement leads to the establishment of a temporal sequence which makes working within a transference context possible.

Making the analyst's presence felt, not simply because he is there, but because he can respond to the patient's needs, becomes a central task which is designed to lead to a firmer distinction between inside and outside. The latter facilitates projections which can be dealt with interpretively.

This type of investigation into the analytic process is facilitated by the study of persons suffering from primitive fixations. It sharpens our analytic focus as well as providing us with a framework and a thread of hope enabling us to deal with patients suffering from misery of such proportions that would otherwise overwhelm us with despair and feelings of futility. There are many reasons to despair, but to some extent they are buffered by the recognition that there is much that has to be done and can be done.

REFERENCES

Bettelheim, B. (1967). *The Empty Fortress.* New York: The Free Press.
Boyer, L. B. and Giovacchini, P. L. (1967). *Psychoanalytic Treatment of Characterological and Schizophrenic Disorders.* New York: Jason Aronson.

Colby, K. (1955). *Energy and Structure in Psychoanalysis.* New York: Ronald Press.

Deutsch, H. (1942). Some forms of emotional disturbances and their relationship to schizophrenia. *Psychoanalytic Quarterly* 11: 301-321.

Ekstein, R. (1966). *Children of Time and Space of Action and Impulse.* New York: Appelton-Century-Crofts.

Fairbairn, R. W. D. (1941). A revised psychopathology of the psychoses and psychoneuroses. *International Journal of Psycho-Analysis* 22: 250-272.

————(1954). *An Object Relations Theory of the Personality.* New York: Basic Books.

Federn, P. (1952). *Ego Psychology and the Psychoses.* New York: Basic Books.

Fields, M. (1975). *Personal Communication.*

Flarsheim, A. (1975). *Personal Communication.*

Freud, S. (1900). The Interpretation of Dreams. *Standard Edition* 4 and 5. London: Hogarth, 1955.

————(1905). Three essays on the theory of sex. *Standard Edition* 7: 135-243. London: Hogarth, 1949.

————(1911). Psycho-Analytic notes on an autobiographical account of a case of paranoia (Dementia Paranoides). *Standard Edition* 12: 9-82. London: Hogarth, 1958.

————(1914). On narcissism: an introduction. *Standard Edition* 14: 73-102. London: Hogarth, 1957

————(1915). Instincts and their vicissitudes. *Standard Edition* 14: 117-140. London: Hogarth, 1957

————(1920). Beyond the pleasure principle. *Standard Edition* 18: 7-64. London: Hogarth, 1961.

————(1923). The ego and the id. *Standard Edition* 19: 12-66. London: Hogarth, 1962.

Giovacchini, P. (1963). Integrative aspects of object relationships. *Psychoanalytic Quarterly* 32: 393-407.

————(1965). Some aspects of the ego-ideal of the creative scientist. *Psychoanalytic Quarterly* 24: 79.

————(1972). The symbiotic phase. In P. Giovacchini, ed., *Tactics and Techniques in Psychoanalytic Therapy.* New York: Jason Aronson.

————(1977). *Psychoanalysis of Primitive Mental States.* New York: Jason Aronson.

Glover, E. (1945). Examination of the Klein system of child psychology. *Psychoanalytic Study of the Child* 1: 75-118.

Kardiner, A., Karush, A., and Ovesy, L. (1959). Methodological study of Freudian theory: I. basic concepts. *Journal of Nervous and Mental Diseases* 11: 129-185.

Kernberg, O. (1974). Further contributions to the treatment of narcissistic personalities. *International Journal of Psycho-Analysis* 55: 215-236.

Klein, M. (1935). A contribution to the psychogenesis of manic-depressive states. In *Contributions to Psychoanalysis*. London: Hogarth.

————(1946). Notes on some schizoid mechanisms. In J. Riviere, ed., *Developments in Psychoanalysis*. London: Hogarth.

Kohut, H. (1971). *The Analysis of the Self.* New York: International Universities Press.

Reisen, A. (1947). The development of visual perception in man and chimpanzees. *Science* 106: 6-20.

Spitz, R. (1965). *The First Year of Life.* New York: International Universities Press.

Strachey, J. (1934). The nature of the therapeutic action of psychoanalysis. *International Journal of Psycho-Analysis* 15: 127-160.

Winnicott, D. W. (1947). Hate in the countertransference. In *Collected Papers: Through Pediatrics to Psycho-Analysis*. New York: Basic Books, 1958.

————(1952). Psychoses and child care. In *Collected Papers: Through Pediatrics to Psycho-Analysis*. New York: Basic Books, 1958.

————(1955). Metapsychological and clinical aspects of regression. In *Collected Papers: Through Pediatrics to Psycho-Analysis*. New York: Basic Books, 1958.

Zetzel, E. (1956). An approach to the relation between concept and content in psychoanalytic theory (with special reference to the work of Melanie Klein and her followers). *Psychoanalytic Study of the Child* 11: 99-121.

WARREN J. GADPAILLE

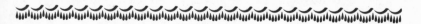

Adolescence is known to be so intimately dependent upon the surrounding culture for the form in which it manifests itself that its very existence as a valid and inevitable stage in human development has often been questioned. This communication examines the evidence that, at least in its sexual aspects, the biological consequences of puberty are not ignored in any recorded culture. It is possible that some form of sexual adolescence may be the only universal manifestation of adolescence, and this may have significant implications for the philosophy of psychotherapy.

Let me indicate the definitions of puberty and adolescence that will apply in this chapter, because these terms are not consistently used in the literature. Puberty is the spurt in biological maturation that eventuates in reproductive capacity and a physically adult body. Adolescence is the psychosocial—the individual and the societal—response to puberty. Puberty is universal; adolescence is individually and culturally variable. Thus, adolescence has a biological onset, but a psychosocial offset. So, to refine the thrust of this discussion, the question is whether or not it is possible for any variety of cultural attitudes to ignore or obliterate the response to puberty, both in the individual pubescents and in their social milieu.

The divergent opinions primarily embody a difference in emphasis; few express the extreme position that one or the other influence is exclusive. As a discipline, psychoanalysis tends to place greater emphasis upon the biological determinants. The more temperate point of view is well expressed by Settlage (1970) in his discussion of the interplay of influences, in which cultural variables act with great force upon an innate and never negligible biological substrate. One may also find the extreme view, as in

Berman's (1970) statement that "The basic dynamics of adolescent psychology are the same for all mankind."

Kiell (1964) has attempted to demonstrate, through autobiographical material from a variety of cultures and times, that the same kind of tumultuous adolescence so often visible in contemporary Western culture is a universal phenomenon. His documentation, however, is notably lacking in examples from vast world areas of cultural diversity in which cultural institutions bear little resemblance to those he includes.

The culturalists minimize the inevitability of biological influences, and describe a seemingly endless diversity of individual and societal behavioral forms at and following puberty. Mead (1928) documents an apparently untroubled negotiation of puberty by Samoan girls; she does not, however, suggest this as evidence against the existence of biological influences, and reports strong cultural response to the puberty of those girls in the social hierarchy deemed worthy of that attention. Keniston (1971) makes a persuasive case for adolescence, as we think of it, having only become possible in Western culture in the nineteenth and twentieth centuries, but he is scrupulous in stating that he is not questioning adolescence as an innate developmental phase, but is postulating the power of culture to negate the opportunity for its young people to experience the phase. Even so, there seems to be some lacunae in the historical perspective behind this reasoning. Judeo-Christian culture is a continuously developing entity over several millenia and includes the Hellenic in its origins; Aristotle in the fourth century B.C. and St. Augustine in the fourth century A.D.—to name but two—both wrote of adolescence in entirely contemporary terms.

A problem inherent in both the historical and the descriptive anthropological approaches to this issue is that inner emotions and responses, when not given easily recognizable expression in a culture, may go unnoticed. Nonetheless, one has no valid license to assume the presence of emotions and societal responses in the absence of demonstrable evidence, no matter how compelling the argument may seem that so massive a shift in every aspect of a person's biological self must be impossible to ignore. The issue will rest ultimately upon verifiable data alone. Salzman's (1974) belief that ". . . adolescence may be passed over entirely," precisely confronts the subject of this discussion.

To address this question, it is necessary to abandon for the moment the consideration of specific adolescent manifestations in particular cultures. Both human biology and the unique phenomenon of culture are common to all mankind; the relationship between the two must first be explored. This calls for operational definitions of society and of culture.

144

The Group for the Advancement of Psychiatry (1968) study states:

> The term *society* denotes a continuing group of people who have developed certain relatively fixed ways of doing things which express their particular ways of viewing reality, and which employ specific symbols embodying these views. The society creates a whole universe of rules, laws, customs, mores, and practices to perpetuate the commonly accepted values and to cope with the various issues experienced by all members. All of these socially patterned ways of behaving constitute the society's *culture*.

Human psychobiology and culture are not two equally self-determining interacting forces. Culture does not impinge independently upon mankind, as it were from above, influencing and modifying and shaping biological and psychological expressions. Without denying the obvious and inevitable culture-to-individual feedback and influence, there is a sequence, a primacy, and a qualitative difference in the operations upon one another of human psychobiology and culture.

The genus Homo and culture evolved concurrently, but not as equivalently independent phenomena. As the human cerebral cortex evolved, mankind created culture, and however much each phase or variety of culture influenced subsequent generations, changes and inventions in culture can only be created by humans. Culture does not have an autonomous life of its own, capable of effecting modifications within itself; culture is manmade. The reciprocal influences are qualitatively distinct: the action of culture upon mankind is static and perpetuates the *status quo* of the institutionalized value systems. (This is true even if one cultural value is change; by itself, culture could not decide to shift that value to one of stasis.) By contrast, the action of mankind upon culture is innovative and determinative.

Mankind's evolving capacities provide the ability for, but probably not the cause of, cultural change and diversity. It is more likely that human biology, and man's psychological responses to both internal and external reality in the effort to adapt and survive, constitute the dynamic source of specific cultural patterns. Ego capacities in general, and the ego mechanisms of defense and adaptation, seem to be common to the species. They define the limits of the presently evolved brain's repertoire for coping with inner and outer reality; cultural differences affect them only in terms of which mechanisms are preferentially employed or rewarded, and to what degree ego capacities are given scope to develop.

All the major biological events of the life cycle—birth, puberty, pregnancy, death—call attention to themselves. Societies tend to take note of them, and cultural institutions evolve around them as shared psychological techniques for coping with them and with the emotional response they elicit. Different cultures do not accord equal attention to the various landmarks in the life cycle, and cultural variability is of such magnitude that it is difficult at first to discern any underlying theme that might be considered universal.

Turning to adolescence and culture, it is noteworthy that (1) puberty is (among other things) an unmistakably sexual event, and (2) the only universal human taboo is mother-son incest. (The limitation is intentional; while father-daughter and sibling incest taboos are generally as strong, there are known institutionalized and ritual instances in which those taboos may be, or must be, violated. Even such rare exceptions never apply in the mother-son relationship.) Is there any inevitable and relevant association between these two facts?

By definition, the young will displace and finally replace their parents and other adults, however much there may be a mutually rewarding joining of forces during part of their shared adult lifespans. Being replaced is difficult to accept. But even though the cycle of generational replacement takes place in every sphere of life, it is only in the sexual sphere that there are universal intergenerational sanctions that admit of no exceptions. This does not hold true for any of the other arenas in which replacement occurs, for example, economic takeover by the young, acquisition of skills, accession to prestige and authority, even replacement by murder. The universality of the incest taboo is persuasive evidence that the replacement by succeeding generations is primarily perceived and guarded against in sexual and family terms. There are many similarities in cultural responses to the sexual implications of puberty regardless of cultural differences, and only the sexual modes of the replacement of parent by child are channelled and limited in universal ways.

It is a task of all adolescents that they must move from their family of origin to a different family of procreation. The institutionalization of its timing may vary, from the enforced segregation of latency age children from one or both parents in some cultures, to an unlimited period of being permitted to live at home as in our own, but the two families of any one person are never the same. And regardless of timing, puberty is the crucial biological instigator of this move because only a postpubescent could functionally (procreatively) replace a parent. Thus, while a parent may be replaced by the child in every other area of life, a father's sexual

146

prerogatives with his son's biological mother remain universally inviolate. A mother's similar prerogatives are only a shade less absolute.

The universality of the incest taboo is also undeniable evidence for the omnipresent existence of the wish against which it defends; it is not necessary to forbid behavior in which no one is interested. The taboo bespeaks the conscious or unconscious recognition of the desire, as well as the corresponding guilt, denial, and avoidance. The question whether or not the universal mother-son incest taboo implies also that the oedipus complex is universal has given rise to differing opinions and has resulted in anthropological reports of cultures in which some of its more classic manifestations are not clearly in evidence. There seems little doubt that the oedipus complex is subject to cultural modifications. But there is one ubiquitous fact that speaks in favor of a biological root underlying all observed cultural variations. Nowhere may a boy marry his biological mother. This holds true no matter what cultural permutations of family structure exist, or whether it is the biological parents or other adults who rear the child. The universal core of the incest taboo applies to biological parents and their offspring, and attests to the existence of the oedipus complex essentially within the nuclear family.

Application of psychodynamic understanding to the majority of puberty rites readily uncovers their oedipal content, as revealed primarily through the behavior of the initiating adults (Muensterberger 1961). For boys it involves separation from mother, termination of oral dependence upon her, and identification with father as an adult. But it is often attainable only after being subjected to considerable phallic aggression and cruelty at the hands of the adult males who project their own unconscious oedipal wishes upon the boys and symbolically castrate them in retaliation, punishing them for what they know they once desired for themselves. Girls are often subject to equal or greater aggressive behavior and sexual and genital cruelties by the adult women, extremes being infibulation and clitoridectomy.

Indeed, cultures may reflect the oedipal dilemma far more broadly than in their immediate ways of responding to puberty, and in their specific controls of coital and procreative options. LaBarre (1969, 1970) marshalls an impressive body of documentation to the effect that many of the major aspects of all cultures may be instructively viewed as differing solutions to the oedipal dilemma, arising as it does from the unique characteristics of the human family, the anthropologically typical sex-specific roles of mother and father, and the human child's long period of dependency. Within the statistically typical family (evolutionarily, historically, and cross culturally), identification with mother or identification with father would result in significantly different characteristics. Individual personalities express a blend of identifications with both parents, and one way of viewing culture is as "a compound of the identifications that are most characteristic of people in a group at a specified time" (LaBarre 1969).

Differences in the preponderance of mother- or father-identification in any culture at any period in history would result in either matrist or patrist societies. Obviously, various combinations and differences in subcultural groups are possible, as are partial or total rejections of the values associated with either parent or sex. These may be regarded as differing oedipal styles in culture because of their clear relationship to intrafamilial oedipal anxieties. Patrist societies are male-authoritarian; they stress unquestioning obedience to authority and are hostile to change or dissent. Women, unless idealized in asexual form, are the objects of suspicion and derrogation; they are the source of trouble between sons and fathers. In consequence, emotion is suppressed, sexual differences are maximized, and sexual guilts and prohibitions, especially for women, are heavy. Even that greater sexual freedom accorded males in a patrist society is surely not an expression of love between two equally valued partners; women are not dangerous to the masculine order of things as long as they can be disregarded. A prime illustration is the patently oedipal preoccupation of medieval patrist Christianity, when the evil role of sexual woman in undermining the loyalty and obedience of earthly sons to their heavenly Father was expressed as official doctrine, just as it was lived out in the culture that spawned it.

In contrast, matrist societies are democratic and liberal; they tend to be progressive rather than conservative. Mother-identification results in greater status and freedom for women. Creative change is sought and welcomed; social reform and concern for the disadvantaged and helpless reveal the association with the archetypal mother's nurturant and non-demanding love for all infants. Sexuality is less guilt ridden and more emancipated for both partners.

The oedipal style of a culture is reflected in many of its traditions and institutions beyond those which are clearly sexual. It is a way of characterizing major attitudes toward intergenerational relationships, religion, and the functions of authority and power toward private and public behavior in general. Thus the entire style of a culture may come to bear upon how it responds to adolescent sexuality, and to express itself in the peculiar conflicts and stresses and options it imposes upon the basic adolescent task of coming to terms with adult procreative sexuality.

In sum, because of the universal preoccupation with avoiding incest, because of the ubiquity of limitations upon adolescents' procreative choices, and because it is in the nature of societies to reflect their particular resolutions of the oedipal dilemma in the evolution of cultural styles with the most far-reaching impact in the lives of adolescents (and, of course, all its members), it is clear that the sexual component of puberty is nowhere ignored culturally. Nor, therefore, could the post-pubescent adolescent totally ignore the strictures and sanctions imposed upon his sexual object choices, or the sexual attitudes and styles that are culturally inherited, even if his sharply different biology and new body would allow him to do so. Even where there is no recognized social phase of adolescence, puberty demands and inevitably receives some form of degree of psychosocial response in the sexual sphere of life. These considerations suggest that, however attenuated or masked, some form of sexual adolescence, as adolescence is defined herein, is innately imperative in any culture. And when one considers that no other aspect of puberty elicits such a universal response, one might speculate that sexual adolescence may be the only aspect of adolescence that has any claim to be regarded as universal.

However valid this hypothesis may prove to be, it leaves serious practical considerations unresolved. Even if puberty inherently evokes some psychosexual response, the coping with which constitutes the bedrock of human adolescence, it is entirely unclear what determines a culture's oedipal style, and why some societies evolve more stringent and prohibitive restrictions upon adolescent sexuality, while others find it unnecessary to do so. It is certainly not related to the degree of complexity or primitivity of a society, nor to the degree of ego development fostered or required, because all gradations from permissive to restrictive attitudes toward adolescent sexuality can be found at all levels of culture (Ford and Beach 1951). I can offer no answers to the etiology of the differences; it is a prime issue for sociosexual research.

Clinically, the options are of necessity usually limited to helping specific adolescents learn to achieve sexual identity and a workable balance between gratification and control within a specific cultural milieu. In these circumstances, it is both easy and appropriate to think in terms of how the cultural mores and institutions are influencing—limiting, facilitating, complicating—that youngster's innate biological task.

Conclusions

One must remember that culture is man-made. It grows, in analogy with the adaptive techniques of individuals, out of unconscious identifications, conflicts, and needs of past generations of fallible human beings in their gropings for solutions to shared problems and anxieties. Because of its significant unconscious component, its institutionalized solutions often bear but tenuous relationship to human realities. Our own culture is only one of many and equally a blind creation of the past, "a phenomenon we might be better able to control if we understood it and to revise if we knew what was needed" (GAP 1968). The ultimate question is not how culture affects its members, but what has impelled a given society to manufacture its particular culture. Therapy of individuals may be no more than a rear guard action in the absence of a concurrent therapy of cultural institutions. But, mindful that mankind does, indeed, make his own cultural bed, "In the quest for custom-made values, beware of what you want, because you will get it" (LaBarre 1971-1972).

REFERENCES

Berman, S. (1970). Alienation: an essential process of the psychology of adolescence. *Journal of the American Academy of Child Psychiatry* 9: 233-250.

Ford, C. S., and Beach, F. A (1951). *Patterns of Sexual Behavior*. New York: Harper and Row.

Group for the Advancement of Psychiatry (1968). *Normal Adolescence: Its Dynamics and Impact*. New York: Scribners.

Keniston, K. (1971). Youth as a stage of life. *This Annual* 1: 161-175.

Kiell, N. (1964). *The Universal Experience of Adolescence*. New York: International Universities Press.

LaBarre, W. (1969). Changing mores in American society. Paper given at the Annual Meeting of the American College of Psychiatry, New Orleans, La., Feb. 1, 1969.

———(1970). *The Ghost Dance*. New York: Doubleday.

———(1971-1972). Authority, culture change and the courts. *Loyola Law Review* 18: 481-492.

Mead, M. (1928). *Coming of Age in Samoa*. New York: Wm. Morrow.

Muensterberger, W. (1961). The adolescent in society. In S. Lorand, and H. I. Schneer, eds., *Adolescents: Psychoanalytic Approach to Problems and Therapy*. New York: Hoeber, pp. 346-368.

Salzman, L. (1974). Adolescence: epoch or disease. *This Annual* 3: 128-139.

Settlage, C. F. (1970). Adolescence and social change. *Journal of the American Academy of Child Psychiatry* 9: 203-215.

11] FILIAL OBLIGATION IN ADOLESCENCE: AN ORIENTATION

MAURICE J. ROSENTHAL

> *It is said that the world is in a state of backruptcy, that the world owes the world more than the world can pay, and ought to go into chancery, and be sold.*
>
> —Emerson

People attach great significance to feelings of obligation toward their parents. To honor one's parents is one of the Ten Commandments and similar injunctions seem to be as conspicuous and familiar in non-western cultures as well. But how do concerns about filial obligation affect younger individuals? How much do we know about the part they play in their emotional lives? What gives filial obligation its power? In this chapter I shall survey the pervasiveness, origins, and significance of feelings of obligations by adolescents toward those adults (usually parents) who had been and often still were active in maintaining their well-being.

It is curious that the subject has received so little clinical attention. Perhaps this is due to the oppressive mood which the subject engenders. There seems to be no opportunity in it for dealing with the latent excitement of unmasking drive disguises and vicissitudes, for flaunting the wit of deft paradoxes, or for creative spontaneity. In recognizing the anhedonia of the countertransference to the subject one is in fact well prepared for the survey. One begins with a feeling that it will be unpleasant and that the more one delves into it the worse the boredom will become. By

Presented to the Chicago Council of Child Psychiatry on October 8, 1975.

empathy we have grasped the emotional undercurrent of filial obligation in the typical adolescent.

The attitudes of filial obligation are specific and are evident whenever the adolescent speaks or acts out of gratefulness or appreciation for what his parents have done for him, or of having to repay them for their devotion. It is apparent also in the frequently explicit struggles against being held to honor these obligations. Still evident, if somewhat less specifically so, is its expression in uncoerced sincere concern for the welfare of the parents and in decisions and acts made because of such reasons. It is one component out of many when the adolescent wishes to please the parent.

Filial obligation, if excessive, may interrupt or distort the process of adolescent individuation. How can the adolescent form intense peer relationships, how much freedom can he have in planning for his future if the oppressive weight of feelings of obligation compels him to put his family first in all things? The indentured servant may not break his contract. On the other hand, absence of such feelings may bespeak such lack of concern for objects as to indicate a grave developmental defect.

The ideas in this chapter are derived primarily from clinical sources. There is, then, stress on the pathological. More specifically, I have followed the spirit of Erikson (1956), Anna Freud (1958), and Blos (1962) in regarding adolescence as a turbulent period. The case material is derived mainly from American middle class adolescents. It is hard to avoid the temptation to make generalizations.

Several recent studies of healthy American adolescents and young adults, as summarized by King (1971), do not view the adjustments of these young people as demonstrating much disturbance or sense of crisis. Their capacity for coping and self-esteem remained high. Of particular relevance are the findings that the relationship between these adolescents and their parents remained good throughout the entire period. Presumably, conflicts between parents and their adolescent children did occur, but were gentler than those described in the psychiatric literature. These findings imply that the parents generally approved of the way their offspring conducted themselves and made no special demands on them to the extent of causing hardship or serious friction. If this interpretation is correct, conflicts over filial obligation were not conspicuous.

The Disentanglement from the Parents

Gould (1972) stated that in observing a group of adolescents aged sixteen to eighteen, he and his coworkers were "unavoidably" struck with this theme,

"We have to get away from our parents." The theme was loudly and repetitively verbalized but not acted upon. They considered themselves more as members of the family than as true individuals. In the age group eighteen to twenty-two, Gould found a continuation of the theme, but from a different position. "They feel themselves to be half-way out of the family and are worried that they will be reclaimed by the family pull and will not make it out completely. They are, however, striving toward separating, living away from home at school, working."

In the following brief summary, the GAP report (1968) has distilled the essence of a number of important contributions on the psychodynamics of the adolescent's attitude toward his parents:

> The detachment from parents is impelled by guilt over the oedipal fantasies re-awakened now in the threatening context of near-adult capabilities for sexual and aggressive behavior, and by the need to discover individual identity, which is felt to be jeopardized by too close an attachment to the adult with his strongly established identity. The need for guidance from adults and for adult models for identification persists, but attachments even to adults other than parents usually are transitory.

This excerpt from an authoritative work on the psychology of adolescence is typical in its disregard of filial obligation. Of course the drives, oedipal, identity, and dependency factors do indeed figure prominently in the changing adolescent parent relationship, but they do not explain enough.

I propose that the commonly observed rebellion and withdrawal from parents may also be reaction formations to free the adolescent from feeling he must devote his life to repayment of his parents for what they have done for him, that is, an attempt to work through his feelings of filial obligation.

Their ensuing mottoes or rationalizations have long been familiar to psychiatrists, but have usually been regarded only as signs of oedipal or identity conflicts. "Since I do not love or because I hate or disrespect you; or because my first duty is to my work (schooling); or to a cause; to my self-development; or to someone else—I do not owe you much or anything at all. I am therefore free to dispose of my affection and favors as I choose." "You say I am selfish and ungrateful but I didn't force you to do anything for me. Anyway, aren't parents supposed to do things for their children?"

CLINICAL EXAMPLE

J was a fifteen-year-old adolescent male whose life seemed to churn in a torment of conflicts centering on filial obligations. In this case, there was much grumbling but no decisive move toward liberating himself from parental authority. J was referred because he was a loner and unhappy. He spent his leisure time in the house where he was generally sullen, complaining about his two younger brothers not carrying their share of chores, and physically abusing them for alleged provocations. He was assigned more chores than they, but while protesting this, performed his household duties in a thorough manner. After he had been in therapy for a number of months, it seemed as if progress in therapy had come to a halt. Thus, I decided on a new tack. I called to his attention that he seemed to spend most of the time complaining about difficulties in the home and always sounding as if he were defending himself in court. I noted also that there seemed to be little fun in that house and yet he did not consider getting out more from such unpleasant surroundings. J agreed and added that he felt squelched by his parents. Did he feel any freer at school, I asked. He did. Yesterday he had worked on "barber shop singing" with his friends. It was as if he led two different lives. I expressed surprise and told him that he seemed so weighed down by responsibility that I found it hard to think of him any other way. He said he didn't know what to say to that, but then told how yesterday he'd felt guilty for staying later at school without notifying his mother. Apparently, mention of the pleasantries at school had been suppressed. Perhaps they were a new development. Following this session, J began for the first time in therapy to report having had enjoyable experiences. These occurred through his membership in the school choir. Shortly afterwards he sought my opinion about asking his parents for permission to attend a choir function instead of going away for a weekend with the family. I told him I saw no reason why he couldn't at least inform his parents what he would prefer doing. This seemed to relieve him. Two sessions later he mentioned without elaboration that his mother had had an operation for varicose veins and was doing well. This was followed in the same session by prolonged accolades for his male choir director who had helped a lot of people in many ways. Among his other admirable qualities he had taught students how to mix fun with work. Also, he would not use any of the money earned by the students to defray his own expenses for a tour the choir was to make. At the end of this session he complained that his mother had kept him from having contact with certain relatives that might have been enhancing.

It was clear that the choir director was a displacement of the therapist and both of us were contrasted with the parents. The two of us permitted fun and were helpful to others without asking for anything in return (the payment of a fee in therapy was not mentioned). The failure to discuss feelings and fantasies evoked by the mother's operation suggested a denial of guilt feelings, the denial aided by an allegiance to someone outside the family who said it was all right to enjoy oneself. Here we can see how the admiration for someone outside of the family is preferable to one in the family because it contributes more to personality growth and is free of the constricting sense of obligation that characterizes the family relationship. Furthermore, a simple inference suggests that he questions the wisdom of his mother's having protected him from the influences of others since he had found that some outside relationships could be very pleasant. This implies that he needed to placate his mother for his limited involvement outside the home. The encouragement and permission of two outside authorities to pull away from the exclusive involvement with the family at first had only a limited effect. He soon clarified that he could not go any further in his individuation because he would have felt guilty about failing to requite his obligations to his mother. His initial moves in this direction had caused this whole issue to emerge.

About one month later J was in a state of acute frustration and expressed his conflict with intense agitation: "Mother feels she spent all her time cleaning up our messes when we were little and now it was our turn to repay her. I've talked with her about this. I don't feel that a child owes anything to parents. The child didn't ask to be born. Along with having children comes the responsibility of parents to look after the children until they're grown. Sometimes, though, I feel like my mother's right. What's right?" J told me that this matter had been the cause of considerable preoccupation and begged me to render a verdict. J's excessive involvement with his family must have been promoted by the needs of the parents. His mother was often ailing, and both parents were miserable in their relationship with one another. Both made use of J's presence and through heavy emphasis on his obligations helped to interfere with the attainment of a maturing level of independence from them.

I believe that the obligation distress in this case is best understood as an existential dilemma. By contrast, the usual clinical discussion of the contention between J and his mother would focus on a number of more familiar psychiatric issues derived from the premise that J was in an obsessive/compulsive state, and that the obligation attitude served multiple functions. The need for justice, the stubborn withholding attitudes, the overt ambivalence of the anal character can be quickly recognized.

As was noted earlier, filial obligation is deeply involved with other intrapsychic matters. The case material suggests that such attitudes arise from feelings of affection and gratitude which have become merged with guilt and shame stemming from a prominent fixation on toilet training.

What was the obligation, in fact, in this family? It meant most immediately a debt of gratitude and love to be paid off with toil and lessened autonomy. The son opposed the parents' claim and pressed his own countersuit.

The overt negotiations between parents and child took place only around the explicit issue of obligation, partly because doing so spared the child from awareness of painful guilt (over hostile, incestuous, and possessive impulses) and shame (over longings for infantile gratifications and insouciance). Simultaneously, for the parents the obligation issue cloaked rejecting and exploiting attitudes. However, there was acceptance by both sides that they had obligations toward one another. In fact, this code is the important constitutional law of family life itself. All members may appeal to its jurisdiction, as it makes possible displacements and rationalizations like those in J's family.

There is another significant advantage for all parties in covertly negotiating treacherous unacceptable matters under the rubric of obligation duties and entitlements, to wit, that it provides a rational method for placing controls on the expression of underlying tensions. The use of filial obligation as camouflage is so impressive it almost causes us to overlook its importance in its own right.

Unfortunately, the compulsive attempt to balance entitlements against obligations indicates that a just resolution cannot be arrived at objectively. Each party to the conflict seeks relief from tormenting superego pressure by trying to use the other as witness or judge. When the others refuse, the issue is left undecided. Unlike ideal legal judges, they are not disinterested and have their own claims to make. From these considerations we can seen that one must always accept a certain amount of uncertainty about whether one has given too much or too little in most relationships calling for emotional commitment. It is only when the giving or withholding is spontaneous and wholehearted that the conflict does not become intense.

I have attempted to illustrate in this section the important and distinctive influence of filial obligation and the problems it gives rise to in the striving for greater independence. It is one factor, among others, which can contribute in an important way to difficulties. Not incidentally, J's therapy went on to a favorable outcome. One sign of this was his ability to josh his mother in an agreeable fashion when she became overzealous in claiming entitlements. I must also mention, however, that the favorable result depended in part also on the successful treatment of the parents by another therapist.

The Persistent Tie to the Parents

Everyone agrees on the desirability of parental assistance for their adolescent sons and daughters. An additional factor which usually is overlooked is that the adolescent feels indebted to the parents. Thus, he may not be able to achieve true independence until he has somehow moderated this particular encumberance.

Some college and family therapists have observed that when the adolescent, particularly when he is the last child, leaves home the relationship between the parents often deteriorates (Elson 1964, Framo 1970, Levenson, Stockhammer, and Feiner 1967). When the parents demand or reveal a need for the child's help (as was true with J), the adolescent may not be able to extricate himself without seeming heartless.

Blos (1967) described some of the intrapsychic obstacles in the adolescent's move toward independence. He pointed out that until the end of adolescence, the "parental ego makes itself available to the child and lends structure and organization to its ego as a functional entity." It is the task of adolescents to disrupt this alliance, but young adolescents cannot do so because continued immaturity of their egos makes them unable to dispense with this support. Blos also emphasized that temporary regressions, one aspect of which involved getting closer to the parents, was necessary for optimal, progressive development at this time. Finally, Blos clarified with case material that the struggle against parental ties involved mainly the tie to an internalized parent whose qualities bore the stigmata of the earliest years of the child's life.

In the contemporary affluence of urban American culture, the adolescent is not compelled to make significant personal or material offerings to the middle-class parents. But in many other cultures the child grows up with the understanding that obligations to the parents may be boundless and obedience to them peremptory.

In such cultures there is a demand for self-abnegation to parents to which the child is expected to submit rather than feeling obligated to do so as in

American culture, which leaves it optional. There, the adolescent does not disentangle himself or herself from the family without explicit permission. From the American middle-class perspective, no doubt the cultural stress on filial obligation as a duty appears as a rationalization for keeping authority in the group with vested interests. As such, filial obligation seems the internalization of oppression.

Anna Freud (1958) has insisted on the pathology implicit in the behavior of the "too-good" adolescent. Zachry (1940) described adolescents who "feared to rebel" and described a number of situations which led to this. One familiar situation, described by her, was that in which one of the parents had a child-like attitude toward the adolescent. In this instance "he may respond to the parental role, serving the parent, caring for and giving his first consideration to him or her, and . . . particularly in the case of mother and son . . . early assuming responsibility for the parent's financial support." This last situation graphically portrays the obligation force in action.

Deutsch (1945) carefully considers the pressure emanating from the mother against the child's wish to become more independent. As her theme statement, she writes: "Every phase of the child's development ends with the intensifed tendencies to liberate himself. The mother . . . every mother . . . tries to keep him attached to herself and opposes the actions that tend to dissolve the tie. She continues these attempts anachronistically later as well." Deutsch considers several forms of mother-child relationships from this point of view. Thus:

> In my opinion, maternal over-protection, in its numerous forms and variations, ultimately serves the purpose of preserving the child's dependence and of averting the separation trauma for the mother. The most direct means to this end is infantilization, that is, the tendency to keep the child childishly helpless as long as possible. . . . The overindulgent as well as the domineering mother lead to the same end, that is, the dependence of the child.

As I stress in this chapter, I agree with her statement, "Many mothers in their attempt to tie their children to themselves appeal cleverly and consistently to guilt feelings: 'You will abandon me, who has suffered so much?' " From the standpoint of the child, growing up and individuating could give rise to a feeling that something has to be taken away from the mother (Modell 1971, Anna Freud 1967, Stierlin 1973).

CLINICAL EXAMPLE

G, a fourteen-year-old girl, was legally removed from her mother and stepfather when she was ten years old because of evidence of severe neglect. She was then placed with affluent, warm, and devoted foster parents, and in this home G flourished impressively. From being almost a nonachiever in a school with low academic requirements, she became an average student at a school with much higher standards. From being heedless of her dishevelled, filthy appearance, she learned to groom herself with care. From a life spent marking time in school and languishing about the apartment without companions her own age, she became interested in her studies, made many friends, developed appropriate social skills, and began to contemplate an agreeable future. But the action of the court had aroused considerable distress in the mother who was determined to get her child back. Finally, when G became fourteen, the mother succeeded in getting the girl to choose to return and live with her. But even before G's actual return, the girl had declared that returning to her mother was her "main goal in life." The girl's decision was unquestionably a response to her sickly mother's strenuous efforts to get her back, although G had been informed that legally she did not have to go if she chose not to. From the available evidence, it seemed that G had given up a much more fulfilling existence out of a sense of filial obligation. That such motivation could be so powerful regarding a mother who had seemingly done so little for her (true, she had not abandoned the girl) was astonishing. The mother, who was sickly and partly disabled, undoubtedly made maximum use of her physical problems to lure the girl to her.[1]

We are compelled to infer that this girl must have yielded to the demands of filial obligation despite great inner protest. Thus, while we can generalize that the adolescent resents a heavy burden of filial obligation, they cannot always disavow it even when circumstances would seem propitious for doing so, if the demands of the original parenting object(s) are insistent enough.

Discordant Filial Obligation

The importance of the obligation problem gains further significance when we find it revealed in persons where we would least expect it.

The notoriously egotistical Cellini (1730) of Renaissance Italy wrote as follows in his autobiography:

When I reached the age of fifteen, I put myself, against my father's will, to the goldsmith's trade. In a few months I caught up with the good, nay, the best young craftsmen in our business, and began to reap the fruits of my labors. I did not, however, neglect to gratify my good father from time to time by playing on the flute or cornet. Each time he heard me, I used to make his tears fall accompanied with deep drawn sighs of satisfaction. My filial piety often made me give him that contentment, and induced me to pretend that I enjoyed the music too.

CLINICAL EXAMPLE

V, a very self-centered, complaining and demanding seventeen-year-old girl was in treatment because of several episodes of superficial wrist-cutting. In one session, she reported her experiences during a weekend spent on a boat with her mother and other adults and remarked: "My mother watched over me to see that I didn't jump off. I liked the attention but felt why should I get it when I hadn't done anything for her?"[2]

Occasionally, one glimpses obligation attitudes even in the sickest of individuals as in a case reported by Boszormenyi-Nagy (1973) of a sixteen-year-old boy considered to be hopelessly psychotic, who looked after his father asleep in the chair in front of the television by picking him up and carrying him to his bedroom upstairs every night.

I have frequently encountered feelings of obligation in adolescents even to parents who had accepted very little responsibility for them. I would like to present a case now where the child's reaction, while still surprising, was more typical than G's in that it did not lead to an act of impressive self-sacrifice.

CLINICAL EXAMPLE

C was a seventeen-year-old girl living in a foster home where she had been placed at the age of four because her alcoholic mother was unable to care for her properly. There was nothing known of the father's whereabouts. Throughout the years, C had maintained infrequent contact with her mother. Recently the mother had undergone surgery for a benign brain tumor and was to have a second operation. A session from C's therapy at this time began with C asking the therapist about her mother's condition. The therapist told her that mother's second scheduled reparative operation had been postponed. C began to weep at this news and wondered if the therapist was withholding something. She had heard that when a tumor is malignant, they cannot do a second operation. The therapist assured her that the mother did not have cancer and explained the reason for the delay on other grounds. C then went on to say: "I'm sorry for my mother. If she dies, I'll feel bad. It is not that I'll be losing a companion because we never were close. Also, it's not that I have such fond memories of living with my mother because I don't have those either. I don't know why I feel this way. Sometimes I feel she expects me to take care of her when she gets older. In some respects I feel that I ought to, but at other times I feel I have my own life to live and I don't know how I'd be able to do it even if I wanted to. My mother has had a rough time of it, but I have a chance for happiness now."[3]

It may be noted that while no action was taken by C to look after her mother at this time, the feeling of responsibility came up quite spontaneously and was deeply felt. Her not behaving accordingly required justification; and she all but admitted that one day she would have to look after her mother, although her mother had hardly ever looked after her.

The paradoxical appearance of feelings of filial obligation, even when by most standards the child would be considered to have been neglected or abused, undoubtedly has one root in the child's need to maintain a fantasy of an all-loving mother as was emphasized long ago by Klein (1932). Traditionally, the child's feelings of gratitude are thought to be based on the recognition of the role of the parents in caretaking and in bringing him into existence. However, there is another ultimate ground for gratitude demonstrated in the following case vignette.

CLINICAL EXAMPLE

An eight-year-old child had been placed in a foster home and then abandoned by her parents. A few months after the abandonment she told the following fantasy: "The baby tiger was rescued by a grown up after its mother didn't want to take care of it. The neck had teeth marks where its mother had carried it." Then the child noted: "The mother could have killed it."[4]

One could be a good parent even if all the parent had done for the child was not to kill it. Such reasoning on the part of the child makes possible strange, depressive, moral positions. Thus, not infrequently, neglect and rejection by the parents leads to greater appreciation of them by the child on the grounds that the parent suffered some because of him. Although obviously preoccupied with their own needs and often openly resentful toward the child, they did allow it to come into existence, to survive, to claim it as their own, and even to tend it after a fashion.

The situation is set where the child readily regards himself as mainly a burden to the parents toward whom he may feel enormously indebted. The need to minimize the burdening of the parents may be an important factor in producing the well known precocious self-reliability of rejected children (Newell 1936, Redl and Wineman 1957, Stierlin 1973). Reese (1962) and Boszormenyi-Nagy and Spark (1973) have pointed out that the enormous hostility which most of these children develop is mainly displaced from the rejecting parents onto other persons or the world in general, manifesting in this way their parental regard. The fact that a child develops filial obligations even toward rejecting parents is well known to clinicians dealing with child placements.

Narcissistic Factors in the Struggle Against Filial Obligation

Most (American, middle-class, disturbed) adolescents are aware of feelings of obligation toward parents, but these feelings are partly unpleasant and if they are felt to be too great, the adolescent attempts to minimize, repudiate, or ignore them. While they do not always succeed, the disavowal of filial obligation seems to be particularly marked whenever narcissistic features are conspicuous.

CLINICAL EXAMPLE

E, a sixteen-year-old male, was considered to be exceptionally callous in his disregard of parental wishes and values. In some ways, he had much in common with schizoid white, middle-class, American, adolescent school dropouts and underachievers (Erikson 1956, Noshpitz 1970). It was striking to see how the boy acted out to free himself from filial and other kinds of obligations. The mother described her son as follows: "E is flunking everything at school and didn't go to school today. Each time there is a crisis between his father and myself, E gets disturbed. How much of this school problem is depression? How much laziness? He irritates teachers because he doesn't turn in his work. He's also been upset at home when he heard that his father was seriously sick. I don't know if this is an adolescent upset or what. Sometimes he says he's self-centered. Father's and my lives are a mess. Salvage E's if you can." When E was in treatment for about a month, he moved to the apartment of the obliging maternal grandparents in another section of the city because "things were no good at home."

This act was overdetermined. In some ways it seemed healthy, but his primary concern was that his home provided inadequate narcissistic supplies. To expect him to cater to the needs of others was too much. Moving enabled him to avoid being directly reproached for not being more sympathetic. Finally, there was the less obvious aspect that, insofar as he was a burden to his parents, removing himself from the scene had the result of easing that burden. The weight of evidence, however, relegates this altruistic motive to a subordinate position.

The case material provides us with the opportunity to examine an important phenomenon, the attempt by the adolescent to rid oneself of all sense of filial obligation. The modern adolescent has enormous mobility, and deliberately leaving home is commonly resorted to for this purpose, among others.

E reported about this time: "Haven't been home. Yesterday was my mother's birthday and I didn't even go then. Yesterday I felt depressed. I have nothing to do. I can't even have a good time anymore. In the last couple of years I can't give presents. I get some from others. I shop but I don't buy. If I buy some things today, I'll feel the gifts are no good. I never do what I want to do. Something holds me back. Sometimes I won't even let myself watch TV. The arguments at home are my fault, because I'd procrastinate with chores I was asked to do." I asked if perhaps he thought he was too selfish. He responded unexpectedly: "But if I did do them, it wouldn't mean anything anyway. If it were my own house, I wouldn't mind." This was followed spontaneously by a new topic. "I try to size people up as to how much guts they have. I wonder how much chance I'd have of winning in a fight with them." Clearly, E's flight did not spare him from depression.

Here we again see the Mobius interweaving of motivations. In this instance the primary emphasis is narcissistic. The patient was aware that he was not fulfilling his filial obligations. It was not the concern for the parents, however, that was making him depressed. Rather, it was that he was dissatisfied with his overall functioning. He realized that he was the cause of much unhappiness in the family and for a moment it seemed that he was expressing mainly guilt. But the inference was wrong in overemphasizing the guilt, even if he had done his chores and thus had helped avoid much of the arguing, "It wouldn't mean anything." What would it take to make it mean something? "If it were my own house (i.e., if he were doing something to maintain what was indisputably his integrated self-cathexis and self-esteem) I wouldn't mind."

The amenities of a mother's birthday had not been observed by him. He had refused to make what would have seemed even a minor effort to honor his mother, an avoidance of a token expression of appreciation or obligation to her. Nor was this primarily an act of deliberate hostility. The reasons for it were mainly narcissistic (Hartmann 1956, Kohut 1971). Only in therapy did he reveal that the idea of going to the party for his mother had seriously been considered by him. Now it is to be recalled that E's not honoring his obligation had given rise to considerable narcissistic distress. He had failed to measure up to the standard of his ego-ideal. Thus, in the end, he had been unable to avoid some aggravation of his feelings of inadequacy.

What, then, is the nature of the narcissistic motive in feelings of filial obligation? Freud (1920) remarked that all children's play was dominated by the wish to be grownup and to be able to do what grownups do. He particularly singled out for careful study an infant's emulation of adult mastery in the instigation and termination of separations in which both the object and the self could be made first to disappear and then reappear. In this discussion Freud came very close to recognizing that the child attributed to the presence of the adult a basic condition for self cathexis. Older infants, toddlers, and nursery school children often play at mothering dolls, other children, and even their own mothers. Tolpin (1971) speaks of the narcissistic cathexis of the mother's functions which causes these functions to be included in even rudimentary self systems. Jones (1913) speculated that feelings of omnipotence may require that one should be able to cater to the needs of others because superiority to the needy ones can be demonstrated in this way. In requiting a filial obligation the adolescent would then be giving proof of having achieved the ego-ideal's goal of emulating the parents.

Clearly, then, the wish to become like the parent is, from the beginning, a basic narcissistic desire. The wish to repay the parent is partly a wish to undo the narcissistic humiliation in having acknowledged one's dependency on another person for fundamental physical and emotional care, as if this constituted an admission of imperfection and inferiority. Partly, it is also a wish to undo the state of vulnerability resulting from such a dependent relationship. One gives the parent the kind of care which had been received from them, thus signifying, by using competence in this way, the attainment of the long sought narcissistic goal of realistically emulating the parent, of having attained emotional independence, and of having thereby mitigated the feelings of humiliation and vulnerability.

I have stressed the importance of narcissistic aspects of obligation conflicts because of their clinical importance. While there is some controversy at the present time concerning narcissistic versus object relationship issues in the understanding of disorders, in our cases sometimes object relations (Cases J, G), at other times narcissistic needs (Cases V, E) seemed to prevail. Correspondingly, sometimes the adolescent gave up too much autonomy, sometimes not enough. What determines whether or not feelings of obligation will be requited depends largely on the relative strengths of opposing libidinous-moral and narcissistic interests. (However, it must be stressed that the intrapsychic situation in regard to requiting of filial obligation is in turn so greatly influenced by family needs and cultural factors that they must also be assessed. For instance E's family was in great need but apparently did not insist on his help, and obliging grandparents helped his evasion.)

The position reached here concerning narcissistic and object oriented distress was anticipated by Jacobson (1964). Guilt feelings, she pointed out, "seem to have particular reference to hostility and harm to others, and in general to the quality of our object relations." In contrast, she feels, shame and related feelings of inferiority and of humiliation have narcissistic-exhibitionistic implications. These feelings refer essentially to the self:

> . . . with regard to its power, its intactness, its appearance and even its moral perfection, but not in terms of our loving or hostile impulses and behavior toward others. It is interesting indeed that to some extent even moral pride and, the opposite, moral shame reactions have this conspicuously narcissistic quality.

Finally, regarding narcissistic forces, their effect in limiting the claims of filial obligation in less severely narcissistically damaged adolescents may be wholesome.

Requiting the Obligation

Of all the ways of diminishing the discomfort of felt obligations, the most direct ways—the expression of gratitude and doing services for the parent toward whom the adolescent feels obligated—would ordinarily seem the most satisfactory. No doubt most adolescents, even the ones we deal with clinically, do perform many small favors in this way daily. To enumerate a few will suffice: helping with household chores, saying thanks on obtaining the car keys, babysitting for younger siblings, etc. The degree of negativism or inhibition over such an ostensibly minor obligation as that felt by E regarding his mother's birthday is infrequent. However, some inconsistency about performing these acts and fluctuation in the willingness with which they are performed is the rule. Particularly conspicuous is the reluctance to keep one's own quarters tidy to the displeasure of the parents.

Doing something for the parents also acquires a significance of "reversal of generations" to use Jones' phrase (1923). The child who once envied the parents, their sexual and other adult pleasures, and hated them for the punishments and restrictions they inflicted on him, now in a measure has become a superior parent—like person to his own parent. The act may be regarded as a proof of having grown up and, therefore, no longer subject to the indignities which are so often the lot of the child (See also Jones 1913).

Of course, kindnesses toward parents may have ulterior motives having nothing to do with felt obligations. I would agree with the maxim of La-Rochefoucald: "Almost everyone takes a pleasure in requiting trifling obligations; many people are grateful for moderate ones; but there is scarcely anyone who does not show ingratitude when it comes to big ones." American culture is generally lenient about expecting adolescents to take much responsibility in regard to requiting filial obligations, so that unless there is strong pressure from the family or from intrapsychic motives, obligation issues may not be prominent in an overt sense. But if the pressure is felt to be strong enough, the sense of obligation and the attempt to requite it may be, even in adolescence, a bottomless pit. An obligation felt as such contains a strongly unpleasant ingredient. It constitutes an interference with the pursuit of more unambiguous selfish aims.

Theoretical Issues

I regard the feeling of filial obligation as an autonomous system providing its own motivation, producing attitudes, behavior, and ultimately conflicts which are distinctive. However, it will never be found in isolation from other more widely discussed psychodynamic issues such as oedipal, dependency, and identity conflicts.

These attitudes are conscious or preconscious as a rule. The adolescent can hardly be oblivious of the concern and efforts made on his behalf by his parents, especially since on suitable occasions the parents are apt to become repetitive and sanctimonious on the subject. But the attitudes also have roots and important connections in the unconscious. There they are deeply involved with other intrapsychic matters and like them are heavily freighted with psychic residues from earlier times.

The main effort of the study has been to describe feelings of filial obligation and to trace their influence in a variety of contexts. It is appropriate now to try to answer the question, Where does its power come from? There are three main sources: intrapsychic, intrafamilial, and cultural, but in this chapter I shall examine only the first, the intrapsychic.

First, there is a wish of the child to do things for the parents, particularly the mother, arising from feelings of love or filial affection. This is the purest source of the feeling. I must hasten to add, however, that the inevitable inconstancy of this love is also of decisive importance. Exactly how this mysterious love arises has been the subject of considerable metapsychological speculation.

Banham (1950) wrote that at about four months of age affectionate behavior is first shown by the infant in an outgoing striving and approach:

> Its gaze is fixed upon the person's face. It kicks, holds out and waves its arms, and tries to raise its body from the crib. The direction of the arm and leg movement is not well oriented or coordinated in the beginning, but repeated attempts to get closer to the attractive person become more successful, and useless movements are restrained. . . . The child responds reciprocally to affectionate cuddling. It reaches for the mother's face and mouth. Possibly, it would feed her if it could. Later, as a toddler, it does try to feed its dolls, carry them about, wrap them warmly, and rock them to sleep. Affectionate behavior, even in its beginnings, as all through life, is that of cherishing, protecting, giving of the self to and caring for another person.

Feelings of filial obligation impel one to love and to behave in a loving fashion. To achieve this the child must have loved and been loved. It will be recalled that similar behavioral features were described as narcissistic strivings. Freud (1931) assumed that sublimated erotic and narcissistic features coexist in a given individual and believed that this coexistence was descriptive of the most common of all personality types. Giving, then, can serve both self and object libidinal interests. The presence of both components makes possible the questions: Do I really love? Am I really loved?

One component of what the adolescent does for the parent is voluntary and arises spontaneously in the course of developing affection for the caretaker. To be sure, acts of love are not subjectively identical with acts of requital, but love is necessary to the development of the commitment to requite. Love also makes one always and precisely (via empathy) aware of the needs and feelings of the object. One cannot, however, completely separate this altruism from selfish reasons such as the concomitant motives of concern for a needed object or dread of offending a feared one (cf. Winnicott 1965).

In the typical passage through adolescence the cathecting of an object outside the family may give rise to guilt feelings over having forsaken parents. This guilt in turn renews filial obligation with new vigor. But if the child has learned to love and be loved, he has also learned in the same relationships to betray this love since hatred toward the parents is an inevitable development. Stated differently, the conflict between narcissistic needs and those of being the lover of another person or of being a dutiful child are present long before adolescence.

A second factor promoting filial obligation is the gratitude the child becomes increasingly aware of as he realizes how much his parents have actually done for him. Klein (1957) traces the origins of feelings of gratitude to experiences in infancy. Her discussion is illuminating and penetrating even if her chronology is debatable. She writes:

> It is enjoyment that forms the basis for gratitude . . . a gratification at the breast means that the infant feels he has received from his love a unique gift which he wants to keep. This is the basis of gratitude. Gratitude . . . includes . . . the ability to accept and assimilate the loved primal object (not only as a source of food) without greed or envy interfering too much. . . . Gratitude is bound up with generosity. Inner wealth derives from having assimilated a good object so that the individual becomes able to share its gift with others.

Gratitude is always coupled with the feeling of obligation.

A third factor expresses the need to redress narcissistic injury. There is more involved in gratitude than the desire to repay the preoedipal mother, to make love to the incestuous object, or to share one's gift. The awareness of dependency on parents is a painful blow to primitive narcissistic pretensions. Here is one of the reasons attempts are so often made to requite and especially to repudiate filial obligations. Even in adulthood the offense to narcissism may rankle.

Emerson (1844) remarked:

> It is not the office of a man to receive gifts. How dare you give them? We wish to be self-sustained. We do not quite forgive the giver. . . . [However] we can receive anything from love, for that is a way of receiving it from ourselves; but not from any one who assumes to bestow. . . . The gift, to be [acceptable], must be the flowing of the giver unto me, correspondent to my flowing unto him.

Interestingly enough, it is from the perspective of redressing a narcissistic offense that Freud (1920) traced the origin of what came to be known as "rescue fantasies":

> When a child hears that he owes his life to his parents, that his mother gave him life, the feelings of tenderness in him mingle with the longing to be big and independent himself, so that he forms the wish to repay the parents for this gift and requite it by one of like value. It is as though the boy said in his defiance: "I want nothing from father; I shall repay him all I have cost him." He then weaves a phantasy of saving his father's life on some dangerous occasion by which he becomes quits with him. . . . The mother gave the child his life and it is not easy to replace the unique gift with anything of like value. . . . He gives her back another life, that of a child as like himself as possible. . . . When in a dream a man rescues a woman from the water, it means that he makes her a mother . . . he makes her his own mother. When a woman rescues someone else (a child) out of the water, she represents herself as the mother who bore him, like Pharaoh's daughter in the Moses legend.

We should note two things about rescue fantasies. First, they are an important class of attempts at discharging feelings of obligation. However, we have seen that in real-life actions the requital usually assumes less picaresque forms than those mentioned by Freud. Second, in psychoanalytic literature they have been described nearly always as vicissitudes of the oedipus complex (Freud 1910, Abraham 1922, Jones 1913). Yet even in Freud's keen but brief discussion of them it may seem that while at every point they deal with oedipally derived factors, other factors, related but different, are also involved: above all the narcissistic injury arising from reflecting on the aboriginal (preoedipal, prepsychic) datum which one comes to appreciate later that one once had to be born. The wish to do something to heal this egotistic wound leads to fantasies and acts of altruism.

Fourth, there appears to be an inherent desire in people to repay devotion received in kind. Boszormenyi-Nagy and Spark (1973) assert that every person carries around with him a ledger in which one records things done for them against repayments made for these favors. The young child accepts many things done on his behalf by the parents as a right, something taken for granted without feeling any need for repayment (Balint 1972). But when adolescence is attained, the child is no longer entirely comfortable in exclusively receiving. He is more apt to feel that whatever favors the parents have done for him will have to be repaid (recall J case).

Fifth, gratitude and especially verbal and nonverbal expressions of it are taught the child ("Say 'Thank you' to Grandma." "Here is your present, give Daddy a big hug."). Thus, feelings and expressions of gratitude are partly extensions of learning to do autonomously what one was urged or forced to do as a child. These learned behaviors must be powerfully reinforced by the increased benefits conferred upon the appreciative child.

Sixth, in the overall identification which the child makes with the parents by sharing their values, the child is encouraged to do things for other people including the parents themselves as the "right" thing to do (Furer 1967). Doing this sort of "right" thing is, of course, esteemed morally. But it is also esteemed narcissistically as evidence of a personality which is self-sufficient, which has energy to spare to help others.

Seventh, filial obligation helps secure a cohesive sense of self (Kohut 1971) since the clinically encountered adolescent often manifests an unstable self-cathexis (Spiegel 1964).

Filial obligation implies that the adolescent has a relationship, and for one with a feeling of having a tenuous existence this is reassuring because a relationship, particularly an enduring one, provides some sense of security. It feels safer to have some kind of human connection, even an oppressive one with a demanding parent than none at all (Searles 1961, Guntrip 1969). In real or even fantasied involvement with another person, the other person confirms one's existence as a distinct and psychologically integrated individual. Kohut refers to the use of objects in this way as "mirroring."

Finally, feelings and acts of filial obligation may be an expression of appeasement, or of a wish to make reparation for real or fantasied damage done to loved or needed objects (cf. Abraham 1922). This concept has been discussed extensively by Klein and Riviere (1964). Klein (1957) states:

We frequently encounter expressions of gratitude which turn out to be prompted mainly by feelings of guilt and much less by the capacity for love. I think the distinction between such guilty feelings and gratitude on the deepest level is important. This does not mean that some element of guilt does not enter into the most genuine feelings of gratitude.

These intrapsychic factors derive from every level of the psyche and from a variety of sources, and help explain why very few adolescents fail to develop filial obligation to a significant degree.

Conclusions

The assuming of marital responsibilities appears to be a major derivative of filial obligation.

It is to be expected that a culture would encourage individuals to perform maximally in their social roles. As a rule, it is in adult life that culture demands the most of the individual, because it is then that the ego has attained the height of its powers. But in American middle-class society, this comes at a time when the individual may have transcended his family of origin. The effect of this circumstance on requiting filial obligation is ironic. When the obligation could be most effectively repaid, the primary allegiance and efforts may be directed elsewhere. Yet, as Flugel (1921), Deutsch (1945), Benedek (1959), and others have noted, the parents find considerable enrichment in later years (and earlier) by identifying with their offspring. Under favorable circumstances, then, adults are able to repay part of their filial debts by providing their parents with continued and strengthened, if vicarious, cathexes in life.

Finally, it seems likely that feelings of filial obligation contribute to one's altruistic social acts and attitudes, whether or not they have an instinctual basis. The social sphere is readily made the displaced vehicle for expressing attitudes derived from the family life of childhood. For the many adults who have never raised children it may provide a mean of requiting debts of filial gratitude in a beneficient manner, which extends well beyond the compass of a nuclear family. Bacon observed all this and left us a striking aphorism: "The care of posterity is most in them that have no posterity."

In a final perspective, then, we see that expressions of filial obligation persist throughout entire life spans, passing from one generation to the next and enriching the social well being of everyone.

NOTES

1. Therapist: Sylvia Telser
2. Therapist: Arnold Samuels, M.D.
3. Therapist: Karen Roin
4. Therapist: Beverly Thompson

REFERENCES

Abraham, K. (1922). Father-murder and father-rescue in the fantasies of neurotics. In R. Fliess, ed., *The Psychoanalytic Reader.* New York: International Universities Press, 1948.

Balint, E. (1972). Fair shares and mutual concern. *International Journal of Psycho-Analysis* 53: 61-66.

Banham, K. M. (1950). The development of affectionate behavior in infancy. *Journal of Genetic Psychology* 76: 283-289.

Benedek, T. (1959). Parenthood as a development phase. *Journal of the American Psychoanalytic Association* 7: 389-417.

Blos, P. (1962). *On Adolescence: A Psychoanalytic Interpretation.* New York: Free Press.

———(1967). The second individuation process of adolescence. *Psychoanalytic Study of the Child* 23: 162-186.

Boszormenyi-Nagy, I., and Spark, G. M. (1973). *Invisible Loyalties.* New York: Harper & Row.

Cellini, B. (1730). *Autobiography.* Garden City, New York: Doubleday, 1946.

Deutsch, H. (1945). *The Psychology of Women,* Vol. II. New York: Grune and Stratton.

Elson, M. (1964). The reactive impact of adolescent and family upon each other in separation. *Journal of the American Academy of Child Psychiatry* 3: 697-709.

Emerson, R. W. (1844). Gifts. In *Essays and Journals.* Garden City, New York: Doubleday, 1968.

Erikson, E. (1956). The problem of ego identity. *Journal of the American Psychoanalytic Association* 4: 56-121.

Flugel, J. C. (1921). *The Psychoanalytic Study of the Family.* London: Hogarth.

Framo, J. L. (1970). Symptoms from a family transactional viewpoint. *International Psychiatry Clinics* 7: 125-171.

Freud, A. (1958). Adolescence. *Psychoanalytic Study of the Child* 13: 255-278.

————(1967). About losing and being lost. *Psychoanalytic Study of the Child* 22: 9-19.

Freud, S. (1910). A special type of object choice made by men. *Standard Edition* 11: 163-176. London: Hogarth, 1957.

————(1920). Beyond the pleasure principle. *Standard Edition* 18: 7-17. London, Hogarth, 1955.

————(1931). Libidinal types. *Standard Edition* 21: 216-222. London: Hogarth, 1961.

Furer, M. (1967). Some developmental aspects of the superego. *International Journal of Psycho-Analysis* 48: 277-280.

Geleerd, E. (1961). Some aspects of ego vicissitudes in adolescence. *Journal of the American Psychoanalytic Association* 9: 394-405.

Gould, R. L. (1972). The phases of adult life: a study in developmental psychology. *American Journal of Psychiatry* 129: 521-531.

Group for the Advancement of Psychiatry (1968). Normal adolescence. 6: 68.

Guntrip, H. (1969). *Schizoid Phenomena, Object Relations and the Self.* New York: International Universities Press.

Hartmann, H. (1956). The development of the ego concept in Freud's work. In *Essays on Ego Psychology.* New York: International Universities Press, 1964.

Jacobson, E. (1964). *The Self and the Object World.* New York: International Universities Press.

Jones, E. (1913). The God Complex. In *Essays in Applied Psychoanalysis.* London: Hogarth, 1923.

————(1923). The fantasy of the reversal of generations. In *Papers on Psychoanalysis.* New York: William Wood.

King, S. (1971). Coping mechanisms in adolescents. *Psychiatric Annals* 1: 10-45.

Klein, M. (1932). *The Psycho-analysis of Children.* London: Hogarth.

————(1957). *Envy and Gratitude.* London: Tavistock Publications.

————, and Riviere, J. (1964). *Love, Hate and Reparation.* New York: W. W. Norton.

Kohut, H. (1971). *The Analysis of the Self.* New York: International Universities Press.

Levenson, E. A., Stockhammer, H., and Feiner, A. H. (1967). Family transactions in the etiology of dropping out of college. *Contemporary Psychoanalysis* 2: 134-157.

Modell, A. (1971). The origin of certain forms of pre-oedipal guilt and the implications for a psychoanalytical theory of affects. *International Journal of Psycho-Analysis* 52: 337-346.

Newell, H. W. (1936). A further study of maternal rejection. *American Journal of Orthopsychiatry* 6: 576-589.

Noshpitz, J. D. (1970). Certain cultural and familial factors contributing to adolescent alienation. *Journal of the American Academy of Child Psychiatry* 9: 216-223.

Redl, F., and Wineman, D. (1957). *The Aggressive Child.* New York: Free Press of Glencoe.

Reese, H. (1962). *Heal the Hurt Child.* Chicago: University of Chicago Press.

Searles, H. (1961). The source of anxiety in paranoid schizophrenia. In *Collected Papers on Schizophrenia.* New York: International Universities Press, 1965.

Spiegel, L. A. (1964). Identity and adolescence. In J. Lorand and H. Schneer, eds., *Adolescents: Psychoanalytic Approach to Problems and Therapy.* New York: Harper and Row.

Stierlin, H. (1973). Interpersonal aspects of internalizations. *International Journal of Psycho-Analysis* 54: 203-214.

Tolpin, M. (1971). On the beginnings of a cohesive self. *Psychoanalytic Study of the Child* 26: 316-354.

Winnicott, D. W. (1965). The development of the capacity for concern. In *The Maturational Processes and the Facilitating Environment.* New York: International Universities Press, 1965.

Zachry, C. S. (1940). *Emotion and Conflict in Adolescence.* New York: Appleton-Century.

12] PARENTS AND ADOLESCENTS: EMPATHY AND THE VICISSITUDES OF DEVELOPMENT

ANDRE P. DERDEYN AND DAVID B. WATERS

Psychotherapy with adolescents has always been perceived as difficult—the adolescent being found a relatively poor subject for analytic types of therapy. Such therapies are quite dependent upon the loyalty of the patient to the process, and the adolescent has difficulty establishing that loyalty. He is all too apt to withdraw from therapy as soon as his psychic pain has diminished or the external pressure for therapy is reduced. Gitelson (1948) described the goal of therapy with adolescents as "character synthesis," implying that the therapeutic role is restricted to that of facilitating psychosocial development. Furthermore, the adolescent's need for social relationships, particularly with peers, has led to the impression that adolescents are relatively inaccessible to the therapeutic process. This has given rise to the idea that adolescents are bad patients, insufficiently amenable to what psychotherapy has to offer.

More recently, the upsurge of ecological psychiatry has led to a change of emphasis from the intrapsychic to the interpersonal sphere. In this change of emphasis, however, a new imbalance may have arisen. We have gone from thinking of the bad adolescent, unavailable for therapy and in a state of turmoil and tenuously controlled impulses, to thinking increasingly of the helpless adolescent, victimized and misunderstood by his environment, and disturbed only as a reflection of the disturbance around him. This notion of the adolescent as victim has to some extent been the product of the systems theory approach to family therapy, according to which the identified patient is thought to express intrafamilial conflict more than any inherent disturbance of his own. Excessive adherence to this concept can lead to the distortion that the adolescent is exclusively the victim, and prevent the therapist from taking a critical look at the adolescent's role in his own and in his family's distress. To consider the patient exclusively as victim, implying polarities of good and bad, right and wrong, active and passive, will not make for helpful understanding of the patient and his family. It is no better to see him as helpless victim than it is as bad patient, for both labels imply distortions in the therapist's view more than they are likely to be descriptive of any adolescent patient.

Therapists who work with adolescents and their parents are subject to another common distortion. We tend to be very responsive to the stresses developmental change places upon our adolescent patients and recognize and are accepting of the difficulty the adolescent experiences in achieving any kind of nominal functioning. This is very different from how we perceive the parents of the adolescent.

Stress and Change in the Adult

The constant stresses and adaptive demands placed upon the parents of the adolescent seem to make less of an impression upon us. Among therapists who work with adolescents a tendency to hold an unspoken and naive assumption that the postadolescent, normal adult will naturally be able to conduct his life in a planned, orderly, and relatively healthy fashion, consistently emerges.

Only recently have we begun to acknowledge the sensitivity of adults to environmental changes. Lindemann's (1944) work on bereavement, Lifton's (1967) studies of survivors of Hiroshima, and studies of the effects of catastrophe, such as the 1972 Buffalo Creek flood in West Virginia, have demonstrated adult vulnerability to major disruptive changes in the enviornment (Erikson 1976, Titchener and Kapp 1976). Recent empirical studies exhibit the stressful effects of common life changes upon adults. Events such as serious illness in one's self or in a family member, death in the family, divorce, and changes in employment has been shown to be followed by increased utilization of medical services (Wilmuth, Weaver, and Donlan 1975), depression (Briscoe 1975, Clayton, Halikas, and Maurice 1972, Paykel, Myers, and Dienelt 1969), and suicide (Paykel, Prusoff, and Myers 1975, Humphrey, French, Niswander, and Casey 1974).

The adult must respond not only to environmental crisis and normative stresses, but also to changes and developments within himself and his own family. The strongest voice against the naivete regarding adult normalcy is that of Erikson (1959) who describes a scheme of life crises or challenges extending from infancy to death. These crises concern not only the internal dynamics and development of the individual, but also his relationships with important others. It is worth noting that Erikson translates and expands the traditional psychosexual stages into specifically interpersonal terms. Every Eriksonian stage implies successul interpersonal adjustments if it ends well and unsuccessful interpersonal adjustment if it ends poorly. Erikson frames the occurrence and resolution of crisis in terms that inherently include emotionally important others. Erikson's terms, such as trust, intimacy, integrity, and others, have a distinctly interactional and interpersonal emphasis.

The Task of the Adolescent Therapist

We have belatedly approached the realization that interpersonal factors are fully as important in our understanding of people's problems as intrapsychic ones, and that the individual's involvement in social and other relationships renders him remarkably vulnerable to changes in any of them. The adolescent therapist must attempt to integrate intrapsychic, developmental, and relationship issues involving all family members.

It will be helpful to review some of the more specific stresses experienced by parents when their children enter and traverse adolescence. The discussion will emphasize the effects upon parents of the adolescent development of their children and the implications of the parental response in terms of the continuing relationship between parent and child. Particular attention will be paid to the interplay of parental and adolescent developmental problems.

The Effect of Their Children's Adolescent Development Upon Parents

DEVELOPMENTAL STAGES OF THE FAMILY

A useful method for looking at the interrelationship between adolescent and parent is the family developmental scheme proposed by Solomon (1973). Deriving significantly from Erikson's work, this scheme conceptualizes the family as having five developmental stages: (1) the marriage, (2) the birth of the first child and subsequent child bearing, (3) individuation of family members, (4) the actual departure of the children, and (5) the integration of loss. Much as in Erikson's scheme of psychosocial

177

development, each stage is conceptualized as a crisis in which resolution by the family is required for successful transition to the next phase. Two stages are of interest to us in looking at the adolescent and his parents.

Stage three, individuation of family members, spans the time from the departure of the first child through the adolescence of the last. It takes into account how the beginning separation of the adolescent may threaten the balance of the family, which often depends upon the dependency of the children. Families may respond to this crisis in either of two unconstructive ways. The parents may attempt to exert greater control over the departing child in an effort to reestablish an earlier state of dependency. The child may at the same time be strongly but unconsciously motivated to stimulate the parents to reestablish him in his previous status of dependency. The other extreme is for the parents to support the departing member's independent strivings only while ignoring the more dependent needs in a subtly hostile way: "You don't need us anymore!" This response may cause premature separation of the child from the family at a time when he is ill-equipped to be autonomous, and the result is often the eventual return of the child in a dependent, defeated state.

Solomon's stage four, which involves the actual departure of the children, requires the parents to modify their demands and expectations and to relinquish the gratification of the parental role vis-a-vis dependent children. The less direct gratification deriving from a relationship with independent young adults is then a necessary substitute. This shift requires that each parent confront the other's needs more directly than he or she may have done for years. In many marriages the capacity of each partner to relate to the other has atrophied, if indeed it ever developed well before the advent and raising of children. In addition, serious conflicts between the spouses may have been deferred, if not actually acted out, in triangular relationships with children; then the departure of the last child necessitates the difficult process of establishing a new marital balance that can be sustained without the gratification of the dependency of children. If the reintegration of the marriage is not taking place and reinvestment is not possible, the family may unconsciously mobilize to hold onto the last child. The family may previously have avoided the problems surrounding separation by allowing one child to leave and subsequently focusing on the next in line. Solomon points out that, in the past, psychotherapists have tended to respond to the problem presented by each child as though it were an isolated phenomenon and, consequently, have not helped families identify their behavior as an expression of family developmental problems.

ANDRE P. DERDEYN AND DAVID B. WATERS

ERIKSON'S CRISIS OF INTEGRITY VERSUS DESPAIR

The parental developmental state at the time of their children's adolescence is usually the seventh crisis, in which Erikson describes the extremes of the outcome as integrity versus disgust and despair. Erikson (1959) says of the concept of integrity, "Integrity is the acceptance of one's own and only life cycle and of the people who have become significant to it as something that had to be and that, by necessity, permitted of no substitutions."

For the adult, who in this life stage must accept as final his choice of work and his choice of spouse, the challenge to his equilibrium posed by the adolescent is considerable. Besides realistically having more options than his parents, the adolescent recapitulates his own fantasies of infantile omnipotence and stimulates similar fantasies in his elders (Pumpian-Mindlin 1965). This is a considerable threat to a person whose major choices in life lie in the past and who, as Erikson says, can permit of no substitutions. At this stage, the strength, freedom, and open future of his own adolescent children can be a painful counterpoint to an adult.

Levi, Stierlin, and Savard (1972) in discussing the intergenerational problem point out that the crises of separation and identity formation in the adolescent boy often coincide in time with his father's climacteric crisis. The presence of an adolescent with seemingly open choices in work and love objects forces the middle-aged father to complete his grieving over lost alternatives and to reaffirm his own life choices. In this study of adolescent boys and their fathers, the fathers seemed unable to mourn adequately their real or fantasied shortcomings and were accordingly unable to come to terms with their lives or to find satisfying new courses of action.

The authors found the fathers to be suffering from a masked depression which typically emerged as envy. Since these fathers saw themselves as weak or impotent failures, they did not enjoy their son's successes or compete with them but were instead primarily jealous of their sons' vigor, sexual vitality, and freedom from tedious work.

As the fathers tended to withdraw, the mothers became more actively involved with their sons, seeking from them the appreciation that their husbands failed to give. The mothers' increased activity, often perceived as unwelcome intrusiveness, aroused in the sons anxiety about infantile dependent and sexual wishes toward the mother; these had to be warded off by hostile and defiant behavior. At first such mothers felt hurt. They then became vindictively enraged at their ungrateful boys, with their anger making them even more intrusive, further intensifying the cycle.

THE BREAKDOWN OF EMPATHIC COMMUNICATION

There is a broader principle at work here than the specific conflict of crises just described. This broader principle signifies the breakdown of empathic communication between parents and adolescents. In contrast to the sharing of feelings in families with children in earlier childhood, most families lack intimate sharing with their adolescent children (Williams 1973). Up to this point in life, most parents perceive themselves as confidently leading or guiding their children to adulthood. At adolescence this parental image is shattered; the adolescent tends to take the initiative and demands that the parent surrender his secure position of the past. Guidance as a parental style must give way to a more equal exchange. When there is an abrupt parting of the ways, it is often related to the conscious feeling of both parties—parents and adolescents—of their being very different from each other. This feeling of difference is more apparent than real; the breakdown of the relationship has at its center a defensive misperception and exaggeration of their differentness. Each stirs in the other acute, if unconscious, awareness of issues that are at the very heart of their own psychological struggles. The adolescent and his parents are struggling with different sides of the same coin, at the same time denying their painful kinship and their commonality.

A clear area of commonality is that of loss. The need for the adolescent to mourn the infantile objects from whom he is separating and to mourn many aspects of earlier childhood is widely accepted (Sugar 1968). Similarly, most parents need to mourn the loss of their role as the parent of a younger, more dependent child. The struggle faced by parents and adolescents is the same: relinquishing a past status that may have had its difficulties, but that has provided a framework and an organizational principle to life ("I am a parent," "I am a child"). In addition, both parents and child are relinquishing each other as primary objects of love and concern and have to face replacing that loss. This is an anxiety-provoking proposition. Change from the known to the unknown (or less known) cannot be without ambivalence. The anxiety of moving on to a new life phase can either be shared or denied. The sharing of that anxiety by either side with the other may lead to mutual disclosure of concern and feelings of loss. The loss may be seen as the end of a happy period that will be missed, or as the end of an unhappy period that could have been better. Either case—lost pleasures or missed opportunities—needs to be mourned. What tends to happen, however, is that mourning is denied, sadness is obscured in intergenerational conflict, and parents and child part emotionally distant from and angry at each other.

From the adult's side, this distancing has been well accounted for by Pumpian-Mindlin (1965). He proposed the omnipotentiality of adolescence—the feeling that one can do anything and everything and do it well—as a vital aspect of ego development. Parents are often indulgent of this, but at the same time, undermine it. He says:

> the adult must depreciate this period in the youth because of the anxiety and feelings of frustration which it arouses in him. . . . This anxiety of the adult is certainly an important aspect of the universal social devaluation of the younger by the older generation—the fear that their renunciation of omnipotentiality may have been in vain, or may have been unnecessary.

Pumpian-Mindlin describes the response of the adult as a kind of defensive emphasis on the difference between his own pragmatic awareness of human limitations and the adolescent's naive self-confidence and feelings of strength. The adult emphasizes the difference and distance between himself and his children in the process of repressing his own sadness at lost potential and abandoned dreams.

From the adolescent's side, we may surmise that the emphasis on the difference between his parents and himself has much to do with the need to believe in himself and to avoid and deny his own inescapable fears that he may not amount to all that he hopes. It is important to deny one's kinship and inheritance from people who are flawed, who have not been extraordinary. The common adolescent complaint that adults, usually including his parents, have sold out automatically includes the unspoken disclaimer, "But I won't; I am not like you, I will never be like you, and I won't end up like you." They tell their parents that they do not and will not have the same values, the same kinds of relationships, the same hypocrisies and shortcomings. They devalue their elders in much the same way as their elders devalue them, and with much the same purpose: to deny their commonality, to avoid the similarity of their struggles. As parents are afraid that "their renunciation may have been in vain" (Pumpian-Mindlin 1965), adolescents are afraid that their omnipotentiality may be mere daydreams.

Parent and child may thus be seen maintaining a wary distance from each other, each defensively preoccupied with the other's shortcomings. They are virtually lost to each other as emotional resources. Their mutual lack of empathy—their inability to feel strongly and subjectively what the other might be going through—is crippling to them both. It is also a defensive rejoinder to the critical and unempathetic response from the other side. They arrive at a stalemate in which any positive move one might make toward the other becomes increasingly unlikely. Each needs the other to suffer to some degree; parents want adolescents to recognize the harsh realities of the world and surrender their omnipotentiality, while adolescents want their parents to recognize and admit to the emptiness of their lives.

On a more immediate level, the challenge by the adolescent of the parents' position of power threatens parental self-esteem, severely limiting parental capacity for empathy for the adolescent. The adolescent, on his part, fears intimacy with his parents because of the regressive pull toward types of relationships which were in earlier life enjoyed, but are now abhorred. The result is a strong tendency for mutual rejection between the adolescent and his parents.

EMPATHY AS A THERAPEUTIC GOAL

The goal of reestablishing empathic relationships within the family appears to be commonly recognized. Anthony (1969), in decrying the stereotyping, deflating, and controlling techniques used by adults with adolescents, speaks of the needs for a person-to-person response to them. This idea is akin to what Paul (1965) has termed "parental empathy." Cohen and Balikov (1974) speak of the need for treatment for parents so that their empathy can be "updated." Our goal is to expand these notions to include reciprocal awareness and expression of empathy between the generations.

Freedom, independence, and separation are legitimate goals for adolescents, but so are empathy, openness to, and acceptance of one's parents as people. As therapists we tend to emphasize separation, perhaps short-changing both generations of the family. In so doing, we contribute to adolescent fantasies of omnipotentiality, and we also perpetuate the conflict between generations when we cast either the child or the parent as winner or loser, a right or a wrong party. Perhaps worst of all, we are not facilitating for the adolescent any valid kind of separation if we provide him only with permission or even encouragement to reject and defeat his parents.

With sufficient attention to the developmental problems of parents, the therapist can support them, help them to achieve a better sense of self, and can enlist their aid in freeing their child from his ambivalent attachment to them. In healthier families, the reestablishing of a close marital relationship may facilitate the adolescent's separation (McPherson, Brackelmanns, and Newman 1974). Treatment of the parents in relation to the development of their adolescent child can offer them a unique opportunity for growth. In support of this latter idea, Schecter (1970) writes, "... the point in time when psychic maturity is most likely to occur is when a parent has allowed his children full separation." A child's successful passage through adolescence offers challenge and reward both to parents and to children.

For both parent and adolescent the task is to relinquish their defensive dismissal of each other and to experience each other more directly as people. For parents this demands that they learn to give up their perception of the adolescent as a child and accept him more as a peer; again, they must surrender guidance and adopt exchange as the basic medium of communication with their adolescent offspring. The realization that they have had their chance to teach, and must let the adolescent do with their teaching what he will, is often painful and difficult for them to accept.

For adolescents the task may be even more demanding and complex. In addition to learning a new view of his parents and a new style of communication, the adolescent must increasingly accept responsibility for what he is and give up his accusatory stance. Often adolescents may be simultaneously demanding adult status while clinging tenaciously to childlike invective against their parents. If they can be helped to give up the latter and to take the step toward true equal exchange, a new and more successful relationship can be forged.

The capacity to see and accept himself as he is, imperfect and less than he might have hoped, allows both parent and child to relinquish their scornful and defensive derision of each other. The parent is entering middle age with most of his choices behind him. His commitments have for the most part been made. Accepting this situation of a diminution of opportunities is the challenge of the crisis of integrity.

The adolescent faces a very similar difficulty. It is only when he confronts the broad opportunities available to him and makes some choices and commitments that he can begin to move forward to adult status and to a more comfortable exchange with his own parents as people. As long as he clings to his omnipotentiality and refuses to deal realistically with the question of what he can and cannot be, he impedes not only his own development, but also the development of empathy between himself and his parents. Identity and integrity, in Erikson's sense, refer to a similar process at two different moments in the life cycle. It is in the discovery of this similarity and shared difficulty that empathy between parent and child can be a basis for a mutual recognition and a new acceptance of each other.

Conclusions

In order to gain an adequate view of the adolescent as a member of his family, the complement of intrapsychic and interpersonal modes and the reciprocal effects of developmental problems on both sides of the generation gap must be appreciated. These concepts play a key role in any practical approach to families.

It appears, then, that our basic goal with an adolescent is to engage with his conflicts, whether they be classically psychopathological or developmental in nature. The second goal, and achievement of this goal can aid immeasurably in achievement of the first, is that of reestablishing empathic communication between the adolescent and his parent. By assisting family members to be of help to each other, we are not only being useful to the family before us but are perhaps teaching a mode of relating which our young patient can take to his adolescent children.

REFERENCES

Anthony, J. (1969). The reactions of adults to adolescents and their behavior. In G. Caplan and S. Lebovici, eds., *Adolescence*. New York: Basic Books.

Briscoe, C. S. (1975). Depression in bereavement and divorce. *Archives of General Psychiatry* 32:439-443.

Clayton, P. J., Halikas, J. A., and Maurice, W. L. (1972). The depression of widowhood. *British Journal of Psychiatry* 120:71-78.

Cohen, R. S. and Balikov, H. (1974). On the impact of adolescence upon parents. *This Annual* 3:217-236.

Erikson, E. H. (1959). Identity and the life cycle. *Psychological Issues* 1:1-171.

Erikson, K. T. (1976). Loss of commonality at Buffalo Creek. *American Journal of Psychiatry* 133:302-305.

Gitelson, M. (1948). Character synthesis: the psychotherapeutic problem of adolescence. *American Journal of Orthopsychiatry* 18:422-431.

Humphrey, J. A., French, L., Niswander, G. D., and Casey, T. M. (1974). Process of suicide: sequence of disruptive events in lives of suicide victims. *Diseases of the Nervous System* 35:275-277.

Levi, L. D., Stierlin, H., and Savard, R. J. (1972). Fathers and sons: the interlocking crises of integrity and identity. *Psychiatry* 35:48-56.

Lifton, R. J. (1967). *Death in Life: Survivors of Hiroshima.* New York: Random House.

Lindemann, E. (1944). Symptomatology and management of acute grief. *American Journal of Psychiatry* 101:7-21

McPherson, S. R., Brackelmanns, W. E., and Newman, L. E. (1974). Stages in the family therapy of adolescents. *Family Process* 13:77-94.

Paul, N. L., and Grosser, G. H. (1965). Operational mourning and its role in conjoint family therapy. *Community Mental Health Journal* 1:339-345.

Paykel, E. S., Myers, J. K., Dienelt, M. N., Klerman, G. L., Lindenthal, J. J., and Pepper, M. P. (1969). Life events and depression. *Archives of General Psychiatry* 21:753-760.

————, Prusoff, B. A., and Myers, J. K. (1975). Suicide attempts and recent life events: a controlled comparison. *Archives of General Psychiatry* 32:327-333.

Pumpian-Mindlin, E. (1965). Omnipotentiality, youth and commitment. *Journal of the American Academy of Child Psychiatry* 4:1-18.

Schechter, M. D. (1970). About adoptive parents. In E. J. Anthony and T. Benedek, eds. *Parenthood: Its Psychology and Psychopathology.* Boston: Little, Brown.

Solomon, M. A. (1973). A developmental, conceptual premise for family therapy. *Family Process* 12:178-188.

Sugar, M. (1968). Normal adolescent mourning. *American Journal of Psychiatry* 22:258-269.

Titchener, J. L., and Kapp, F. T. (1976). Family and character change at Buffalo Creek. *American Journal of Psychiatry* 133:295-299.

Williams, E. S. (1973). Family therapy: its role in adolescent psychiatry. *This Annual* 2:324-339.

Wilmuth, L. F., Weaver, L., and Donlan, S. (1975). Utilization of medical services by transferred employees. *Archives of General Psychiatry* 32:85-88.

13] THE "JUVENILE IMPOSTER":
SOME THOUGHTS ON
NARCISSISM AND THE DELINQUENT

RICHARD C. MAROHN

Since Anna Freud (1958) emphasized that the study of adolescence has been neglected in psychoanalytic investigations, this neglect has diminished. It was held that by the time the child passed into latency little more would be added to or subtracted from his psychological development. Adolescence was seen as a reworking of earlier conflicts and traumata. Of course, later stages of development must of necessity build on earlier stages, but more and more the importance of adolescence as a unique developmental phase has been emphasized in the literature. Blos (1972b) recently challenged the concept of the infantile neurosis. He described the contributions of adolescence to the formation of the adult neurosis and stressed the important psychic restructuring that takes place in adolescence, exerting "a decisive influence on the adult personality, regardless of whether the outcome of this process is a normal or a pathological one."

Work with a specific kind of adolescent patient, hospitalized delinquents, has touched upon many of these issues. Numerous children function quite adequately until confronted with the developmental tasks of adolescence and the family turmoil associated with this separation-individuation process. Adolescence can be understood as the interaction of a number of different phases of development, and delinquency can be understood as resulting from problems in superego development, ego deficiencies or distortions, object searching, disordered defensive constellations, deviant libidinal development, a failure of socialization, substitute

First presented before the Society of Medical Psychoanalysts, October 10, 1973, New York; and in a revised form before the Chicago Society for Adolescent Psychiatry, February 23, 1974.

libidinal gratification, severe guilt, a disease of the psychic structure, and the like. In addition, some of the newer ideas on narcissism and the self contribute greatly to our understanding of the adolescent process, and in particular the delinquent process. This chapter describes our work with delinquents and traces some of our current ideas back to the early contributions of Aichorn.[1] The patients described are not "imposters," though such is at times part of their repertoire. Aichorn's "juvenile imposter" was his springboard for understanding the narcissistic transference; this study attempts to develop his ideas.

August Aichorn died at the age of seventy-one in 1949 (A. Freud 1951). He began his work as a teacher in the elementary schools and attempted to rehabilitate delinquent children from the streets of Vienna. Later becoming the superintendent of a Viennese reform school, his experiences there induced him to join the psychoanalytic movement and undergo a training analysis (Eissler 1949). His landmark work, *Wayward Youth* (Aichorn 1925), documents in nontechnical language, with abundant clinical vignettes, his intuitive approach with delinquent boys. This "intuitive gift" was acknowledged by Freud in his Introduction to that work. Psychoanalysis gave Aichorn a theoretical framework around which he could organize his clinical experiences. He was not doing analysis, for as Freud (1925) remarked:

> The possibility of exerting influence through psychoanalysis depends on quite definite conditions, which may be described as the "analytic situation"; it requires the formation of certain psychic structures and a certain attitude toward the analyst. When these factors are lacking, as in the case of children and young delinquents and, as a rule, in criminals dominated by their instincts, the psychoanalytic method must be adapted to meet the need.

Aichorn's pioneering work initiated considerable psychoanalytic interest in the field of delinquency (Aichorn 1964, Eissler 1949). Viewing delinquency as the result of an early childhood deprivation (the genetic point of view), Aichorn (1925) attempts to find the psychic imbalance responsible for delinquent behavior (the economic point of view), searches for the unconscious conflicts responsible for the symptom of delinquency (dynamic point of view), visualizes the delinquent's behavior as the interactions of ego and superego (structural point of view), and focuses on the delinquent's attempt to master external reality through his behavior

187

(adaptive point of view). Psychic trauma causes delinquency. "Our task is to remove the cause rather than to eliminate the overt behavior."

Aichorn demonstrates that the underlying causes of delinquency can be brought to light only in the context of the transference and describes a form of narcissistic transference. In making several references to the grandiosity of the delinquent, he mentions that delinquents cannot be reformed without there being "a strong bond of feeling" between the director and the staff and between staff and delinquents, and emphasizes the struggle in the treatment relationship for "mastery of the situation. . . . My attitude from the very beginning lets the boy feel that I have a power over him." This omnipotent posture by the therapist is detailed when Aichorn (1964) describes how in treating a neurotic delinquent it is necessary for an identification with the therapist to emerge from an object relationship. In other kinds of delinquents, however, he notes that after a considerable period of time the delinquent begins to perceive the therapist for the first time as a separate object and as an independent person—indicating that previously the therapist served as a narcissistic object. The implication of this, Aichorn says, is that the delinquent is still unable to identify with the therapist because he has not yet developed an "object libidinal relationship to our person." He states that this kind of relationship is frequently seen in working with delinquents of the "imposter" or "mountebank" variety. The delinquents possess "a peculiar psychic structure which makes them well nigh incapable of forming object-libidinal relations of any kind." He describes a young man who boasted about his being in demand by so many girls that he could finance his sexual affairs only by stealing. Aichorn determined from the history that this was an imposter and, from the beginning, he employed several omnipotent gambits to throw the young man off guard. Aichorn would not argue whether or not the youth had stolen a sum of money from his mother; he simply demanded to know what he had done with it. The youth soon found himself coming under some sort of spell of cooperation which he felt as "silly," a transference phenomenon. On occasion, Aichorn would also point out to the delinquent how some of his schemes could have been more successfully and brilliantly executed, but cautions against encouraging or directing the youth toward further crime.

He describes in theoretical terms that these delinquents are not capable of an object-libidinal relationship, but that libido is focused entirely in the person's love of self, following Freud's (1914) formulation of the antithesis between narcissism and object relations. In such a state, the other person has taken the place of the ego ideal and is "loved" as one might love oneself, and in working with these delinquents it is this situation which the therapist should attempt to recreate.

> When we meet the type of juvenile delinquent described, then we do not attempt to establish an object-libidinal relationship at all. We behave from the beginning in a manner which incites the youngster to let his own narcissistic libido flow over to our person, so as ultimately to create that dependence of his total personality upon us, a situation parallel to the ego's dependency upon its ego ideal. [Aichorn 1964]

At times the therapist would appear to engage in role playing and transference manipulation to "provoke" the necessary state of tension.

Aichorn emphasizes that deficiencies in the ego ideal cause delinquency. If a child is capable of moving from the period of autoerotism to a period of object relating, then narcissistic libido has been converted into object libido and, in the context of an object relationship, identification can take place. If satisfactory identifications take place with the parents, then an ego ideal can develop; if on the other hand such object relating and identification are not possible, the ego ideal is "weak or non-existent." Consequently, without parental identifications there can be no healthy ego ideal; without ego ideal formation, there is no principle of socialization and the child is directed only by his own self-love.

Aichorn is witness to the grandiosity of the delinquent. His delinquent charges attempt to embarrass and intimidate the staff, complaining to their parents that they were being mistreated. They play one parent against the other, try to impress the therapist, conceal what they are really like, misrepresent themselves, lie, and deceive the adversary. Even some delinquents who appear neurotic or "nervous" may simply be engaging in a power struggle and attempting to escape the demands of reality. With these delinquents it is necessary to "work fast" because one is dealing with an "emergency." From the start one must make the delinquent "emotionally dependent upon us." When this has been achieved, treatment can begin.

Hoffer (1949) summarizes Aichorn's and his own techniques. He alludes to what we presently call a mirror transference in treating a delinquent and sees the idealization of the therapist by the delinquent as a defense against frustrated grandiosity, just as a child's dependence on his own parents is a blow to his narcissism. He pinpoints Aichorn's purpose—to intrude in the ego ideal, to unmask it, and prove its inferiority by proving his own superiority.

These ideas, the formulations of empathic and intuitive therapists, have been enhanced by the theoretical and clinical contributions of Kohut (1966, 1968, 1971, 1972a). Kohut, like Freud (1914), sees the infant progress from a state of autoerotism to primary narcissism to object love, but disagrees with the idea that there is an antithesis between narcissism and object relations. He differentiates object relationships from object love. Object relations, a social or interpersonal concept, may be characterized by either narcissistic or object libidinal ties. In a narcissistic relationship, the object is sought for the maintenance and cohesion it provides the self; in an object libidinal relationship, the object is sought for the gratification of instinctual drives and the relief of tension. A person with many friendships may be relating on a narcissistic basis; conversely, a solitary person engaged almost totally in a creative work may be capable of the highest levels of object love. Kohut posits a specific development for narcissism, emerging from the stage of primary narcissism, as does the object libidinal development, but separate from it. He emphasizes that there are transformations of narcissism which are no longer primitive and are consistent with the most sophisticated forms of psychic development. One's self-esteem, enthusiasm, ambitions, empathy, and wisdom are transformations of narcissism, in a general sense secondary narcissism. For Freud, secondary narcissism is a narcissistic regression away from object love as a result of a painful experience; for Kohut, this is still primary narcissism, for the person had never progressed beyond self-object relating.

Kohut postulates, in the stage of primary narcissism, two primitive structures: the grandiose self and the idealized parental imago. These coexist and neither has prior status. These two structures originate in the self-object relationship of the child-mother symbiotic pair. Kohut's viewpoint is the transference in working with adult patients. His formulations are not derived from direct observation of children and do not refer to the real interpersonal relationship, but rather to the mental constructs which emerge from this primitive stage of life and which are later reactivated in the transference. The narcissistic transference is not the reactivation of an infantile neurosis, but the reactivation of the two primitive narcissistic structures. The grandiose self may emerge in the treatment relationship in one of several forms of mirror transference, in which the analyst or therapist is treated by the patient as though he were a reflection of the patient's own unconscious grandiosity, exhibitionistic or omnipotent. The idealized parental imago is reactivated when the patient idealizes the therapist and attributes to him the omnipotence and perfection of the early parent, and its soothing and regulating functions.

Kohut explains that these two primitive structures are gradually modified as the normal child develops, provided the parenting figures are capable of responding empathically, either to the child's request for narcissistic reassurance or to the child's attempts to idealize the parent. The empathic parent will realize that the child needs to be seen at certain times in his life as wonderful, pure, and simple. The empathic parent realizes that the child also needs to see the parent at certain times as close to divine. Kohut believes that as the child develops greater reality testing, these primitive structures will be gradually modified, though some remnants of primitive narcissism may persist throughout life. However, if the parent does not respond empathically, and either severely frustrates or disillusions the child, a traumatic state may result which causes the child to repress the archaic structures (the grandiosity or the idealization), such that they remain active but walled off during adult life. Hence, they may emerge later in a transference, as already described, or they may reveal themselves in certain kinds of personality configurations.

The grandiose self may remain active consciously but disavowed as a result of what Kohut calls a "vertical split." Here, grandiose behavior in certain areas of the personality is blatant and exists simultaneous with a person's more realistic appraisal of himself and his abilities, or even with some self-depreciation. The grandiose structure may also, however, be repressed but remain active unconsciously through what Kohut calls a "horizontal split"; here the person depreciates himself and feels worthless, because no matter what he does or how much he accomplishes, he never lives up to his primitive and archaic concept of wonderfulness. The repressed idealizing structure may result in a person readily idolizing others, as in an infatuation where the lover easily overlooks the faults and deficiencies of the beloved. It may show itself in a fanatic devotion to a religion, a political or social movement, or an ideology. Such idealizations may be quite conscious, but the person may also experience a chronic state of disillusionment and frustration when, every time he involves himself in a new relationship or activity, he finds himself unsatisfied because reality and the real relationship never measure up to the repressed, idealized parental imago.

Kohut points out that a frequent problem in treating patients with narcissistic problems is the therapist's difficulty in tolerating narcissistic transferences. Therapists frequently do not permit mirroring or idealization to develop because of their own unresolved narcissistic problems, or, because of their ignorance of these issues, they interpret material in the object instinctual line of development. Kohut recommends that first of all the vertical or horizontal split be removed so that the observing ego can be brought to bear on the primitive narcissistic structure; this can only occur after the narcissistic transference has been permitted to unfold. Then, gradually, the narcissistic structures are modified and transformations occur in the narcissistic development leading to enhancement of self-esteem, an increase in the capacity for object love, and an increased capacity to empathize.

Kohut (1971) refers to Aichorn's active techniques to establish a narcissistic transference and cautions that in working with narcissistic personality disorders the active encouragement of an idealizing transference through artifical means would be a contaminent and not analysis. Yet, he agrees that in working with certain delinquents we are in need of "emergency measures" to keep the patient in therapy. He, himself, wonders whether the narcissistic transferences that Aichorn described and that are seen when working with many delinquents are reactivations of the grandiose self or the idealized parental imago. He recognizes that the therapist who presents himself in a grandiose manner encourages mirroring on the part of a grandiose delinquent. Kohut's belief is, however, that the grandiosity of the delinquent, which he attempts to mirror in the therapist, is really serving a defensive purpose against a more painful complex; the emergence of the delinquent's chronic and frustrating search for the idealized parent. Because the grandiosity of the therapist does not interfere with the delinquent's grandiose defense but actually permits mirroring to occur, it is not threatening to the more deeply repressed structure, the need to idealize, which will emerge later in treatment.

Kohut also describes how certain patients regress to a state of threatened fragmentation of the cohesive self. They do not actually fragment to the stage of autoerotism as in the psychotic, but maintain a relatively stable self though fragmentation is threatened. Many such patients exhibit behavior which would suggest an oedipal neurosis, but the excitement of an oedipal struggle is really serving to defend against a loss of cohesion. Such patients require a self-object relationship for cohesion, self-soothing, and self-esteem regulation. When the relationship is broken or disappointing, they are unable to soothe themselves, their self-esteem drops, and fragmentation may occur.

Delinquency as Narcissistic Pathology

Just as adolescence as a developmental phase involves significant transformations of primitive narcissistic structures in the movement from primary to secondary narcissism, so does delinquency involve significant pathology of this progression in the narcissistic development. My own impressions of the delinquents we have seen is that both primitive structures, the grandiose self and idealized parental imago, are important determinants of delinquent behavior. Sometimes one or the other predominates; sometimes both appear with equal intensity.

The grandiose ways of a delinquent are many. He tries to defeat the therapist's best efforts. He boasts of his accomplishments in an exhibition of unmodified grandiosity reminiscent of Kohut's vertical split. The decreased self-esteem and the self-depreciation which he denies or against which he rebelliously acts are reminiscent of the horizontal split. And much of his delinquent behavior protects him from fragmentation.

He searches for his ideal parent and tests the strength of that parent-therapist, his knowledge, his omnipotence, and his therapeutic skill, while trying desperately to idealize him. He expresses disillusionment in his real parents by disobeying their rules, by searching for an alternate omnipotent authority, and by provoking authority to respond irrationally. He seeks omnipotence in the gang leader, drugs, or the automobile. If he is unable to control his environment or to manipulate others, he may rage helplessly, expressing his impotence or attempting to control and provoke a powerful response, for which he then feels responsible. Such behaviors are an important part of the delinquent process, and incessantly confront the therapist and the treatment staff.

CLINICAL MATERIAL

The Delinquency Unit at the Illinois State Psychiatric Institute, the training and research hospital of the Illinois Department of Mental Health, is a ten bed intensive treatment unit for delinquent adolescents providing a full complement of mental health services.[2] The inpatient treatment program is organized around a structured day including school, activities, community meetings, limit setting, and interactions with a milieu staff, all of which are designed to provide externally those kinds of ego functions which are lacking internally. Simultaneously, the milieu emphasizes the need for self-observation, all of which point toward the development of those ego functions needed to engage in an individual psychotherapeutic relationship. Group therapy and family therapy are provided on the unit when indicated, and a therapeutic aftercare program is made available to all patients. The average length of stay is from six to eight months, although some patients stay as long as two years.

The following four cases are illustrative of the kinds of delinquents treated on the unit:

Case 1. Nick was thirteen years of age when first admitted to the program. He had a long history of disruptive behavior as far back as kindergarten. Around age twelve he began having increasing difficulty with his school work, was inattentive in class, and truanted. He sneaked out of the house at night, roamed the neighborhood, and engaged in petty theft. About six months prior to admission, he had left home and was apprehended as a Peeping Tom, an act for which he denied any sexual motive. He was seen by a private psychiatrist in a once-a-week individual psychotherapy, and was described as an impulsive and hyperactive youth who tended to act out in order to evade feelings of depression, related to an early separation from his father at age two, when the father was convicted of pederasty. The mother, an extremely infantile person, continually turned to Nick and their other children for gratification of her own needs. She saw Nick as organically damaged and as perverse as his real father. Nick's relationship with his stepfather was an extremely distant one in which the patient resisted whatever efforts the stepfather made to reach out and engage his stepson in meaningful activity. At the same time the patient idealized his maternal grandfather who had encouraged the patient's interest in building a minibike, although such activity was prohibited by his parents. In the course of his prehospitalization office therapy, he had boasted of his sexual "exploits," talked about his "tough" friends, described his older brother as an idol, and would frequently entertain the therapist with slight of hand tricks; for example, he would frequently take items from the therapist's office and conceal them as if he were planning to "steal" them when the session was over. Initially, his attempts to steal these items was quite obvious, but as the therapy progressed, he became more and more skillful and deceptive, so that only at the end of the session when he turned in his loot, did the therapist realize how he had successfully eluded detection. When Nick was arrested for more serious breaking, entering, and theft, inpatient treatment was decided upon, and he was admitted to the delinquency program. He was described, on admission, as a behavioral disorder of adolescence, giving no evidence of a psychotic process. Psychological testing confirmed his feelings of incompetence, struggling as he was between imminent decay on the one hand and a grandiosity which told him that he could fulfill whatever impulses he experienced. In addition, there was evidence of marked depression over the loss of a meaningful father. He was described by one senior consultant as a person who only internalized objects that were gratifying to him and only as long as they were gratifying; someone who communicates primarily through actions rather than words, and someone who in the course of a treatment relationship gave evidence of a "narcissistic idealized transference." Nick described his father as "the greatest chess player in the world," assumed that his therapist knew everything, but at the same time attempted to undermine the authority of the therapist through clever manipulation. After thirteen months of hospitalization, he demonstrated increased self-control, greater ability to delay gratification, and increased attention span and was discharged. He weathered the death of his favorite grandfather, became increasingly aware of his search for his real father, and continued in twice-a-week psychotherapy following discharge. As affectionate feelings for his therapist became more obvious, his thievery returned. After several runaways he became aware of his fantasy to return to a far state where he had last lived with his father. As the therapist tried to explore these fantasies in the transference, the patient disturbed other waiting patients, physically damaged the waiting room, stole liquor from his stepfather's locked cabinet, and engaged in homosexual prostitution with an older man. At no time did the therapist explore the meaning of the patient's grandiose challenges or his hunger for an omnipotent father—narcissistic issues—but continually interpreted depression and sadness over the early loss—object libidinal problems. He was referred back to the Juvenile Court and was placed in another treatment program where he was interviewed one year later. He had just been returned from a runaway to that distant state of his fantasy where he had been apprehended for theft. He was to be discharged in a few months and hoped to live with his therapist. He returned home, lost his therapist who moved to the state of our patient's dreams, was arrested for vandalism, theft, and drug possession, resisted arrest, escaped while being returned to the treatment program, went to the opposite end of the country, was rearrested for further criminal activity, and placed in a correctional facility. He was eventually released, and on last report was living with a roommate and engaging in homosexual prostitution.

Nick demonstrated not only the need to idealize significant men in his life such as his stepfather, his older brother, and his therapist, but also the need to test out and defeat that omnipotence through a variety of clever delinquent schemes. His own grandiosity was quite overt at times, while at other times marked feelings of worthlessness, the failure to live up to such standards of perfection, were evident.

Sometimes his behavior served to deny and relieve him of feelings of depression. As the repressed fantasy of searching for the idealized but lost father became more and more conscious in the transference, he could not tolerate the intense stimulation of achieving that relationship and instead needed to act out to discharge tension and to destroy the relationship. The intensity of the emerging transference was also discharged in homosexual activity with the resurrected perverted father. In many ways, the therapist served as a self-object and the patient attempted to utilize him for self-soothing and regulation. Other relationships, for example in the hospital, were utilized to maintain or even establish a sense of cohesion and boundaries. None of this was readily apparent at the time, and had the therapist viewed the patient's need for self-object relating more clearly, and not focused on the homosexual aspects of the transference, the outcome of this case might have been different. However, this patient, unlike others, was unable to utilize people as self-objects without considerable anxiety. Whether the anxiety resulted from a fear of merger and therefore fragmentation, or whether, indeed, the stimulation of having found the long lost and idealized father was more than he could handle must remain speculative.

Case 2. Theresa, fifteen years old, was admitted because "everybody says I am crazy." Since early in grade school, she had viciously assaulted other people either on her own or in gang activity. Just prior to admission she had been caught carrying a gun on a school playground. She boasted that she frequently carried a gun, had shot one person, and had fired at many others. She described herself as being the "chief" of a gang of seventy-five girls as old as twenty-one years of age. She maintained her leadership position through aggressive, hostile attitudes and behavior. The gang warred with other black girls' gangs while at the same time abusing, humiliating, and assaulting white teenagers. Her parentage troubled her; her mother was white, her father was black, and she was raised by a black woman to whom she had been given. She saw herself as black, but the daughter of a "white bitch." Occasionally she would have contact with her black father.

In the unit she showed a marked intolerance of anxiety, which she usually mastered by a defensive toughness and bravado. For example, during a teaching conference when a staff member left the room while Theresa was being interviewed and was visibly anxious, she shouted "she can't do that, walk out of my meeting. I am the one to walk out." She was described by one consultant as "really falling apart with nobody to fight against." Sometimes she would hold her head, and at others her entire body while rolling around on her bed as if she were "going to explode." She was exquisitely sensitive to the problems of other patients and frequently found herself getting mixed up in their difficulties and conflicts.

Her self-revulsion was evidenced not only by her frequent attempts at self-mutilation, but also in the alleged statement of her father: "I wish you had never been born." At other times her grandiosity was shown in her attempts to control the unit, openly defy staff, intimidate other patients, and in the alleged statement of her white mother which she quoted, "Gee I wish I had never given Theresa up. I want to come back and claim her. Sometimes I go to bed at night and I can't stop thinking about her." After several episodes of running away from the hospital and being readmitted, the patient was transferred to a white female therapist toward whom she had shown a marked affinity. During treatment sessions she would wrap herself in a blanket and present numerous somatic complaints, many of which were the result of self injury. She was described by one consultant as someone who manipulates people into giving her direction, structure, and identity, and that when she is unable to achieve an identity from those about her she panics. Gradually during her two-year hospitalization, she moved from panic and fragmentation, through omnipotent struggles with her therapist, to a capacity for self-observation, if not overwhelmed by internal stimulation. Eventually, the patient expressed concern about whether or not she would serve certain needs of the therapist, like being a therapeutic success or failure, as indeed she had so often fulfilled the ambitions and needs of her foster mother. She began recognizing that she had changed and was unable to return to her life of violence even though her current adjustment was in some ways more painful. Repeat psychological testing demonstrated that the patient could now experience and tolerate affect, recognize that she was a troubled person, and have conscious ideas and fantasies yet poorly integrated. A sense of self had evolved which enabled her to engage in relationships with people rather than break away. Yet, she could separate from her "white bitch" therapist in only a most abrupt manner, running away from the hospital and returning twice. The third time she stayed away. Later, she returned, on drugs, pleading to be readmitted. She was refused, and began seeking an outpatient therapist in another facility.

The patient's overt grandiosity exhibited itself in violent gang behavior and attempts to control and manipulate the hospital environment. Yet she responded quite readily to staff interventions to limit her omnipotence and readily reverted to feelings of worthlessness. She idealized her therapist, but at the same time defended herself against a merger for which she desperately wished. At times it appeared that her delinquent behavior, her stirring up of other people, and her manipulations for power on the unit, served simply to prevent her own internal panic and probable fragmentation. Her special relationship with the staff was evident to any visitor, and her approval or disapproval became crucial for any new patient on the unit.

As she gradually modified her own omnipotence and began to idealize the therapist, a depression became evident, which was however more manageable and resulted paradoxically in less and less destructive activity. At this time she began demonstrating a capacity to care for other people. She now kept secrets, not in rebellious withholding, but as someone who respected her own integrity. As the anxiety of discharge planning approached, she questioned whether or not the therapist would rescue her should she involve herself in serious delinquent activity. Her final departure from the program was a painful blow to a heavily invested staff.

The patient utilized her therapist as a self-object in order to maintain cohesion and defend against fragmentation. Simultaneously, however, she experienced the anxiety of fusion and merger. Separation was equated with annihilation and destruction, removed as she was from the nurturing self-object. She did not seem to have the capacity to separate gradually in a stepwise fashion, and when she returned several weeks later readmission was refused. The therapist did offer to work with her on an outpatient basis, but the patient was unable to follow through on this, immersing herself heavily in narcotics, again recreating the merger experience for which she hungered. Eventually, however, with the help of another therapist of her own seeking, she was able to emerge from this situation. When seen approximately a year later, she was relatively symptom free, was involved in no delinquency, and was preparing to marry a man with a young child, about whose care and discipline she was quite concerned. Her relationships then continued to be of a self-object nature, serving to maintain and soothe her, but it is significant that her delinquency has disappeared completely.

Case 3. Lorraine, seventeen years old, somewhat childlike in appearance, gave no reason for her admission other than her need to be in a "stable environment" because of her inability to get along with her mother. She had dropped out of high school a year before and was living with her boyfriend, with her mother's permission. Three months prior to admission her mother moved her back home because she had forged some checks. The patient's parents had separated when she was six. The patient had frequent contact with her father who lived in another city; her mother's life was unstable, with several subsequent marriages, one psychiatric hospitalization, and several psychotherapists. Lorraine was extremely bright and precocious. She exhibited marked feelings of depression with periodic episodes of crying and recurrent suicidal thoughts, but no suicidal attempts.

During her hospitalization the patient would occasionally act superior to certain staff members and many patients. For the most part she was aloof, served as a mother-therapist for some of the other patients, and had great difficulty seeing herself as a delinquent. At one point, in the course of her hospitalization, staff discovered that drugs were being used on the unit. It was only with great difficulty that Lorraine admitted that she had herself brought the drugs in on admission; her reason for concealing this was not a fear of punishment or loss of privileges, as was the case with several other patients, but rather a dread of disapproval, that her reputation on the unit, and particularly with her therapist, would be besmirched. On psychological testing, she scorned certain tests as obvious or trivial, while at the same time she attempted to achieve perfection on other tests and became quite angry when she was unable to control the testing situation or respond comfortably. Her unconscious fantasy was that she was admired by other people while at the same time she sought everywhere for affirmation of her own worth. Because she demonstrated little sense of self worth or self confidence, she would rarely risk failure by actively and constructively striving for success. Her standards for herself were very high, and she felt quite depressed about her failure to live up to them. Her choice of boyfriends was comparable to her personality structure; she sought out boys who were narcissistic, defiant, and status oriented, hoping through them to realize ambitions of her own. She treasured her individual treatment relationship, stayed in the hospital for one year of her own volition, achieved considerable self understanding, and confronted the reality of a symbiotic relationship with her mother. In occupational therapy shop, she "carressed" her work, labored meticulously, and permitted no intrusion, almost as if she was fusing with her artifacts. In school she looked upon other classmates with disdain, frowned on their work, participated only with the teacher and not with her peers, but eventually became more realistic and peer oriented in the classroom. When interviewed in a case conference, she commented several times on the number of people that were there to see her. She readily became angry when her mother would not do what she wanted or when people around her would not satisfy her needs. Within six weeks after discharge, she discontinued individual therapy, reaffirming her inability to sustain a relationship without considerable ongoing gratification.

This patient exhibited conscious and overt grandiosity in her disdain of other people, but also a repressed grandiosity in her constant feelings of worthlessness and self-depreciation, feeling as she did that she always failed to be successful. She also avoided those situations that might challenge these ideals and her performance. Her need to idealize exhibited itself with her mother and her therapist. She was enraged with her mother because she could not live up to the patient's expectations for perfect mothering, and she sought substitute gratification and numerous heterosexual relationships. The ready idealization of her therapist, which had pushed her into a treatment relationship almost immediately, was eventually terminated on discharge from the hospital when the therapist was no longer part of an all encompassing, all nurturing milieu. One year later the patient had left her mother's home, was living nearby with her boyfriend, and was functioning satisfactorily at school. It would appear that she had been able to make the shift from clinging to an idealized but frustrating mother to a more appropriate peer relationship without significant or continued delinquent involvement.

Case 4. Barry, fourteen years old, was referred for admission by his family and his parole officer for recurrent runaways, drug abuse, and resistance to authority. This behavior had been going on throughout his grade school years but had become increasingly intense in the two years prior to admission. His behavior was unaltered by parental controls or external authority, and he demonstrated a flagrant lack of anxiety or conflict over the behavioral situations in which he found himself enmeshed. He was the illegitimate son of his mother and was adopted by his stepfather at age two and one-half, both of which facts were unknown to him. His parents insisted that he not be told. This trust was respected by the staff, but considered a serious handicap to treatment. It was discovered after discharge that these details were known to the patient and apparently he too participated in the deception. He was a waiflike, frail youth, who readily became defensive and belligerent when attempts were made to empathize with him. In addition to his runaways, he had been out of control at school, threatening teachers, threatening to burn down and bomb the school, and becoming so disruptive in class that he had been expelled. His bomb threat was taken seriously because he was known to make bombs as a pastime and was alleged to have in his possession a blueprint of the school building. He had been detained by the police for marijuana possession, and on admission to the unit brought in posters and other symbols depicting his fascination for marijuana and the psychedelic culture. He remained on the unit approximately seven months, first being discharged after one month because of repeated assaults on the staff, but readmitted, until six months later he was finally discharged for further violence to staff. His therapist described him as seeing people only in terms of his own needs and unable to relate to others if his needs or wishes were denied. He pictured himself as a powerful scientist who constructed a vehicle that could penetrate steel. His mother described a secret nonverbal mode of communicating with him which excluded his stepfather, a virtual outsider in the mother-son relationship. On visits to the hospital the mother would monopolize Barry's attention totally. He boasted of his sexual exploits, frequently attempted to have sexual contact with one of two female patients, and on many occasions pranced about like a young stud. When drugs were discovered, he concealed the fact that he had brought marijuana to the hospital after a home visit, and at the same time flagrantly smoked marijuana in his room, participating in ward meetings and other activities while stoned. For several days while stoned he wrote a diary about the "merits of grass." He saw this as a clever deception and victory over the staff who would frequently visit him in his room and never detected either his intoxicated state or his preparation of his diary. Several months later when his behavior on the unit became so flagrant and his violations of rules so persistent that he was finally discharged administratively, he triumphantly presented his therapist his "grass autobiography," ultimate proof of his victory over his therapist and staff who had strived unsuccessfully but diligently to achieve with him some kind of treatment alliance.

In his autobiography he boasted of participating in meetings, therapy sessions, and other encounters with staff while stoned without being detected, though he feared getting "busted." He drew a picture of a long road leading to a sunny horizon with a stop sign placed midway along the highway, which he ignored. The autobiographical notes were meant for his therapist, for he wrote, "I think of what you will say to me if I show you this or not." He boasted of power against the staff and of encouraging people "to follow me to fight the staff." Even after he was "busted," he continued to write and to smoke surreptitiously while complaining, "People are not paying attention to me. I feel like I am not even here." Following discharge he maintained no contact with the program except through several other patients whom he had encouraged to run away from the hospital in a continuing assault on the therapeutic efforts of the staff. Within nine months he had been placed in a correctional facility. Interviewed in a youth camp one year after discharge, he had matured considerably, but still tended to externalize his problems and saw little that he needed to change in himself.

Barry's grandiosity was unquestionable. His alliance with his mother was never dealt with successfully nor was his cleverness in evading the rules and deceiving the therapist. Perhaps one reason no progress could be made in treatment is that the deception the staff entered into at the time of admission only perpetuated a fantasy of a powerful and successful scientist yearning for and seeking out an omnipotent and lost father. The deception and its universal acceptance never permitted treatment to become a realistic experience. His unconscious grandiosity was exhibited in his marked defensiveness when anyone attempted to empathize with him, help him understand a problem or painful affect, or simply inquire about him. There then erupted a barrage of defiant rejection, stemming from the realization that he had not lived up to unconscious goals of perfection and omnipotence. Frustrations of his own grandiose ambitions would lead to outbreaks of narcissistic rage, while, concurrently, his yearning for an idealized parent caused him to test the therapist at every turn while at the same time attempting to destroy the therapist should he prove too human. One must question whether someone with Barry's characterological configuration can really engage in psychotherapy, where the narcissistic pathology and preoccupations flood and seriously interfere with the establishment of a therapeutic alliance.

Discussion

These four cases demonstrate disturbances in the narcissistic line of development shown by many delinquents. Aichorn (1964) saw quite clearly that some delinquents, the "imposters," who boast about their exploits, yearn for an omnipotent therapist. Their grandiosity needs to be confronted quickly by an opening therapeutic gambit which demonstrates that the therapist is more brilliant or powerful. This provides a safe framework wherein the delinquent's grandiosity can be expressed without fear of overwhelming the therapist. The therapist mirrors the delinquent's grandiose self-expression while simultaneously encouraging and fostering his idealization of the therapist. It is this narcissistic transference that Aichorn emphasized as so important in the treatment of certain delinquents. Because of impaired object relating ability, these adolescents cannot yet identify with an external object, the therapist, and internalize some of his values. In order to achieve a more socialized adolescent such identification and internalization are necessary.

Aichorn agreed with Freud's (1914) ideas on the antipathy between narcissism and object relations; object libido had been converted back to narcissistic libido. What was loved by the grandiose delinquent was an ideal projected onto the therapist, not the therapist himself. When the therapist fostered the development of such idealization, it was then possible for narcissistic libido to be transformed into object libido. With the development of an object relationship and object love, identification and ultimately internalization of the therapist-object could be achieved.

Kohut (1972a), however, offers an alternate explanation. Though it is true that many delinquents engage in object relations more characterized by narcissistic ties than object love, such as Lorraine's and Barry's relationships with their mothers, his perspective is a more precise attempt to determine the internal representations and the kinds of structures that are transferred onto the therapist in the transference. As a developmental stage, adolescence represents a significant way station in the transformations of narcissism wherein the adolescent tests out his grandiosity, idealism, and ambitions against the demands and constraints of reality. At the same time he deidealizes those previously omnipotent parents and idealizes other adults, heroes, ideas, or movements, gradually modifying his idealistic view of the world into an outlook that cherishes certain values and respects certain people.

Wolf, Gedo, and Terman (1972) emphasize "that a change in the self emerges as the pivotal focus during adolescent development." They suggest that deidealization of archaic parental imagos requires the use of peers or real or historical heroes as self objects to help the adolescent maintain cohesion and facilitate the shift from an archaic parental idealization to one's own ego ideal. Acquiring new idealizations can be seen in those adolescents who join secret academic societies, a process that is relatively quiescent; but the delinquent's struggle is considerably more tumultuous, and his deidealization or disillusionment may lead to rebellion, criminal activity, gang behavior, drug abuse, runaway, or premature heterosexual commitment. The delinquent's yearning for the omnipotent parent is seen in Nick's devotion to his grandfather, the minibike, and his runaway search for the lost father, Theresa's almost immediate attachment to the long-lost white mother, Lorraine's virtual merger with her therapist who feeds and sustains her on the unit, and Barry's ecstasy and devotion to the marijuana experience. When a youth has externalized the internal idealized parent, he may strive fanatically to achieve a perfect world, or may experience painful disillusionment if society is imperfect. In some, disillusionment may appear in the narcissistic rage of an irrational violence (Blos 1972a). Theresa's threats and assaults before and during hospitalization and Barry's threats to destroy his school are such examples, as well as attempts to conform the external world to one's internal imagos.

Some adolescents may not be able to utilize self object relating either with the therapist through heroes, or in peer relationships, to achieve deidealization and the establishment of new idealizations and eventually one's own ego ideal. Instead, self object relating may raise anxieties over merger and fragmentation which not only become serious problems to manage as a transference, but also seriously interfere with the therapeutic alliance. Indeed, they may even interfere with the establishment of a therapeutic alliance. Such delinquent adolescents are probably psychotic, prepsychotic, or borderline in nature, and more than likely are unable to engage in an intense psychotherapeutic relationship. Treatment relationships in which the intensity of the transference is minimized, such as group, family, milieu, or supportive psychotherapy, might be considered more appropriate.

It is the excitement and enthusiasm of adolescence that reveals that love of self is resurgent, only too soon to wane. The unmodified grandiosity of Nick who deceives the therapist by stealing and hiding things during the session, of Lorraine who looks upon other patients with disdain, of Theresa who boasts of her aggressive and sexual prowess, and of Barry who flaunts his violation of unit rules are all examples of failures to modify primitive narcissistic structures. But the grandiosity does not seem simply a defense against the emergence of a painful, ungratified wish for the omnipotent parent. It represents one aspect of that primitive self object state, a point of fixation, a state of relative cohesion, which may express itself in omnipotence, a wish to idealize, or frantic efforts to prevent fragmentation and loss of cohesion.

It seems that all adolescents struggle with resurgent grandiosity, some derived from sexual prowess. Klumpner (1972) suggests that "the increased self-aggrandisement during early adolescence is also focused primarily upon the rapid increase in sexual feelings, with their accompanying fantasies of sexual grandiosity, and upon the developing secondary sexual characteristics, with the accompanying changes in body image." Kohut (1972b) emphasizes that it is important to examine adolescents from the point of view of both the sexual drives and the vicissitudes of the self, and suggests that the major task of adolescence in its narcissistic development is "re-forming the self [which] may evoke in us temporarily old fragmentation fears until a new self is again firmly established." Fragmentation of the self is threatened in some adolescents not only by the increase in sexual and aggressive drives, but also by the grandiosity which accompanies these; not only by a changing and therefore bewildering body, but also by the fright of new found prowess or beauty; not only by object removal and separation from the infantile love objects, but also by the accompanying deidealization. The resurgent grandiosity and idealization of new objects seen in many delinquents may be denial of ego depletion and threatened disintegration, or regressive attempts to cling to those relatively stable structures of a cohesive self, serving to defend against fragmentation.

Frantic acting out may also serve a similar defensive purpose. Blos (1962), for example, has described "pseudoheterosexuality"—heterosexual behavior as an attempt to achieve individuation from merger with the mother. This might be better described as heterosexual activity in order to prevent fragmentation, insofar as sexual stimulation provides one with a sense of self and cohesion. It served this purpose for Theresa, as did other kinds of defiant, challenging, and agitated behavior, expressing both impending disintegration as well as activity to fill a void and maintain cohesion. Whether it be Lorraine's haughtiness as she attempts to prevent merger with the maternal self object or Theresa's bravado which she clings to in defense against further regression to a stage of somato-psychic fragmentation, the grandiosity represents a relative state of stability. Though some of our delinquents may experience temporary states of fragmentation and struggle constantly against fusion and merger, they still maintain for the most part a sense of self, albeit primitive and archaic.

Some grandiosity is not experienced consciously, but rather as a nagging sense of failure to live up to the repressed grandiose perfect self. Lorraine is constantly unsure of herself and avoids situations which might open her to failure; Theresa, when confronted with the spuriousness of her bravado, becomes readily depressed, withdrawn, isolates herself, and even injures herself repeatedly. Much delinquent activity has been viewed as a way of eliminating painful depressive affect. The delinquent act may accomplish this by bolstering self-esteem temporarily through a transient defiance of reality, defeat of the omnipotent parent, or criminal achievement of the greatest magnitude. Or the delinquent act may temporarily excite and fill an internal void and reestablish self-cohesion.

In the hospital, the vicissitudes and transformations of these two archaic structures present interesting challenges. The period of depression sought for in the treatment of many acting out adolescents, which has been seen as the successful conversion of alloplastic behavior to internal conflicts (Friedlander 1947) and which Rinsley (1971) describes in the hospital as separation from parents and investment in therapy, may also be the disillusionment the delinquent confronts when his search for the idealized parent has failed him and his own grandiosity begins to be tempered by reality.

Easson (1966) emphasizes the adolescent's need to see his therapist as omnipotent and omniscient and warns the therapist neither to destroy this nor to treat it as reality. He states that such idealization is part of the process of separation from parents, and the adolescent's own ego ideal is crucial to the success of this phase. Our delinquent needs to see his therapist, the milieu workers, the social worker, and the unit director as omnipotent and omniscient. He believes that his therapist, though only one member of the team, really has the power to grant certain privileges, but chooses not to do so. He exaggerates his therapist's clinical skills into a capacity to read his mind when the therapist anticipates his wish to break hospital rules, use drugs, or run away. He tests the firmness and certitude of the milieu worker, the consistency and agreement between staff members, in order to reassure himself that his own grandiosity will not run rampant. He is exquisitely uncomfortable when staff is uncertain, confused, or indecisive (Marohn, Dalle-Molle, Offer, and Ostrov 1973), for then his need to idealize or mirror cannot be realized. He sees the social worker who works with his parents as someone who manipulates and controls them, and then tries to divide and conquer by convincing his parents that he is being mistreated and should be removed from the hospital, as Theresa and Barry tried on a number of occasions.

It has long been said that the person who works best with delinquents has some kind of charisma, although Kohut (1971) suggests that the therapist's charm should be replaced by rational tools of interpretation and reconstruction. Such charisma may indeed be related to comfort with one's own narcissism, a sense of humor about it, and a ready acceptance of the idealization of the delinquent. On our unit the leader is ascribed with superhuman qualities. At times his insistence on truthfulness and the therapeutic process may result in admissions and self observations surprising to an outsider. A confession following a correct interpretation to a delinquent, who has been lying about some plot, may not be the result simply of having addressed the unconscious complex. The surface symptom is laid bare, yet the delinquent finds comfort in the leader's (to him) omniscience, and feels safe to talk openly about his painful concerns. Only when a patient was asked about his anguish over his therapist's departure and his transfer to a new therapist, could he talk about his plan to obtain drugs from a visitor. It is essential then not that staff be omnipotent, nor the leader charismatic, nor the therapist omniscient, but that the leader, therapist, and staff have resolved some of their own self-esteem disequilibria, have a certain amount of confidence in their work, maintain a certain level of suspicion, and not rely on the delinquent's words, promises, or behavior—or therapeutic outcome—for their own gratification. Such relatively comfortable people, who are capable of respecting others, and are simultaneously fulfilling their own goals in life, permit the emergence of certain idealizations by the delinquent as well as create an atmosphere where the delinquent's own grandiosity can emerge without fear of overwhelming an incompetent staff. It is in this atmosphere that the mirroring and idealizing transferences described by Kohut can unfold.

Tendencies to mirror or to idealize, arising from resurgent adolescent grandiosity and the search for an ideal parent, and the need for self objects, arising from the upheaval and threatened fragmentation of adolescence, are perhaps more obvious in adolescent patients than those of other age groups. Adolescents are characterized by a certain openness and bluntness. Much of the anxiety of the beginning therapist (Hendrickson 1971) in working with them may be related not simply to countertransference problems such as unresolved adolescent conflicts, particularly about heterosexuality, but may be related specifically to discomfort with one's own unresolved narcissistic struggles. The therapist who cannot be decisive, or set limits, or ask a direct question about suspected delinquency because he does not want to be omnipotent had best turn his attention to his own unresolved, but unconscious grandiosity.

The management of acting out behavior by the delinquent and adolescent in therapy is a difficult problem both in and out of the hospital. Traditional acting out in the context of the therapeutic relationship has been viewed as a defensive maneuver designed to avoid painful recall. The adolescent has been characterized as particularly prone to acting out because adolescence itself involves action and discharge rather than contemplation of fantasy. Blos (1966) reiterates four roots of acting out behavior: oral conflict, heightened narcissism, intolerance of frustration, and inadequate grasp of reality. He describes a state of precocious ego development which enables acting out children very early in life:

> to read cues, to manipulate the environment, to know well what other people like, dislike, or fear, how to present themselves endearingly if need be, how to get adults into rages in order to effect a response on the level of sado-masochistic object relations.

This clinical description is quite comparable to what one sees in a narcissistic personality disorder, and one must now consider how much acting out behavior is indeed an attempt to control the external environment and the parental other in a grandiose, omnipotent style.

Newman (1973) specifies that some disruptive behaviors may be attempts to overcome feelings of self-fragmentation and emptiness, some may be the use of grandiosity as a defense against narcissistic injury, while others may be outlets for grandiose exhibitionism. Whether the therapist serves then as a self object to help the delinquent maintain or reconstitute cohesion and defend against fragmentation; or whether the therapist functions as a self object to soothe hurt feelings or as an ideal object to reverse feelings of disillusionment in the other; or whether the therapist mirrors the primitive or exhibitionistic grandiosity of the delinquent— these questions are crucial in formulating the proper psychotherapeutic approach.

But these ideas partially explain the acting out behavior of our four patients. Kohut (1971) describes a specific regression in the narcissistic development to what he calls a "pathogenic fixation point" where there is a "lessening of the differentiation between self and not-self and thus to a blurring of the differentiation between impulse, thought, and action. In other words, what appears on superficial scrutiny to be alloplastic action is, in reality, not action, but the autoplastic activity of a stage of psychological development in which the external world is still cathected with narcissistic libido." Thus, Kohut suggests that we look for the explanation of acting out behavior not in the interpersonal relationship of its effect on the family or the environment, but rather internally, viewing the narcissistic regression the patient has experienced. This may amplify what I described in an earlier paper (Marohn 1974), that a considerable amount of "acting out" behavior of hospitalized delinquents does not have specific transference determinants, but is the result of a traumatized and overwhelmed psychic apparatus. What appears to be violent behavior is in reality a massive discharge phenomenon, the result of an ego overwhelmed by internal stimulation. Gedo and Goldberg (1973) suggest that different models of the psychic apparatus are more useful in some situations than others; here they would propose the reflex arc model. In Kohut's terms, this can be restated as a severe regression to a period in life when impulse, thought, action, self and non-self, and inside and outside blur and cannot be differentiated.

Conclusions

Have I been discussing problems in the narcissistic line of development as they confront and are exhibited by many adolescents, or have I been saying something more relevant to that psychopathology of adolescence we call delinquency? First of all, adolescence does seem to involve significant struggles with narcissistic issues: fragmentation fears, attempts to maintain cohesion through activity, deidealization of parents, idealization of others as well as of ideas and social movements, disillusionment, fear of merger in intimacy, repeated and fickle infatuations, and many other crises to be mastered, hopefully resulting in the transformations of ambition, goals, ideals, self-esteem, respect and admiration for others, creativity, and empathy. Delinquency as a diagnosis is a collection of adolescents with varying pathology: some depressed, some impulsive, some with antisocial values, some following parental delinquent urges, others defying parental ambition, some psychotic, some not. If there is anything unique about delinquency it is a propensity for mischief or unacceptable activity, but even this can be said about most adolescents. And so the difference may be a matter of severity, degree, and emphasis—as is often the distinction between the normal and pathological. And while an understanding of narcissistic development is important in working with any patient, and perhaps more so in working with adolescent patients, most of our delinquents show serious problems in these areas—low self-esteem, little ambition, no sense of future, an inability to distinguish inside from outside, self from non-self, thought from action, callous use of others, severe disillusionment in others, brutal grandiosity, rage when the world does not conform, periods of fragmentation and frantic activity, and unique countertransference challenges for the therapist. Our delinquents are not experiencing conflicts over how or whether to seek gratification; they are looking for ways to soothe themselves and to hold themselves together.

These challenges are neither hopeless nor insurmountable. Winnicott (1958, 1973) has succinctly related the antisocial tendency to narcissistic trauma, to attempts to control the other and the world, and to search for the "mother over whom she or he has rights" (1956). He describes the antisocial tendency as a hopeful sign, and emphasizes that the delinquent has not given up hope and is still anticipating some final payoff. The wayward youth pushes the therapist in the right direction, plagues him with his demands for help, and does not relinquish easily his need to correct the internal archaic disarray.

The juvenile imposter's presentation may be blatant grandiosity or naive idealization, but it is the delinquent's best prognostic sign.

This chapter is an attempt to reassess what Aichorn described as the narcissistic transference of the juvenile imposter in the light of the contributions of Kohut and our work at the Illinois State Psychiatric Institute with hospitalized delinquents. The importance of self and the narcissistic line of development to an understanding of adolescence, and more particularly, the pathology shown by delinquents is stressed. The grandiosity of the delinquent, his need to idealize, problems with fragmentation, and acting out as a regression as well as the delinquent's use of the therapist as a mirror, as an idealized object, and as a self object are all described.

NOTES

1. This study is supported in part by Illinois Law Enforcement Commission Grant A70-15.
2. The unit serves as the site of a research project conducted in cooperation with the Psychiatric and Psychosomatic Institute of Michael Reese Hospital. (Marohn, Offer, and Ostrov 1971, Offer, Marohn, and Ostrov 1972, Ostrov, Offer, Marohn, and Rosenwein 1972, Marohn, Dalle-Molle, Offer, and Ostrov 1973).

REFERENCES

Aichorn, A. (1925). *Wayward Youth*. New York: Meridian, 1955.

———. (1964). *Delinquency and Child Guidance—Selected Papers*. New York: International Universities Press.

Blos, P. (1962). *On Adolescence*. New York: Free Press of Glencoe.

——— (1966). Discussion, In E. N. Rexford, ed., *A Developmental Approach to Problems of Acting Out—A Symposium*. New York: International Universities Press, pp. 68-71.

——— (1972a). The function of the ego ideal in late adolescence. *Psychoanalytic Study of the Child* 27:93-97.

———. (1972b). The epigenesis of the adult neurosis. *Psychoanalytic Study of the Child* 27:106-135.

Easson, W. (1966). The ego ideal in the treatment of children and adolescents. *Archives of General Psychiatry* 15:288-292.

Eissler, K. R. (1949). Editor: *Searchlights on Delinquency*. New York: International Universities Press.

Freud, A. (1951). Obituary: August Aichorn. *International Journal of Psycho-Analysis* 32:51-56.

——— (1958). Adolescence. *Psychoanalytic Study of the Child* 13:255-278.

Freud, S. (1914). On narcissism: an introduction. *Standard Edition* 14:73-102. London: Hogarth, 1953.

——— (1925). Introduction. In A. Aichorn, *Wayward Youth*. New York: Meridian, 1955.

Friedlander, K. (1947). *The Psychoanalytic Approach to Juvenile Delinquency*. New York: International Universities Press.

Gedo, J. E., and Goldberg, A. (1973). *Models of the Mind*. Chicago: University of Chicago Press.

Hendrickson, W. J. (1971). Training in adolescent psychiatry: the role of experience with inpatients. In D. Offer and J. F. Masterson, eds., *Teaching and Learning Adolescent Psychiatry*. Springfield, Ill.: Charles C Thomas.

Hoffer, W. (1949). Deceiving the deceiver, In K. R. Eissler, ed., *Searchlights on Delinquency*. New York: International Universities Press, pp. 150-155.

Klumpner, G. (1972). Discussion of Wolf E. S., Gedo, J. E., Terman, D. M., On the adolescent process as a transformation of the self. Unpublished, presented 5/23/72 before the Chicago Psychoanalytic Society.

211

Kohut, H. (1966). Forms and transformation of narcissism. *Journal of the American Psychoanalytic Association* 14:243-272.

——— (1968). The psychoanalytic treatment of narcissistic personality disorders. *Psychoanalytic Study of the Child* 23:86-113.

——— (1971). *The Analysis of the Self.* New York: International Universities Press.

——— (1972a). Thoughts on narcissism and narcissistic rage. *Psychoanalytic Study of the Child* 27:360-400.

———(1972b). Discussion of Wolf, E. S., Gedo, J. E., and Terman, D. M., On the adolescent process as a transformation of the self. Unpublished, presented 5/23/72 before the Chicago Psychoanalytic Society.

Marohn, R. C. (1974). Trauma and the delinquent. *This Annual* 3:354-361.

———, Dalle-Molle, D., Offer, D., and Ostrov, E. (1973). A hospital riot: its determinants and implications for treatment. *American Journal of Psychiatry* 310:631-636.

———, Offer, D., and Ostrov, E. (1971). Juvenile delinquents view their impulsivity. *American Journal of Psychiatry* 128:418-423.

Newman, K. (1973). Some applications of concepts of the self to management of adolescents in the hospital. *Bulletin of the Chicago Society for Adolescent Psychiatry.*

Offer, D., Marohn, R. C., and Ostrov, E. (1972). Delinquent and normal adolescents. *Comprehensive Psychiatry* 13:347-355.

Ostrov, E., Offer, D., Marohn, R. C., and Rosenwein, T. (1972). The impulsivity index: its application to juvenile delinquency. *Journal of Youth and Adolescence* 1:179-196.

Rinsley, D. B. (1971). Theory and practice of intensive residential treatment of adolescents. *This Annual* 1:479-509.

Winnicott, D. W. (1956). The antisocial tendency. In *Collected Papers.* New York: Basic Books, 1958.

——— (1973). Delinquency as a sign of hope. *This Annual* 2:364-371.

Wolf, E. S., Gedo, J. E., and Terman, D. M. (1972). On the adolescent process as a transformation of the self. *Journal of Youth and Adolescence* 1:257-272.

14] DISCUSSION OF
DR. RICHARD MAROHN'S CHAPTER:
A CRITIQUE OF KOHUT'S
THEORY OF NARCISSISM

PETER L. GIOVACCHINI

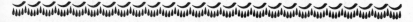

It may seem odd that a discussion of an article by one author should also include a critical examination of another author's work. This unusual combination, however, is the outcome of a phenomenon that deserves study. I am referring to the fashion among many clinicians, psychoanalysts, psychiatrists, social workers, and psychologists of totally and uncritically embracing Kohut's (1966, 1971) theory of narcissism, making it fundamental to all their concepts and observations.

I will anticipate the question of why I want to embark on such an endeavor at all, since criticism and review can be tedious at best. The fact is I do not relish such a project; but the pervasive impact of Kohut's ideas, especially in Chicago but in many other areas as well, compels sober appraisal. The need for such an appraisal was forced upon me at the May 1974 meetings of the American Psychoanalytic Association in Denver. I had just presented a paper dealing with narcissistic transference (Giovacchini 1975). One of the formal discussants took all of my formulations and translated them into Kohut's terms. During my rebuttal, I retranslated Kohut's terms into Freud's, hoping to demonstrate that there was neither advantage nor innovation in using this new language. Numerous members of the audience, especially the younger ones, flocked around me afterwards and with considerable relief confessed that they also did not find Kohut's ideas revolutionary; but because they had been fervently accepted by so many, they felt they had missed the point and attributed it to their ignorance and inexperience. They were pleased to find a senior person who echoed their doubts. Following the meetings I received over eighty letters expressing similar views.

213

I discuss Marohn's chapter because it affords an excellent opportunity to bring important dissent into the open. This is the essence of scientific discussion; communication should be free and ideas should be examined from various perspectives. Marohn's exposition is clear and direct. He presents interesting clinical situations and makes keen observations and skillful formulations. At times, I feel disappointed that he did not develop his own ideas further. Perhaps putting Kohut's framework in its proper perspective may stimulate investigators to develop their own concepts, using earlier work such as Kohut's, of course, but as stepping stones rather than as universal explanatory systems.

Since there is so much merit in the work of Kohut's followers, I believe it proper to begin with one of them with the hope of demonstrating that a more critical acceptance would have resulted in a more creative contribution rather than a reflection of someone else's creativity. Marohn achieves both, but I believe that in the future his emphasis can be more on the former than the latter.

Comments on "The Juvenile Imposter"

When dealing with new theoretical constructs, it behooves the reader to determine whether new formulations represent revisions or extensions of existing constructs, or whether they are only restatements of established principles. Furthermore, one also has to inquire whether an alleged innovation is based upon a misinterpretation of an existing concept, and is, in essence, a statement of definition which differs from the traditionally accepted one.

For example, after briefly mentioning Kohut's separate lines of development of narcissism and object libido, to which I will return later, Marohn makes the following statement: "For Freud, secondary narcissism is a narcissistic regression away from object love as a result of a painful experience; for Kohut, this is still primary narcissism, for the person had never progressed beyond self-object relating." This is an important statement and most of Kohut's subsequent formulations and treatment recommendations hinge upon it.

Let us examine what Marohn (following Kohut) attributes to Freud, that secondary narcissism is the outcome of regression away from object love. True, any developmental stage can be a result of regression from a more advanced stage. But is secondary narcissism only that? Is it only a pathological construct, a result of regression which differs from the corresponding developmental stage, much in the same way that some symptoms act as foreign bodies and have no counterpart in the normal developmental hierarchy (Freud 1926)? This point is crucial because if it is not, then the second clause in this sentence becomes an imprecise definition.

Jones (1955) reports that as early as 1909 Freud postulated that narcissism was a necessary intermediate stage between autoerotism and object love and described this progression in his discussion of the Schreber case (Freud 1911). In 1914 he stated: "Thus we form the idea of their being an original libidinal cathexis of the ego, from which some is later given off to objects, but which fundamentally persists and is related to object-cathexis much as the body of an amoeba is related to the pseudopodia which it puts out" (Freud 1914). Freud thus subdivides narcissism into primary narcissism, an original libidinal cathexis of the ego, and secondary narcissism, the extensions and retractions of the pseudopodia which are necessary stages on the way to object relationships. Clearly, Freud did not consider secondary narcissism only a regression away from object love; he viewed it also and more fundamentally as a phase of developmental progression.

Secondary narcissism and later object relations stem from a primary narcissistic stage but are differentiated from it by their later accretions. This brings us to the second clause of Marohn's statement which refers to what Kohut continues to call primary narcissism. Kohut defines primary narcissism as not having progressed *beyond* the self-object relating which Freud called secondary narcissism. But if one is going to postulate the existence of a self or a self-object, there must be some self-object differentiation even if there is not much progress beyond that. Autoerotism is a stage where there is, as yet, not sufficient operative ego for self-object differentiation. Primary narcissism postulates the existence of an ego toward which libido flows, but this is still a very rudimentary ego. Remember that Freud made his formulations when he was discussing megalomania and omnipotence where the external world, as such, is not discernible. Objects as objects are not distinguishable; one's ego encompasses the universe. Once the pseudopodia make contact with something in the external world, then there is, at least, a dim awareness of that segment of the external world and the concepts of self and object and self-object become meaningful. This awareness is by definition an aspect of secondary narcissism and represents an advance in libidinal organization. There is no advantage to changing this definition since it is consistent with the concepts of progressive differentiation of the self and the perception of objects.

This definition would not have been worth expounding if it were not decisive for a point made earlier concerning separate lines of development of narcissism and object libido, and what is to follow, the concepts of grandiose self and idealized parental imago.

Marohn mentions the separate lines of development of narcissism and object libido only in passing, so I will postpone discussing this concept until I discuss Kohut's writings directly. I will proceed with Marohn's article where he discusses the grandiose self and the idealized parental imago.

Marohn states: "In the stage of primary narcissism, Kohut postulates two primitive structures: the grandiose self and the idealized parental imago. These coexist and neither has prior status." Again, one would question the feasibility of putting such constructs in the framework of primary narcissism. In particular, the idealized parental imago requires some awareness, not only of an external world, but of a specific aspect of the external world, the parent: an important and decisive step beyond primary narcissism. The formation of such an imago implies the achievement of the capacity to project, which must be present if the type of transference described by Kohut is to occur. To be able to project requires a definite distinction between inner and outer worlds, a level of structure beyond primary narcissism but certainly compatible with secondary narcissism.

The same considerations apply to the concept of grandiose self, which is highly sophisticated and beyond the structural capacity of the neonate who has not progressed beyond the stage of primary narcissism.

It is well known that constellations identical to those described by Kohut are regularly found in the transferences of patients suffering from characterological problems. Freud (1911, 1914) wrote of megalomanic, omnipotent stages and how these are often projected into a person in the external world. Klein (1932) frequently described similar phenomena and stressed that in primitive ego states the elements that are projected in the transference are parts of the self—elements of psychic structure rather than discrete libidinal impulses.

It is appropriate here to comment about Klein because in some quarters the very mention of her name is considered ample evidence to invalidate an argument. This is unfortunate because many of her descriptions and formulations are extremely helpful in providing insight about the mental processes involved in severe psychopathology. If she has not been read carefully, it is understandable that one might feel tempted to discredit her contributions. I would agree that many of her formulations sound like the fantasies or the products of psychopathology of adult minds. But to reject everything she says is tantamount to throwing out the baby with the bath water. For our purpose, it suffices to acknowledge that the transferences described by Kohut were well known to Klein and her followers and did not necessitate the assumption that the discovery of these clinical interactions were based upon a new and unique theory of narcissism.

I acknowledge that I am concentrating on microscopic details in order to help the reader evaluate whether we have a new theory of narcissism, or for that matter, one that sheds light on a different perspective that can facilitate work with adolescents and patients suffering from severe character problems.

Marohn continues to elucidate how the grandiose self and the idealized parental imago affect the transference of narcissistically fixated patients. First, he alludes to the mirror transference, then to what is presumably the projection of the grandiose self into the therapist resulting in the formation of an idealized parental imago.

In the mirror transference, the patient expects the therapist to reflect back his self-aggrandizement. He wishes to be acknowledged. Is this not again a matter of definition? Did not Narcissus admire his beautiful image in the mirror of a pond? To want to be admired by others is the essence of narcissism. This would, of course, have its effects upon the transference of narcissistic patients. The mirror transference is simply a narcissistic transference, a well-known and well-described phenomenon that routinely occurs in the treatment of such patients.

Regarding the idealized parental imago, Marohn writes: "The idealized parental imago is reactivated when the patient idealizes the therapist and attributes to him the omnipotence and perfection of the early parent, and its soothing and regulating functions." Again, it must be acknowledged that this type of idealization of the therapist is very common, especially in helpless, dependent patients seeking magical salvation (Giovacchini 1965) or paranoid patients who enlist the aid of the therapist in supporting their megalomania and, by so joining forces, think they can keep all badness in the world outside the consultation room (Strachey 1934).

It suffices to emphasize that Kohut has made a valuable contribution by calling attention to these transferences and by reminding us that a large group of patients, whom many analysts consider unanalyzable, such as adolescents with severe psychopathology, can be treated psychoanalytically. However, there are important questions about the developmental basis of his formulations and about his technical exposition.

Up to this point, Marohn has confronted us with concepts where, at least, the language is familiar. In discussing the vicissitudes of such structures as the grandiose self and the idealized parental imago, he introduces us to new terms, such as *horizontal* and *vertical splitting*. Sometimes, new terms express either novel ideas or a different, overlooked aspect of an already established and useful concept, representing an advancement which usually expands clinical understanding. Let us see how vertical and horizontal splitting augment our conceptual scaffold.

According to Marohn:

The grandiose self may remain active consciously but disavowed as a result of what Kohut calls a vertical split; here, grandiose behavior in certain areas of the personality is blatant and exists side by side with a person's more realistic appraisal of himself and his abilities or even with some self-depreciation. The grandiose structure may also, however, be *repressed* but remain active unconsciously through what Kohut calls a horizontal split [italics mine].

Does this explain anything more than the familiar defense mechanisms of splitting and repression? That various parts of the psychic apparatus, even though polarized, can coexist was noted by Breuer and Freud (1895) and was later described by Freud in many different contexts. Psychoanalysts who dealt with primitive mental states quickly learned the value of the structural hypothesis and have repeatedly encountered clinical situations where patients have effected ego splits to protect one part of the ego from another. *Splitting* refers specifically to psychic structure and not to instinctual impulses, although split-off structures are associated with specific impulses, such as destructive feelings. What advantage is there to bringing geometry into the picture, as exemplified by such adjectives as *vertical* and *horizontal,* especially since we are not supplied with a consistent and relevant spatial model?

Furthermore, the concept of horizontal splitting creates some confusion. According to Marohn, horizontal splitting is clearly the same as repression. The very word *repressed* is used in the definition. Something, in this case, a psychic structure, the grandiose self, is made unconscious and is incapable of becoming conscious, but still continues to affect feelings and behavior. This is a description of the dynamic unconscious, the conceptual basis of psychoanalysis which led to the concept of defenses as repressing forces. Here there is some confusion, because it seems Kohut is describing the repression of psychic structure, in this case, the grandiose self. If one considers psychic development and structure as psychoanalysis does in terms of a hierarchy, then such a formulation is inconsistent with the immaturity of the mental apparatus at the time Kohut says this repression occurs.

The primitive mental apparatus proceeds from the global to the discrete, a progression which is the essence of structuralizing processes. Consequently the distinction between structure and function does not exist during early stages of development. Impulses and needy parts of the self are not differentiated from one another. These discriminations develop when the psychic apparatus has achieved a high degree of organization and perceptual sensitivity. Similarly adaptive and defensive processes can be ordered on a hierarchical continuum, and particular defenses are specific for certain degrees of ego organization. Repression, as Freud discovered, is associated with an ego that has attained a relatively high degree of sophistication, and it is libidinal impulses that are repressed, not psychic structure.

That parts of the psyche, such as defensive megalomanic structures which Kohut refers to as the grandiose self, can be barred from conscious awareness is well known. The mental mechanism involved in keeping megalomanic aspects separate from the reality-attuned ego is commonly known as splitting. Horizontal and vertical really have no meaning in this context, because when one deals with parts of the self rather than libidinal impulses, only one mechanism is involved. Division into horizontal and vertical implies two different mechanisms, but they would both be assigned the same task, that of defending against parts of the self. The outcome of a particular defense, of course, can vary.

True, Freud (1938) did not, as did his followers, directly refer to parts of the self when describing splitting. He described how certain perceptions were disavowed, in particular those involved with the female genitals. The ego, a psychic structure, defensively splits. The disavowed portion contains a bodily part which the rest of the ego does not want to recognize. Fundamentally, this still involves the person's concept of himself as someone who can be castrated. Thus, a brief extension of Freud's ideas quickly leads us to the present-day concept of splitting, which involves keeping different parts of the self *dissociated,* a term that goes all the way back to Janet.

It becomes apparent that horizontal and vertical splitting are the same process, splitting, and have the same consequences. Splitting prevents integration and cohesion, and split-off portions may, on occasion, dominate consciousness and behavior. To bring repression into the picture is a theoretical error, and adds nothing to our understanding of clinical processes.

Marohn next calls attention to therapeutic implications in the treatment of the delinquent and, with Kohut, initially questions the feasibility of actively encouraging an idealizing transference. I strongly agree that any such role-playing on the analyst's part is "a contaminant and not analysis." However, a few sentences later, Marohn seems to mitigate the contaminating quality of the analyst's grandiosity when he writes: "Because the grandiosity of the therapist does not interfere with the delinquent's grandiose defense but actually permits mirroring to occur, it is not threatening to the more deeply repressed structure, which contains the need to idealize and which will emerge later in treatment."

Therapeutic considerations are dependent upon our formulations of the patient's psychopathology. A vagueness in one area is a reflection of a similar vagueness or imprecision in another. The above statements about treatment follow this formulation: "Kohut's belief is, however, that the grandiosity of the delinquent, which he attempts to mirror in the therapist, is really serving a defensive purpose against a more painful complex, the emergence of the delinquent's chronic and frustrating search for the idealized parents." What is minimized here is that the "chronic and frustrating search for the idealized parent" is, in itself, an attempt at establishing a compensatory defense against the miserable feelings of helplessness and vulnerability that overwhelm the self-representation of these delinquent adolescents. A defensive need, as is true of any defense, does not transform into a normal structure by being projected into the therapist.

I will return to these themes in the next section since Marohn does not go beyond these points. Further discussion is necessary, however, since Kohut's ideas of development are very definitely related to issues of technique and treatment, the concern of every clinician.

Marohn devotes the rest of his paper to clinical issues and gives us illuminating and sensitive descriptions of fundamental characteristics of the delinquent adolescent. He describes the consequences of a lack of self-esteem and of a chaotic self-representation consumed with hatred and self-hatred. As would be expected, primitive defenses such as splitting, denial, and projection are used and are accompanied by considerable acting out. The need for salvation by magical rescuing is frequently manifested in the transference characterized by the projection of an overcompensatory omnipotence. There are numerous variations of this theme, and Marohn reveals some enlightening and useful examples.

Critique of Kohut's Theory of Narcissism

Before undertaking a discussion and critique of Kohut's theory of narcissism, it would be germane to briefly outline the main concepts which represent the foundations of his theoretical system. I acknowledge that different readers may choose to emphasize other aspects, but I hope to refer to those facets which are often stressed by his followers. Furthermore, the areas that are frequently discussed can be arranged in a systematic fashion.

Kohut delves into three separate but interrelated areas. He presents us with (1) a theory of development, (2) a conceptual scheme aimed at explaining the psychopathology of patients suffering from characterological problems, and (3) technical considerations about the psychoanalytic treatment of these patients. He progresses from general theoretical issues to specific clinical situations, a method often useful in psychoanalysis.

However, as also frequently happens in ventures of this type, concepts blur. As they are further and further removed from the clinical setting, they become increasingly abstract. Kohut's *The Analysis of the Self* (1971), is not easy to read; his style is ponderous. I have heard analysts state that they find it difficult to understand this book and prefer the writings of his followers, who have been able to cogently summarize his ideas. I agree that the reader is confronted with stylistic difficulties, but I also believe that these partially reflect a basic conceptual imprecision and vagueness. The language is often unique, but one has to examine carefully whether the corresponding ideas are also unique.

DEVELOPMENTAL FACTORS

Let us begin with what are, for me, the most difficult parts of Kohut's work, his ideas about psychic development in general and the development of narcissism in particular. According to Ornstein (1972), Freud's developmental model is a single axis theory which actually hinders theory formation. Freud does not include the concept of the self in his model while Kohut offers us a new theory of narcissism which is based upon two separate lines of development and makes major contributions to the psychoanalytic theory of the self.

Before discussing a double axis theory, let us consider what is meant by a single axis theory and examine the restrictions inherent in Freud that require rectification. The formulation of a new theory is not necessarily a favorable event. Simply because something is new does not mean that the old must be supplanted. The implications of the old theory have to be studied and its usefulness constantly measured as new data are accumulated. Its expansion and modification are the tasks of the theoretician who works in the clinical realm. If the theory cannot accomodate itself to the necessity of making various clinical entities comprehensible, then perhaps a new theory is warranted. Still, what constitutes newness is also a question that requires careful deliberation.

Perhaps single axis means that Freud postulated a line of development based upon a progressive hierarchal structuralization. He outlined a movement from an undifferentiated id to a complex ego organization with many functions (Freud 1900, 1920, 1923). He also postulated a corresponding progression and hierarchal elaboration of the drives.

This might be considered a linear approach, but Freud constantly called attention to interactions with the outer world and how such relationships either developed structure or led to psychopathology. Although Marohn took issue with Freud's concepts of ego-libido and object-libido, it seems apparent that Freud's model has a multiplicity of dimensions that encompass psychopathology based both upon faulty structure and intrapsychic conflict. When the balance between ego-libido and object-libido becomes upset, then one encounters psychopathology, the extremes being megalomania or ego depletion. Psychic processes determine both the direction and the outcome of various relationships with external objects. True, Freud's developmental scheme is, in one sense, linear or single axis, as Ornstein would say, but its allowance for reciprocal interaction with the environment and its structure-promoting effects stresses the fact that other dimensions are included as well. Perhaps my dilemma can best be summarized by admitting that I am not entirely clear as to what a double axis line of development means. Before exploring this dilemma further, I believe it germane to bring more of Freud's ideas concerning narcissism into focus.

Freud's theory of narcissism is mainly a drive theory. As such it neither augments nor hinders the development of structural concepts. The latter belong to another dimension which has been forced upon us by the innumerable patients, such as adolescents, whose psychopathology cannot be conceptualized in terms of conflictual drives. Freud was aware of this and was the first to build a structural scaffold (Freud 1923). What is required, of course, is that structural theory and drive theory be consistent with each other, much in the same way that anatomy must be consistent with physiology.

Much of my critique of Kohut's ideas is based upon a comparison with Freud. This should not be construed to mean that this is a reactionary approach which refuses to acknowledge anything of value beyond Freud. On the contrary, I believe many analysts have made fundamental contributions since Freud, particularly in the areas of ego psychology and characterological psychopathology. I believe further that Freud's attitudes about psychoanalytic treatment are unduly restricted and pessimistic, perhaps in keeping with a basically depressed personality. Some of his theoretical formulations such as the energic theory and the tension-discharge hypothesis have been frequently called into question. Still, simply because a theory is introduced as new does not make it so, and it always behooves us to make comparisons with what has been traditionally accepted.

Freud (1915) had much to say about early developmental positions, grandiosity, narcissism, and their vicissitudes and progressions. In numerous works, he described the development of sexual and self-preservative instincts as they progressed from autoerotic to narcissistic stages and finally to external object relationships. He postulated that the reality principle forces the infant to abandon his early omnipotent position. *Some sexual instincts can remain autoerotic and others require an object.* Kohut (1966) restated this thesis when he described narcissistic elements as instrumental in determining the development of sensitive and empathic reactions, the so-called transformations of narcissism which revealed his formulation of a separate narcissistic line of development. Let me explain further.

According to Freud (1915) all self-preservative instincts require an object and are not subjected to the same vicissitudes as those of the sexual instincts. To repeat, sexual instincts may develop in the context of object relationships or differentiate within the ego sphere without objects. In this regard, one could state that he also had a double axis theory insofar as he is describing a separate line of development for self-preservative and some sexual instincts. However, he emphasized the interrelationships between these two groups of instincts more than their separateness.

Freud directed himself to structural aspects when he described an initial reality ego. This developed when the psyche was able to discriminate the external world from the inner world on the basis of whether motor flight from a noxious stimulus is possible. A painful stimulus from which one cannot escape is recognized as originating from within oneself and distinguished from impingements from the outside. There is a progression from this original reality ego to a pleasure ego and then to another reality ego, but this one involves objects. Freud (1915) wrote: "Those sexual instincts which from the outset require an object, and the needs of the ego instincts which are never capable of autoerotic satisfaction, naturally disturb this state (of primal narcissism) and so pave the way for an advance from it."

The original reality ego cannot proceed directly toward the final reality ego. Instead, it is replaced, under the influence of the pleasure principle, by a pleasure ego. Autoerotic libidinal instincts encourage diversion to a pleasure ego, whereas self-preservative instincts impel the psyche toward the establishment of the adult reality ego. All of this occurs under the influence of the gratifying or nongratifying aspects of the external world. He uses Ferenczi's term, *introject*, at this point and discusses how the introject can be assimilated and lead to further psychic structure, or, if it is a destructive introject, how it is expelled by projection. He discusses the development of love and hate and assigns them to their proper developmental levels. In view of the constant interaction of instinct and external world, introjection and projection, the dominance of pleasure or unpleasure, and the effects of all these processes upon the development or maldevelopment of the ego (psychic structure), it is once more difficult to understand why Freud's theory is a single axis theory that must be modified by introducing a double axis theory.

In many respects I believe that Kohut is simply paraphrasing Freud's ideas of development, and this would be perfectly justifiable if it were emphasized. Kohut, however, seems to underplay Freud's work, which gives the impression that he is postulating something momentously original. If new vocabulary is less cumbersome and more clinically relevant, then paraphrasing Freud's work can be very valuable, but does Kohut's language achieve this?

Before becoming involved with the structural details of Kohut's developmental formulations, I believe a methodological point should be stressed which brings us back to such concepts as separate lines of development. As Marohn asserts at the beginning of his chapter, Kohut (1971) thinks in terms of separate lines of development of narcissism and of object relations. Narcissism leads to what might be considered reality-attuned higher functions such as sensitivity and the capacities for introspection, empathy, and intuitiveness. He sees these functions as stemming from a different developmental path than that which leads to commitment and object love. If one is to be consistent within this theoretical framework, there *must* be a part of the ego that develops certain capacities and another part which relates to objects, and these two parts *have to be kept separate* from each other. Otherwise the concept of separate lines of development is both superfluous and meaningless. At best, this describes splitting, an adaptive and frequently primitive psychopathological defense, rather than ordinary development. Kohut describes a cohesive self, the outcome of primary narcissism, from which development proceeds along two different axes. He believes that there are interactions between his two developmental lines, but if this interaction is as much as it seems to be, then what is the value of making separations? Freud, as just discussed, concentrated on a variety of interactions without artificially isolating developmental vectors. It is easy to see where separate lines of development merge, as is the case when component instincts are subjected to genital dominance—an integrative and cohesive process. But once such integration has been achieved, it is not conceptually consistent to postulate that separation once again occurs as part of normal development. At best, this would be a defensive and regressive process.

In psychoanalysis, insofar as the elements of the mind are ordered in an hierarchal sequence, all theories are, in a sense, single axis. There can be only one line of development, a progression from the global and amorphous to the discrete and structured. The structured end of the spectrum may encompass areas which involve all types of interactions and relationship between various parts of the psyche, and between the ego and external objects. *This may be compared to branches radiating outward from a main stem or trunk, but they are not separate trunks.*

If the mind develops from a state in which it cannot recognize or acknowledge anything outside of itself to one in which it is intimately involved with a well-perceived external world, it is plausible that earlier modalities may continue to operate alongside more sophisticated adaptations. As is so often the case with the soma, such earlier structures as embryonic rests may become amalgamated into higher systems and contribute to their functioning. In the psyche, narcissistic self-involvement may continue to operate and even determine the quality and direction of very sophisticated object relationships.

A theory can be allowed a certain degree of complexity only as long as it can be reduced to basic fundamentals (Cohen and Nagel 1934, Giovacchini 1967). Object relationships can be traced to their early precursors, to ego states and adaptations that lacked the structure and discrimination to distinguish between inner and outer.

As the psyche develops, its capacity to discriminate between parts of the self and between the self and the outer world increases. The perception of and ability to relate to reality depends upon how well the mind can perceive itself. Without sufficient energy, in this case one can call it narcissistic energy or ego-libido, object relations are not possible. Object relations can be traced back to their narcissistic precursors. The latter make development possible and, in turn, continue to develop. As involvements with the self become more sophisticated, they make possible more sensitive, intimate, and complicated object relationships. There is a reciprocal interaction between the self and the outer world, where the self becomes enriched by object relationships, and object relations are in turn enhanced by a progressively structured self. To speak of separate lines of development tends to obscure these subtle structuralizing relationships.

Continuing further, Kohut describes autoerotism, from the viewpoint of the developing self, as the stage of the "fragmented self or self-nuclei." During the next stage, that of primary narcissism, these self-nuclei achieve cohesion. Glover (1930) wrote of ego-nuclei being at first unintegrated and achieving cohesion with emotional development. The only difference is that Kohut uses the word *self* rather than *ego*. However, in these early phases of development, there is no need to distinguish between ego and self, because the concept of self, more accurately the formation of a self-representation, can occur later only when there is considerable intraego differentiation. The concept of self is prematurely introduced and Glover's terminology is more appropriate.

Kohut then states that the child wants to preserve the original experience of perfection by attributing it to a grandiose self which under optimal conditions becomes integrated into the adult's personality. Having undergone structuralization, what was once grandiose, exhibitionistic libido now supplies the instinctual fuel for ego-syntonic ambitions, enjoyment, and self-esteem. The child also attempts to retain original perfection by assigning it to an admired self-object, which is considered a transitional object.

Here, two comments are appropriate. The first concerns general issues and is fundamentally important to psychoanalytic theory. The second involves a specific detail which does not involve basic principles.

Regarding fundamental constructs, I believe Kohut attributes certain qualities to early development that are inconsistent with the neonate's biological and psychological organization. I further believe that many other analysts, including Freud, did the same thing by adultomorphizing, early mental operations. Essentially, Kohut is discussing the same sequence Freud postulated. Freud used the word *grandiosity* although he seemed to have preferred the terms *omnipotence* and *megalomania*. In discussing the projection of grandiosity Kohut added the word *self*. Freud also spoke of the projection of megalomania on external objects and within the transference and saw such reactions in adult life as recapitulations of early developmental stages. Thus, both Freud and Kohut attribute rather complex feeling states, such as grandiosity or megalomania, to the infantile ego. An infant is hardly capable of making even a rudimentary discrimination between the psyche and the external world. I discuss this in detail in chapter 9 and will not pursue these distinctions further except to mention that if megalomania or grandiosity is considered an aspect of development, then it will color and complicate the therapeutic approach.

Both Freud and Kohut agree that the psyche progresses from a fragmented state (autoerotism) to one where some cohesion has been reached (primary narcissism). Yet, this is still a very rudimentary and primitive cohesion and is incompatible with the production of such complex combinations of cognition and affect as grandiosity or megalomania. Insofar as developmental progression leads to states of higher and greater synthesis, it is once more difficult to conceive of separate lines of development, indicative of a lack of cohesion, stemming from an earlier unified state. This would be a regression rather than a progression. True, well-integrated ego states can relate to different facets of the external world and parts of the self, but this is the outcome of development and not its cause. Furthermore, in Kohut's developmental scheme we lose the concept of psychopathology as a regression from higher states of equilibrium. According to his concepts, megalomania or grandiosity become psychopathological in the transference and are still somehow part of normal self-esteem.

The more superficial second point involves the equation of the projected, primitive, admired self-object, which is then known as the idealized parental imago, with the transitional object. It should be apparent that everything that has been said about the grandiose self also applies to the idealized parental imago, since the latter is simply the former projected onto an external object. Its being a transitional object can be disputed if

Winnicott's (1953) concept of the transitional object remains our basic model.

Winnicott found the concept of the transitional object a useful clinical construct as well as valuable for developmental theory. Today, it has found wide acceptance in psychoanalytic circles. He specifically meant that the child creates his own transitional object or phenomenon, a process he called "primary psychic creativity." The transitional object represents the maternal breast, and the child, because of satisfactory experiences with the mother, establishes a particular balance which can be sustained by an internalization of the mothering relationship. Because the child is so well acquainted with the functional aspects of mothering, he is enabled to create an internal construct without being aware of having taken the external object as a model. When everything progresses smoothly, one is often not aware of subtle interactions. In good health, the various parts of the body are not particularly noticed as, for example, would occur with a diseased or painful limb. The external object does not disturb the illusion of self-creation and self-sufficiency. The mother is, so to speak, congruent with the transitional object and reinforces it.

I asked Winnicott if it would be proper to conceptualize something within the ego that could be called a functional modality, the mothering or nurturing function which the infant accepts as part of the self. When elements of this function are attributed (projected) to an external object, then we have a transitional object. Winnicott agreed and then went on to elaborate the nature of the space from which the transitional object is selected. These ideas have been published (Winnicott 1967).

From this discussion, it is strikingly clear that the concept of the idealized parental imago bears little resemblance to Winnicott's concept of the transitional object. Quite the contrary, it is the outcome of a projection of a part of the self which results in the aggrandizement of an external object, whereas with the transitional object the sense of omnipotence remains within the psyche. The transitional object, although an external object, simultaneously remains part of the self and even though it has to be present it is not idealized. It is simply a reflection of internal stability, whereas the idealized parental imago defensively preserves a shaky and vulnerable integration.

CONCEPTS ABOUT PSYCHOPATHOLOGY

The preceding discussion has serious implications for our views about the psychopathology of patients suffering from characterological or structural defects. The immediately apparent issue is related to the assertion that the cohesive self which embodies the grandiose self is part of normal development. Kernberg (1974) has challenged this position and I have already indicated why I believe such a pronouncement theoretically and clinically infeasible. I will now discuss the consequences of such an orientation, as they are related to our understanding of patients suffering from what some have called narcissistic personality disorders.

Kohut calls our attention to a group of patients who are not neurotic and have a fairly stable personality organization. Nevertheless, they often are very sick and form characteristic mirror and merger transferences.

Unfortunately, and this happens so frequently in Kohut's work, these transference states are presented to us as if they were original discoveries. True, the juxtaposition of words may be new, but the phenomena have been observed and reported many times.

Again I refer to Freud, although I could have mentioned scores of analysts after him who acknowledged and extended his ideas. But I believe it is easier to limit the discussion to Freud because he was the first to expound these ideas.

During the mirror transference, the patient insists that he be admired. Here we have an interesting combination of ideas that deserve examination in order to ascertain exactly what is being described. In his early technical papers, Freud described the analyst's role as similar to a mirror so the patient can project his infantile feelings onto the analyst and then have them reflected back to him.

In the case of the mirror transference, Kohut is referring specifically to the reflection of the patient's grandiosity. If one gives this statement some thought, it becomes apparent that the reflecting back of grandiosity is included in the definition of narcissism. Recall that in the original legend of Narcissus the handsome youth has his image, his beauty, reflected back from the mirror pond. Freud used this ancient myth to define narcissism. Narcissistic patients regularly form narcissistic transferences during psychoanalytic treatment and the mirror transference is simply a different way of referring to what has usually been referred to as the narcissistic transference.

The same type of comment can be made on the merger transference and one of its variants, the twinship transference. These are described in terms of an extension of the grandiose self, that is, the establishment of what Kohut calls a primary identity in which the analyst becomes the carrier of the patient's grandiosity, a function once attributed to the mother. Twinship transference is similar, but lesser in degree. There is no question

229

as to the existence of such phenomena in treatment. They have been regularly observed in the therapy of patients with structural defects and have been referred to as fusion or omnipotent fusion. The analyst recognizes that the patient projects his megalomanic orientation onto him and then fuses with him. This represents a regression to a psychopathologically distorted symbiotic phase. I believe it valuable to call attention to this type of transference, but it should be put in proper perspective.

TECHNICAL CONSIDERATIONS

Kohut's (1971) therapeutic principles are based upon the fundamental assumption that narcissism, in this case the structures associated with it, the grandiose self and the idealized parental imago, is intrinsic to normal development. He proposes that the patient relives these stages during treatment, then progresses beyond them. Analytic technique is directed to fostering the merger transference that is the outcome of such a developmental phase and then to helping the patient develop further, something that is accomplished through the help of "transmuting internalizations."

As already discussed, it is theoretically incorrect to assign such complex feelings as grandiosity to such early primitive states. Consequently what follows can be called to question. Kernberg (1974) makes the same criticism about development and also views such orientations as grandiosity as pathological distortions. He also believes that Kohut does not sufficiently emphasize the negative transference, though Kohut does emphasize, during early stages of treatment, the fostering of positive transferences. Kernberg believes that the negative transference should not be evaded and that both negative and positive transference should be analyzed rather than encouraging the latter and discouraging the former.

Kernberg is describing the fundamental principles of analysis. One might venture the rejoinder that Kohut is introducing us to a new technique that will now make the analyses of these patients possible. But how the fostering of a specific defensive and pathological adaptation can lead to resolution and promote structure is by no means self-evident, so it behooves us to look at Kohut's technique in greater detail.

Kohut emphasizes that the analyst, by tuning in on the patient's demands for attention and admiration, provides the required mirroring for analysis. The walling off tendency of the reality ego is opposed by a well-established mirror transference manifested by the emergence of grandiose and exhibitionistic fantasies.

This can be restated in the following fashion. If the patient receives narcissistic gratification within the transference context, then perhaps splitting mechanisms will be used less extensively, and this could lead to structuralization and development. Kohut acknowledges, however, that there will be some inevitable frustration of the patient's grandiose needs, and this may lead to regression to more primitive fusion-like states. Still, there is much to know about the nature of the structuralization process.

If, as emphasized so often in this chapter, the transference states Kohut describes are manifestations of psychopathology rather than ordinary developmental levels, then it becomes difficult to understand how fostering such a state or gratifying the patient's narcissistic needs can lead to developmental progression. True, in any psychoanalysis one expects the patient to regress and to manifest within the transference the various elements of his psychopathology. But this is something that occurs spontaneously and the analyst neither encourages nor discourages the patient. Nor does he respond to the patient's demands within the transference context such as by mirroring back his grandiosity. No matter how understated it may be, the analyst's mirroring is still role playing and, as is true of all role playing, it will make the analysis of the transference difficult if not actually impossible.

Thus, Kohut has introduced a parameter (Eissler 1953), a deviation from classical analysis. This should be acknowledged, and the introduction of a parameter is justified if it can be used for later analytic gain by helping the patient be less restricted and to develop further so that analysis can take place.

Still, how does supporting a patient's defensive narcissistic orientation foster emotional development? As stated, from a technical viewpoint, it will only make the analysis of the transference difficult. From a structural viewpoint, one is dealing with two primary process factors. The patient is displaying primitive aspects of himself, and the analyst, by supporting him, is reacting in the same frame of reference. *A primary process-oriented need and a primary process-oriented response cannot, by themselves, lead to secondary process structuralization.*

The question of whether one should attempt to gratify the patient's infantile needs when the aim of therapy is to achieve further psychic structure is unsettled. Even though the analyst's reaction to the patient's material is largely a response to primary process elements, it usually still contains more secondary process than the patient's orientation. One can think in terms of a gradient and symbolic gratification (Giovacchini 1969). Still, the conscious intent to reinforce psychopathologically distorted developmental stages mitigates the structuralizing potential of the analytic interaction, causing the patient to view himself primarily in terms of his fixation rather than helping him understand why parts of himself, for the moment, require particular adaptations. Such a therapeutic maneuver also makes the analysis of the transference more difficult because of the analyst's deliberate participation.

Kohut correctly warns us that one should not attempt to admonish the patient or to guide him. He stresses that one should not prematurely confront the patient with reality, otherwise the therapeutic setting will upset the proper climate for the remobilization of the grandiose self. He agrees with Freud that the analyst should not be an educator. These are useful and well-known principles which apply to all analytic patients and not just to narcissistic disorders. However, Kohut strongly implies that this classical analytical attitude has its temporal limits, because if one does not prematurely confront and, as Ornstein (1972) more emphatically stated, prematurely "debunk," it must mean that at some point in time one introduces reality and is critical of the transference manifestations of the patient's psychopathology. Again, this is a deviation from analysis, for to encourage first and then to discourage, no matter how gentle one may be in either stance, is manipulative and managerial. Perhaps as supportive therapy such an approach may be effective, but if one ascribes the acquisition of psychic structure to analytic resolution, as Kohut also does, then it is difficult to comprehend how analytic resolution can occur in these circumstances.

Kohut is also concerned about the problem of the acquisition of structure, acknowledging that narcissistically fixated patients, because of early trauma, lack the psychic structures that would maintain intrapsychic balance and self-esteem. In this context, he introduces us to "transmuting internalization."

Transmute means to change, and internalization refers to something that was once outside being inside. If an external object or experience is to lead to a structurally progressive change within the psyche, it has to be smoothly incorporated and integrated. I have referred to this process as the amalgamation of the introject in order to view it in a somewhat microscopic, ego-psychological frame of reference (Giovacchini 1965). The processes involved have been called introjection, incorporation, internalization, and identification (see Schafer 1968). In all of these mental processes, the assumption exists that what is inside differs from what it was before, which means there has been change (transmutation). More clearly elaborating the process by which change occurs is far more desirable than introducing a new catchphrase more descriptive than explanatory.

Conclusions

Kohut has introduced ideas about narcissism which cover a wide area. He directed us to a group of patients who are increasingly coming to the attention of therapists. His contributions have stimulated considerable interest and have created an atmosphere of optimism about the psychoanalytic treatment of patients suffering from severe psychopathology.

Marohn employs Kohut's concepts to deal with adolescent patients, especially delinquents. Marohn is one of many who have embraced Kohut's ideas enthusiastically and who believe that they have been enriched both in their understanding and technical treatment proficiency.

Since Kohut's ideas have been so influential and since they can be directed toward such clinical populations as adolescents and those suffering from characterological problems; it is apparent that, these ideas should be carefully examined. In this chapter, there is a critical discussion of Kohut's ideas about psychic development, concepts of psychopathology, and technical recommendations. I hope that this evaluation will prove useful in helping the clinician put Kohut's frame of reference in proper perspective. I also hope that others will be stimulated to make similar studies to either support, modify, or revise his concepts rather than simply to accept or reject them without serious investigation of their place in the structure of psychoanalytic concepts.

REFERENCES

Breuer, J., and Freud, S. (1895). Studies on hysteria. *Standard Edition* 2. London: Hogarth, 1955.

Cohen, M., and Nagel, E. (1934). *An Introduction to Logic and Scientific Method.* New York: Harcourt, Brace.

Eissler, K. (1953). The effect of the structuring of the ego on psychoanalytic technique. *Journal of the American Psychoanalytic Association* 1: 36.

Freud, S. (1900). The interpretation of dreams. *Standard Edition* 4/5. London: Hogarth, 1955.

——— (1911). Psycho-analytic notes on an autobiographical account of a case of paranoia (dementia paranoides). *Standard Edition* 12:12-82. London: Hogarth, 1967.

—— (1914). On narcissism: an introduction. *Standard Edition* 14: 73-102. London: Hogarth, 1957.

—— (1915). Instincts and their vicissitudes. *Standard Edition* 14: 117-140. London: Hogarth, 1967.

—— (1920). Beyond the pleasure principle. *Standard Edition* 18: 7-64. London: Hogarth, 1955.

—— (1923). The ego and the id. *Standard Edition* 19: 12-66. London: Hogarth, 1961.

—— (1926). Inhibitions, symptoms and anxiety. *Standard Edition* 20: 87-156. London: Hogarth, 1959.

—— (1938). Splitting of the ego in the process of defense. *Standard Edition* 23: 275-278. London: Hogarth, 1964.

Giovacchini, P. L. (1965). Transference, incorporation and synthesis. *International Journal of Psycho-Analysis* 46: 287-296.

—— (1967). Methodological aspects of psychoanalytic critique. *Bulletin of the Philadelphia Association for Psychoanalysis* 17: 10-18.

—— (1969). The influence of interpretation on schizophrenic patients. *International Journal of Psycho-Analysis* 50: 179-186.

—— (1975). Self-projections in the narcissistic transference. *International Journal of Psychoanalytic Psychotherapy* 4: 142-167.

Glover, E. (1930). Grades of ego-differentiation. *International Journal of Psycho-Analysis* 11: 1-26.

Jones, E. (1955). *Sigmund Freud: Life and Work*, Vol. 2. London: Hogarth.

Kernberg, O. F. (1974). Further contributions to the treatment of narcissistic personalities. *International Journal of Psycho-Analysis* 55: 215-238.

Klein, M. (1932). *The Psychoanalysis of Children*. London: Hogarth.

Kohut, H. (1966). Forms and transformations of narcissism. *Journal of the American Psychoanalytic Association* 14: 243-270.

—— (1971). *The Analysis of the Self*. New York: International Universities Press.

Ornstein, P. (1972). On narcissism: beyond the introduction. Presented October 9, 1972 at the divisional meetings of the Western Psychoanalytic Societies, San Diego, California.

Schafer, R. (1968). *Aspects of Internalization*. New York: International Universities Press.

Strachey, J. (1934). The nature of the therapeutic action of psycho-analysis. *International Journal of Psycho-Analysis* 15: 127-160.

Winnicott, D. W. (1953). Transitional objects and transitional phenomena. *International Journal of Psycho-Analysis* 34: 89-98.

——— (1967). The location of cultural experience. *International Journal of Psycho-Analysis* 48: 368-372.

PART III

PSYCHOPATHOLOGY AND ADOLESCENCE

EDITORS' INTRODUCTION

The scientific formulation of psychopathology must be phrased in a consistent conceptual system aimed at explaining how certain behavioral changes occur. To establish causal sequences one proceeds from the surface, the phenomenological, to the inner recesses of the personality. This is a psychodynamic approach characterizing the psychoanalytic frame of reference, which many regard as the only existing approach that attempts to understand psychopathology in terms of etiological processes.

In the behavioral sciences, the understanding of the pathological vicissitudes of psychic processes includes drives and structure as well as developmental factors. In many conditions, it is the empathic reactions of the therapist that stimulate metapsychological formulations which eventually extend our knowledge of psychoanalytic psychology. In this part, we present chapters that will add to our clinical armamentarium through a delicate balance of etiological focus in a consistent conceptual system, and through the additional insights that might extend this understanding derived from various therapeutic approaches.

Moses Laufer, in the 1976 William A. Schonfeld lecture, discusses adolescent development and pathological outcome in adulthood. He is concerned that many professionals view pathology as part of the youth culture and unwittingly dismiss the seeds of future breakdown or mental illness as transitional reactions of adolescence. Dr. Laufer defines adolescent pathology as a breakdown in the process of integrating one's physically mature body into a self representation. This interference with the developmental process then results in failure to form a clear sexual identity which may lead to adult psychopathology and breakdown.

William M. Easson outlines the general symptoms of adolescent depression manifested by mood variations, self-esteem and self-concept actions, and psychomotor, psychosomatic, and social manifestations. He describes depressive syndromes in adolescence, differentiating the normal, depressive-like states (emancipation, mourning, and age-specific moodiness) from pathological depressions (endogenous, object loss, anhedonic, anaclitic, and secondary), and discusses treatment approaches with some emphasis on cultural influences.

Philip S. Holzman and Roy R. Grinker, Sr., from a larger study of schizophrenia, review the impact of this serious illness on the adolescent. Differentiating between schizophrenia (long-standing withdrawal, apathy, poor object relations, thought disorder) from schizophrenic psychosis (overt schizophrenia with secondary features of psychosis), the authors conclude that adolescence imposes severe demands for social, interpersonal, and intrapersonal competence on the biologically and psychologically vulnerable adolescent.

Anorexia nervosa, as a paradigmatic entity, assumes a significance that supersedes its clinical importance and difficult clinical course. As a serious condition, it serves as a model for studying other severe characterological and even psychotic problems commonly associated with adolescence. The deadly course of this disorder warrants a multiplicity of treatment approaches and, consequently, we have included various types of treatment modalities to present a panorama of therapeutic efforts. In part, however, this was editorial largesse. We have our commitments and find techniques which stray from intrapsychic factors, devoting themselves to environmental manipulation in order to change behavior, contrary to our clinical and scientific orientation. Granted, one's ideals may have to recede into the background when faced with a life and death crisis, and that is why we have accepted some of the following articles. Yet, understanding the patient in terms of etiology in a consistent conceptual system is still the most hopeful and meaningful approach to patients with a disorder which, in spite of or because of its gravity, demands such understanding in order to survive. This theme could be developed further and lead perhaps to a comparative analysis of different treatment modalities, but, for the moment, that is not our purpose.

Hilde Bruch presents an overview of her well-known studies on eating disorders in adolescents. She describes primary anorexia as a state of pitiful emaciation characterized by disturbance of body image, misperceptions of body functions, a sense of ineffectiveness, and conflict in family transactions. Atypical anorexia nervosa, on the other hand, presents feeding problems secondary to other psychiatric conditions. Dr. Bruch discusses the treatment of anorectics, dividing the tasks into two integrated phases: restoration of normal nutrition and resolution of underlying psychological conflicts. She describes her approach, which recognizes developmental, ego psychological defects as the underlying cause of the specific reactions.

Alan Goodsitt examines disturbances of narcissistic development in anorexia nervosa. He states that it is only after one has achieved a stable, cohesive sense of self that one can process external stimuli and maintain a sense of wholeness and integrity. A lack of cohesiveness is evident in the anorectics' feelings of body helplessness and fear of fragmentation of the self. Faced with this threat, the symptoms of anorexia nervosa are seen as an attempt to regulate control. Therapeutic efforts should be directed toward minimizing narcissistic injuries and establishing a more stable equilibrium.

Bernice L. Rosman, Salvador Minuchin, Ronald Liebman, and Lester Baker contribute an account of their use of a family therapy model for the psychological treatment of anorexia nervosa. (The nutritional aspect is treated in a traditional medical fashion.) Applying a structural approach to the family, these authors recognized that familial functional patterns were quite similar for anorectics as well as children with other psychosomatic problems. These families, described as highly enmeshed, overprotective, rigidly resistant to change, and manifesting inadequate conflict resolution techniques, involved the child in the parental conflict in particular ways, reinforcing a continuation of the symptom and the peculiar aspects of the family organization.

Katherine A. Halmi and Linda Carson present (by invitation) an overview of the use of behavior therapy in dealing with the nutritional aspects of anorexia nervosa. Part of a National Institute of Mental Health study, the authors describe their research and methodology. The authors believe that their follow-up study revealed that the careful use of behavioral contingencies is not harmful. Patients are encouraged to pursue psychotherapy, but many parents are resistant.

Bertram J. Cohler discusses transference difficulties in the treatment of anorexia nervosa which make it difficult for the therapist to maintain perspective on the adaptive significance of the patient's symptoms. Psychotherapy with anorectic patients leads to intense emotional reactions, perhaps the most intense encountered in any therapeutic relationship. The therapist's problem is to develop the capacity to bear and sustain these painful feelings and to accept the discomfort which develops as an inevitable consequence. Cohler believes that feelings of anger and hopelessness aroused by the anorectic patient are a genuine and intrinsic part of treatment process and not only an element of countertransference. When the patient can attribute these feelings to a therapist who can accept and endure them, the patient first becomes able to achieve personality change and experience a greater sense of intrapsychic integration.

15] A VIEW OF ADOLESCENT PATHOLOGY

For some time now I have attempted to define the developmental function of adolescence and the interferences during adolescence which result in pathological outcomes in adulthood. I have pursued this work in two related endeavors: my own analytic work with adolescents, and a recently completed five-year pilot study at the Centre for the Study of Adolescence in London. Entitled "Mental Breakdown in Adolescence," this study generated clinical material which conveyed something different in meaning from the material afforded me by analytic contact with children and adults.

When I considered the theme of this Conference—"Youth in Transition"—I was faced with a dilemma. My first wish was to purview a variety of problems with which I have been confronted in my work with adolescents. This soon changed, mainly because it seemed inappropriate for one now living in London to comment on a range of psychological, social, and cultural problems, and questions related to youth in the United States. But in thinking more carefully about the Conference theme, I realized there was another danger, one which I feel has permeated much of our thinking about the adolescent, and perhaps our work as well, and which can certainly be detected in much of the recent professional literature on adolescence.

With our increasing respectability as professional people who work with adolescents, and with the wider acceptance, over a period of years, of some psychoanalytic and dynamic psychiatric principles as guides to our work and thinking, there has emerged a tendency to use our clinical experience as

William A. Schonfeld Distinguished Service Award Address presented at the 1976 Annual Meeting of the American Society for Adolescent Psychiatry, Miami Beach, May 9, 1976.

243

the basis for generalizations about the nature of man and, more specifically, the nature of youth. As an exercise in philosophical or peripheral scientific thought, some of these efforts have produced a variety of interesting speculations, including commentaries on aspects of social and political life, on the central turmoil facing youth, and on the relationship between opportunity and internal development. Such generalizations or speculations may help us comprehend what is taking place in the external world, and may at times be able to direct attention to trends in social, educational, or political life which may be detrimental or dangerous to personal freedom, equality, or the integrity of people. The problem is not that those who work with disturbed or ill adolescents have looked to some of these ideas to aid comprehension of what is going on around them; instead, the problem is that some of us have begun to equalize a whole range of social, cultural, and personal conflicts and pressures as a way of understanding psychopathology and its meaning for the suffering adolescent.

Although this is a view shared by many people who work with adolescents, it is one which enables us to withdraw from recognizing the presence of pathology among adolescents. It is not at all uncommon, for example, to meet colleagues who see no special pathological significance in severe depression, attempted suicide, homosexuality in older adolescents, promiscuity, drug dependence, and so on. Some who work with adolescents extend this doubt to assessment in general and consider inappropriate any diagnosis of established pathology in adolescence.

As a group of professional people who work therapeutically with adolescents, it is not sufficient to acknowledge various theories of adolescence and varying views on the pros and cons of certain types of intervention. Instead, it is of prime importance to consider what our aims in adolescent therapy are, what it is that we use in our work which enables us to judge the success or failure of our efforts, and what it is that we use as a theoretical model to enable us to decide what we mean by normality and pathology. This then confronts us with the need to define our views about the function of adolescence as a developmental period; and only then can we be clearer about what is meant by transition—where the person was, is, and is going.

Restated in developmental terms, we may ask: what is the nature of the psychic structure, the quality of the conflicts, and the relation to external reality at the time of puberty? What is or is not taking place during adolescence developmentally? What are the main factors or observations during adolescence which enable us to predict the manner in which a person reaches adulthood, sexually and socially? Such a precise view of the function of adolescence enables our assessments and our therapeutic interventions to be more directed toward the needs and the internal crises which disturbed adolescents face. It also makes it more possible to define the specific nature of adolescent pathology, and to begin to define those forms of adaptation which can be included within the wide range of normality.

This rather extended introduction contains a concern or an anxiety about the wish or need which some professional people have to try to redefine pathology in adolescence, with the result that some of us avoid seeing pathology when it is staring us in the face. Organized, private pathology in adolescence becomes instead something which is part of youth culture. Personal suffering or acute breakdown is dismissed because a number of adolescents share the same manifest behavior. The seeds of future breakdown or mental illness may be there, but we may still prefer to dismiss it as transition, or as change in social expectation.

Adolescence and the Final Sexual Organization

My intention is to concentrate totally on the internal life of the adolescent, and I will describe his life as if nothing else but his internal world exists. I am well aware that every adolescent, whether his development is progressing normally or in a pathological direction, responds to a whole range of pressures which affect his day-to-day life—family, friends, expectations of contemporaries, and expectations within the community. I believe, however, that pathological development is finally determined by the adolescent's internal world, whatever the external pressures. It is an aspect of this internal world which I will concentrate upon, elaborating fundamental factors within adolescent development and pathology, factors which can have some bearing on our work with adolescents— whether that work is therapy, education, rehabilitation, or assessment.

In *Three Essays,* Freud (1905) wrote that it is after puberty that the person shapes (what he there described as) the "final sexual organization." The references to Freud's writings on puberty and adolescence more often emphasize his belief that adolescence is a recapitulation of one's earlier life, but that during adolescence this recapitulation is experienced within the context of physically mature genitals. This insight, of course, still remains a significant guide to the understanding of behavior and disturbance, but the lesser emphasis on the final sexual organization and on the understanding,

245

theoretically and clinically, of what this means for the adolescent's present and future life has created confusion in the thinking of some of us who work with adolescents—a confusion which can be observed in the ease with which we are ready to accept any and all new explanations about psychological life, explanations which often have little bearing on the understanding of adolescent pathology.

Viewed developmentally, the assumption of the establishment of a final sexual organization in adolescence means that the part played by this period of psychological life in the person's future mental health is much more specific than is often believed, I would like, then, to extend Freud's remarks and simultaneously introduce my thesis: Although the individual reaches adolescence with his main sexual identifications fixed and with the core of the image of his body established (this already takes place with the resolution of the oedipal conflict), it is only by the end of adolescence that we can speak of the person's irreversible sexual identity having been established (that is, irreversible without therapeutic intervention). By the end of adolescence this sexual identity represents the manner in which the person has been able, during his adolescence, to integrate a physically mature body as part of the representation of himself. My view, then, of adolescent pathology is that it represents a breakdown in the process of integrating one's physically mature body as part of the representation of oneself, and the breakdown in this process occurring at puberty has a cumulative effect throughout adolescence. Whatever may be contributory or explanatory ingredients to this breakdown—preoedipal, oedipal, or preadolescent—the essential component of adolescent pathology is a breakdown in the developmental process whose primary or specific function is to establish a sexual identity. In the course of the chapter, I will elaborate this in clinical terms.

I referred earlier to the person's irreversible sexual identity being established by the end of adolescence. By this, I am implying that the three developmental tasks of adolescence: (1) the change in the relationship to the oedipal objects, (2) the change in the relationship to contemporaries, and (3) the change in the attitude to his own body can be subsumed under this main developmental function of establishing sexual identity. I am also implying that once the person's sexual identity is established by the end of adolescence, there is no longer the choice for any kind of internal compromise; instead, what we see after adolescence, that is, in young adulthood, at least in pathology, is the result of the breakdown in the developmental process which took place in adolescence. If what I say is correct, then it has some bearing on assessment in adolescence and on our aims of treatment.

I have repeatedly used the phrase *by the end of adolescence*. The end of adolescence is that point in development, following physical sexual maturity, at which methods of dealing with anxiety have become fixed and structural rearrangements have finally taken place. From my clinical work with adolescents and young adults, it seems that this has usually taken place by the age of twenty-one. After that time, it is necessary to assess behavior differently and not to dismiss too lightly any behavior in young adults which may contain carry-overs from adolescence. With young adults, we should question whether what we are observing represents the pathological outcome of a breakdown in the developmental process of adolescence.

Ownership of the Physically Mature Body and the Central Masturbation Fantasy

With physical maturity, with the actual ability to impregnate or become pregnant, body sensation and fantasy take on a meaning developmentally different. It forces the adolescent and, simultaneously, enhances the adolescent's wish, to become totally separate from oedipal objects, especially the mother. This separation from oedipal objects is contained in and experienced via the adolescent's relationship to his body. He feels that he owns his body and is responsible for its sensations, actions, and the fantasies which it stimulates. Blos (1967) was referring to this when he wrote that "adolescent individuation is the reflection of those structural changes that accompany emotional disengagement from internalized infantile objects." Although I agree with Blos' description of the process, I hesitate to refer to it as individuation. The main difference is that I place more specific emphasis on the part played by the relationship the adolescent has to his own body by which this process is experienced and resolved.

Still we must ask what the force from the past is which takes on such new significance with physical sexual maturity? What is it that makes the period of adolescence, even for those developing normally, so laden with anxiety, turmoil, and forms of acting out which often give the impression of loss of contact with reality? And what is it about adolescence which precipitates the breakdowns, the suicides, the psychotic-type depressions, the anorexias, and the range of behavior where the adolescent feels compelled to act or behave in a specific way, without, at that moment, regard for the actual consequences of behavior?

Here I will introduce a concept about psychological development which I believe has a bearing on our understanding of development during adolescence, and which may enable us to make sense of what pathology in adolescence is about. I refer to what I can best describe as the *central masturbation fantasy*. I wish, however, to place emphasis on fantasy rather than on masturbation. It is relevant to include the word masturbation because the fantasy is experienced through autoerotic activities. In adolescence the range of feelings and body sensations is attached to physical sexual maturity.

We assume that, as part of normal development from infancy onward, the person finds means through the use of his own body or with an object to gratify his instinctual demands. The preoedipal child may have available a whole range of autoerotic activities, games, and daydreams which help to recreate and relive the relationship to the gratifying mother. However, following the resolution of the oedipus complex and the internalization of the superego, we can no longer refer in the same way to the child's ways of gratifying his instinctual wishes or demands in relation to the first love object, the mother. Instead, the resolution of the oedipus complex means that all regressive satisfactions will, in the future, be judged by the superego as being acceptable or not. But, in terms of future sexual orientation and of the final sexual identity which is established by the end of adolescence, the resolution of the oedipus complex establishes the central masturbation fantasy, the fantasy whose content contains the various regressive satisfactions and the main sexual identifications (Laufer 1976). This central masturbation fantasy is, I believe, a universal phenomenon—it is not dependent for its existence or for its power on whether the child actually masturbates or not. Instead, it takes into account the fact that the body is a constant source of feelings and sensations, and that it also is an object in its own right to which the person must have a relationship.

During latency the content of this central masturbation fantasy remains unconscious, but is expressed in a disguised way through daydreams, fantasies which accompany masturbation, or games or fantasy activities and relationships (A. Freud 1965). Although the latency child's and preadolescent child's reactions to this fantasy and to various forms of autoerotic activity will be determined mainly by the reaction of the superego, it is only with the physical maturing of the genitals that the content of this fantasy assumes a new meaning and makes demands on the ego which are qualitatively different from what previously occurred.

Although the content of this central masturbation fantasy does not normally alter during adolescence, the fact that it is experienced within the context of physically mature genitals means that it now assumes a new significance in psychological life. It also means that the person's physically mature body becomes the primary vehicle through which this fantasy is experienced or lived out, and, as such, it adds a special and new meaning to the relationship which the person has to his own body. The body is no longer the property of the mother (as it was in childhood), but following puberty and throughout adolescence it becomes the arena within which and through which conflict is experienced, and also the means by which the new representation of the body is established.

Before adolescence, the fantasy acts as a reference for the meaning of body sensations and feelings, and it enables the child, via the experiencing of fantasy, to begin to experience body ownership separate from the mother. But it is only by the end of adolescence that we can speak of the adolescent's ownership of his body. The central masturbation fantasy is the constant force which propels this development in one direction or another.

Although I want to place emphasis on fantasy rather than masturbation, the fact is that body sensations, the active stimulation of fantasy through the physically mature body, and the living out of fantasy by the body during adolescence are significant because of their integrative function. They enable the adolescent normally to try out, in the safety of thought, which fantasies are acceptable to the superego and which must be rejected. Normally, by the end of adolescence, the person will, through various forms of trial action, have found a solution to varying regressive wishes and demands, while simultaneously finding it possible to feel that his gratifications, actions, and sexual body are his own and for which he is responsible. It means for the male that by the end of adolescence he feels that he can actively seek a sexual partner, that he can actively desire to penetrate her without feelings of remorse or of overwhelming guilt, and that various regressive fantasies do not interfere in his ability to identify actively with the father. For the female, it means that by the end of adolescence she feels that she has a relationship to her own sexual body which enables her to express her active wish to be penetrated and to grow a child in her body, and for whom being a woman does not mean passive overwhelming by the mother, but an active identification with her.

Adolescent Pathology

Adolescent pathology is a breakdown in the process of integrating one's physically mature body as part of the representation of oneself. It is a breakdown which occurs at puberty and has a cumulative effect throughout adolescence. Implied in this view is that adolescent pathology has a beginning and an end, and that it interferes in a specific way in the developmental process. The range of pathology in adolescence is vast, and each has its own explanation and meaning for the individual. We know that in each of these specific disturbances there are core fantasies which play a part, and that each disturbance or outcome of conflict contains both the unconscious living out of a wish as well as the defense against it. From the point of view of the function of adolescence developmentally, one must redirect this explanation to explain the specific nature of adolescent pathology.

With puberty, the adolescent is suddenly faced with the fact that his body is not only an extension of his relationship to his oedipal objects, especially his mother, but that it also can be the source of physical pleasure, or can be experienced as the source of fantasies and thoughts which endanger his psychic equilibrium. His body, and the feelings coming from it, now begin to define sexual normality or abnormality. Now, for the first time in his life, it is the relationship to his own body—to the gratifications coming from it, and to the fantasies and thoughts which are attached to it or stimulated by it—by which all experience is judged and measured. Normally, progressive development in adolescence means that genital as well as pregenital wishes, contained in the central masturbation fantasy, can be used actively to help establish equilibrium between these varying wishes; but it is an equilibrium in which genitality is the final arbiter.

There are, however, those adolescents who feel they cannot defend against the regressive attraction of pregenital wishes. Their sexually mature bodies become the source of their suffering. It is as if the living out of their central masturbation fantasy is experienced as a repetitive overwhelming of themselves. The consequence of this is that their relationship to their body must be seriously impaired, affecting object relationships, the means by which they seek and find sexual gratification as well as their relation to reality. Instead of actively being able to use the feelings and sensations coming from their bodies, as well as the fantasies stimulated by these feelings and sensations, to help integrate their genitals as part of their body representation, they experience their bodies as the constant representative of that which will overwhelm them. The manner in which they may deal with this conflict may vary from that of asceticism to that of feeling compelled to behave in specific ways, but the result will be, by the end of adolescence, that they will feel their sexual bodies as enemies or, at best, representing a hindrance to their achievement of genital aims.

What happens with these adolescents can be described as a feeling of "deadlock" (which still contains the fight against giving in to pregenital wishes). This is followed by a feeling of "surrender" (Laufer 1976). The predominant wishes are regressively pregenital for these adolescents, and their bodies are experienced by them as constant proof that they have surrendered their sexual bodies and feelings to the mother who first cared for them. It is as if they have accepted the fact that a choice no longer exists for them.

CLINICAL EXAMPLE 1

John, who is now twenty, first came for treatment at sixteen after being asked to leave school. It was a school with very high standards, and students who did not meet them were asked to leave. Previously, at thirteen, he had left a note in which he described how he would kill himself and why. Before this crisis, John was considered to be a quiet, polite, and highly intelligent person, but with sudden moods of remorse and withdrawal.

In the course of his treatment with me, he described a fantasy which had been conscious since the age of seven. He would enjoy thinking of girls, or of his mother, with a pained facial expression. This fantasy stayed with him, and although he felt ashamed of it at times, he said that he was quite able to live with this secret without having to invite too much punishment or threat. Suddenly, with puberty, he found that he began to have to organize his activities around observing girls or women with pained facial expressions. He felt compelled to visit sports arenas so that he could observe girls straining themselves and tightening their faces. He became especially alarmed when he found that he felt compelled to have to hit his mother, at times to such an extent that he and his family became very concerned that he might seriously harm her.

In addition to the therapeutic task of understanding the specific meaning of this fantasy and of the need to live out this fantasy in a compelling way, it indicated that there was no progress in his ability to integrate which would enable him to experience his body as free. In terms of the thesis of this chapter, I could predict that unless I could help him through treatment, he would have to reject his sexual body, and, instead, he would invariably have to return to the safety of the relationship to his mother. In other words, the present fantasy tied him more firmly rather than enabling him to separate himself from the mother who first cared for him.

CLINICAL EXAMPLE 2

Helen first came to treatment at the age of eighteen. She had been obese, but she came because she felt that she lived with a thread of hopelessness going through everything she experienced. Her excessive eating began, she said, soon after a boy tried to touch her breasts when she was fifteen. She recalled how he tried to arouse her sexually by kissing her and fondling her breasts, and how she reacted to this with disgust. She was astonished by this reaction, and then felt that she must keep away from boys. Separately from this event, she found she had begun to eat excessively, and at one time weighed nearly two hundred pounds.

Within the treatment, the need to understand the specific meaning of the obesity, with its underlying fantasy, its superego component, and its relation to the oedipal father, were all of central significance. From the point of view of the relationship to her own body and of the establishment of her sexual identity by the end of adolescence, there was another factor to take into account. Her disturbance was, at this point, removing her from friends. It isolated her to a great extent and she felt forced to do things in a highly organized and unyielding way.

In the course of treatment, she found to her surprise and horror that she had begun again to masturbate in a rather compelling way. She had, before adolescence, masturbated quite regularly, and although she felt ashamed and frightened of what would happen, she was able to "fool herself and her parents" by always remaining cheerful. She found that, now, the fantasy she had during masturbation was of a man having intercourse with a woman and then killing her. She again now, as she had previously when she first started to menstruate, actively thought of killing herself. Previously, that is, before her treatment, she felt able to keep these fantasies under control, but now she felt that there was no choice but to kill herself—to kill what she felt to be the source of these fantasies, her body. My impression is that, had she not been in treatment, and had this fantasy continued to be allowed to have its force, she would very likely have attempted suicide.

From the point of view of her relationship to her sexual body, she now felt completely stuck, without knowing how to go about changing. She was implying that she had no choice now but simply to give in, to reject her body, and to regressively remain the child who would be loved simply for being good. Developmentally, had she been left to her regressive wishes, the outcome might have been disastrous. The guilt, because of her fantasies and the gratification she obtained from them, was such that she felt that alone she could do nothing else but die.

CLINICAL EXAMPLE 3

I will now refer to an adult patient. Aged twenty-seven when he first came to see me, his initial reason for coming to treatment was that he was told that he might have to be asked to resign his academic post unless something was done about his absences and his constant and sudden cancellation of classes. He had been very highly regarded in his post, and both the head of the institution and his colleagues there tried very hard to help him seek treatment, which he finally agreed to reluctantly.

He described himself as totally isolated, unable to have any friends, completely unable to accept any social invitations, and spending all of his time alone in his room or alone in his office at the academic institution. He was engrossed in his work, but he had to cancel lectures or go on sick leave regularly because he would suddenly feel unable to see people, frightened that somebody might attack him. He might, in the course of ordinary observation or description, be considered to be a suspicious, withdrawn, shy man. He walked with a peculiar gait—he did not swing his arms, he kept his body erect, and he walked very quickly.

He recently had begun to dress as a woman, and to masturbate while looking in the mirror. He did this in his room, and although he thought of walking in the street, he never did. Again, I want to avoid discussing the specific meaning of the symptomatology, in this case the transvestism, but instead focus on what this pathological organization did to his life.

He grew up with the belief that his mother would have preferred him to be a girl. He sometimes thought of changing his name to sound like a girl's, but he was able somehow to overcome this wish. At puberty, he found that he had the wish to cut off his penis. He became so frightened by this thought that he would not remove his trousers when sleeping. In masturbation, he would hide his penis between his legs, and at times he would masturbate anally to the point of orgasm. He often would hit himself on his buttocks (this gave him great pleasure) and at times he would ejaculate while doing this. He secretly continued to live out this beating fantasy during adolescence by masturbating. He also secretly continued to dress up in his mother's clothes (he first did this when he was about thirteen). At the university he was totally isolated, and when he once tried to go out with a girl, he found that he suddenly had to leave the party for fear that some of the men there might attack him.

By the time I saw him the developmental damage had been done. He found that he could not have any relationship, especially to a woman, for fear that his penis would somehow be destroyed. His present life revolved almost totally around the pathological solution which he had found. In terms of his sexual identity, the pathological outcome by the end of adolescence could be seen in that he had given up any thought that he could ever change anything. He believed there was nothing to be done except to go on living this way, to go on with the unconscious awareness that he had surrendered his sexual body to his mother or, in terms of his masturbation fantasy which was still the only vehicle for sexual pleasure, that he could go on offering his infantile body to the oedipal father who could do to him what he believed the father did to his mother, to beat her (Freud 1919).

The clinical examples presented are intended primarily to show what I mean by the developmental function of adolescence, and to define more clearly what is meant by adolescent pathology. I chose to include in the clinical descriptions an adult patient, because I wanted to show the repercussions in adult life of the pathological solutions found during adolescence.

I also wanted to describe some of the criteria which can be of use in the assessment of adolescent pathology. I place the greatest importance in assessment on the adolescent's relationship to his own body because, as has certainly been clear from what I have said, I believe that a detailed description of this can enable us to be more certain about the direction of the move toward adulthood. As the main means for the living out of the central masturbation fantasy, the body in adolescence becomes the vehicle by which the new representation of self is established by the end of adolescence. Detailed knowledge of the adolescent's relationship to his own body must therefore make it possible to know whether progressive development is taking place or whether we are seeing signs of a pathological outcome in the establishment of one's sexual identity.

Intervention in Adolescence

During the past few years, there have been many different views about therapeutic intervention during adolescence. Some have stated that adolescence is a time when intervention should be avoided or kept to a minimum. There are those who intervene only where there is gross pathology or interference in the adolescent's life, so that treatment is the only alternative. My view, in contradistinction, is that intervention in adolescence is not only desirable, but that it may be crucial in a person's future life. But when I speak of intervention, I refer to therapy which takes into account the primary task of adolescence, which works toward undoing the feeling of deadlock or surrender which some adolescents live with, and works toward enabling the adolescent to feel that a choice exists in the establishment of sexual identity.

There are many therapies which are considered suitable for the adolescent. Some therapies contain the belief that with support the adolescent will somehow find his way toward a sexual identity which will be acceptable. Others believe that social factors or, more specifically, environmental changes, may enhance the adolescent's life. The issue is not whether intervention can help the adolescent, but whether our aims of intervention also have contained in them a view of the function of adolescence and of the nature of adolescent pathology.

In my own work with adolescents, whether it is analysis, intensive psychotherapy, or nonintensive work, I am constantly assessing in my own mind what is or is not changing in the adolescent's relationship to his own body. In optimal circumstances, I will therefore want to know about the adolescent's relationship to people of the same or opposite sex, his relationship to his parents, his masturbation activity (including his masturbation fantasies), and generally about the way in which he takes care of or ignores his body. Of course, the developmental model, the use of reconstruction, the use of transference interpretations, and when necessary the use of certain parameters, are all part of my work with adolescents. My primary focus continues to be, however, throughout my contact with the adolescent, the nature and direction of the adolescent process as observed through his relationship to his own physically mature body (Laufer 1975, 1976).

Conclusions

If the thesis put forward about adolescent pathology is correct, then it may enable us to see more critically how the various contributions and views about development can be used in understanding adolescent development in general and adolescent pathology in particular. Hopefully, it may also enable us to feel somewhat less confused about the range of contradictory views not only about the function of adolescence, but about the various pathologies encountered during adolescence and beyond.

I have not, in this presentation, made use of the classical psychiatric categories of disturbance or illness. Instead, I have tried to describe a developmental process and the breakdown which takes place in this process. This still enables us to define severity of interference or extent of pathology which is present. By placing pathology within a developmental model, it becomes possible to see what is going wrong, and it avoids seeing pathology as something static, unmoving, or simply as a classification. It also may enable us to begin to be more critical not only of our own efforts in work with adolescents, but also of the various explanations which exist about the nature of adolescent disturbance. There are some who, working with adolescents, hesitate to see certain forms of behavior as signs of pathology, preferring to view or assess some behavior as reflecting social or cultural change, or as a change in our attitudes to what is acceptable and what is pathological. But if we continue to ask, What is going on in the adolescent's present life and What is the future of this adolescent, then the narrowing of the gap between normality and pathology may be more difficult to accept.

REFERENCES

Blos, P. (1967). The second individuation process of adolescence. *Psychoanalytic Study of the Child* 22:162-186.

Freud, A. (1965). *Normality and Pathology in Childhood.* New York: International Universities Press.

Freud, S. (1905). Three essays on the theory of sexuality. *Standard Edition* 7:125-243. London: Hogarth, 1953.

—— (1912). Contributions to a discussion on masturbation. *Standard Edition* 12:239-254. London: Hogarth, 1958.

—— (1919). 'A child is being beaten.' *Standard Edition* 17:175-204. London: Hogarth, 1955.

Laufer, M. (1975). Preventive intervention in adolescence. *Psychoanalytic Study of the Child* 30:511-528.

—— (1976). The central masturbation fantasy, the final sexual organization, and adolescence. *Psychoanalytic Study of the Child* 31:297-316.

WILLIAM M. EASSON

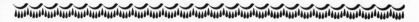

Carefree youth—or was it really so?

Adolescence is a period of growth and excitement, of pain and often of much sorrow. The anguish of the growing adolescent sometimes seems to be ignored by adults and is frequently not recognized by clinicians or helping professionals. Depression is a very common symptom in the teenager. Yet the literature on depression is limited and sometimes contradictory (Malmquist 1971). The standard textbooks in child and adolescent psychiatry do not mention depression or merely discuss the topic briefly, and then most often as preliminary to a discussion of suicide (Teicher 1973). There is no agreement on the clinical frequency of adolescent depression and statistics vary widely. Frommer (1968), in England, states that depressed children and adolescents constitute at least one-quarter of her child and adolescent clinic population, while Schachter (1971) comments that, in the 30,000 children and adolescents seen in his Marseilles clinic, depression is rarely diagnosed. Poluan and Cebiroglu (1972) noted that depression was the primary diagnosis in 4.5 percent of all teenagers seen in their Istanbul clinic in 1970 while Masterson (1967) found that 40 percent of his adolescent psychiatry outpatients were symptomatically depressed. Yet the average American or European teenager readily admits that depression occurs frequently in his peer group. High school counselors talk with concern about the depressed youngsters they see. Work supervisors know from repeated experience that their young workers get "down in the dumps." Why then is so little written about depression in adolescence?

Firstly, there is no predictable measure against which the effect of adolescent depression can be evaluated. During the adolescent decade, teenagers are constantly growing and changing. Since depression affects this growth and change by modifying the rate and degree of development, depression is usually manifested by what does not happen rather than by what happens. The depressed adolescent will temporarily grow and develop emotionally and intellectually at a slower rate. Sometimes, in retrospect, it is obvious that there was a developmental slowing, but it is impossible to gauge just how much an adolescent might have grown during a given period. Only when depression is very severe is the adolescent's emotional and intellectual growth stopped; rarely is depression severe enough that there is definite, recognizable regression in the teenager's psychological status.

Depression in adolescence may not be recognized because depression, like obsessive-compulsive neurosis, makes the adolescent more predictable, more tolerable, and thus, in many ways, more acceptable to adult society. A teenager who is quietly depressed gives less trouble. Challenge to adult authority is muted. Strivings for independence and emancipation are quieter or absent. Adults and teachers may note, "He is much nicer to be around now." When parents feel a sense of relief because their teenager is more manageable, this period of family quiet may have been bought only at the price of a teenage depression.

Depression may go undiagnosed because depression, or part of the depressive syndrome, occurs normally during adolescence (Anthony 1970). A pathological depression may be considered by the teenager and by those around to be merely a manifestation or exaggeration of normality. Only later will it be obvious that the depth of depression was not normal and the precipitating factors and the symptoms were more serious than was realized (Gallemore and Wilson 1972).

For an adolescent to admit openly that he is depressed is often felt strongly by the teenager and equally strongly by the adults around to mean that the adolescent is overly dependent or too childlike. Any admission of depression, of hurting, or of needing help is usually considered by a teenager to indicate, "I am weak."

Teenage depression may be undiagnosed because, when the adolescent admits or openly recognizes and shares the fact that he is depressed, this action in itself may go far to alleviate or to cure the depression. If a teenager trusts himself enough to admit his pain and trusts others enough to expose himself, the closeness and the resulting support that can develop may relieve the teenager's depression and provide a natural cure.

General Symptoms of Adolescent Depression

The effect of depression in the teenage years is similar to that in adult life but, in diagnosing adolescent depression, the clinician must always keep in mind the normal adolescent mood and behavior patterns and how this age-appropriate behavior might be affected by depression.

MOOD

When the adolescent is depressed, the teenager's emotional mood is low or, and this is most important, it is lower than the teenager's normal high emotional mood. Many adolescents live in a state of moderate hypomania, constantly active and energetic, always feeling, doing, and reacting. When measured against adult standards, a depressed youngster may appear merely normal or average. "She has become quite grown up." The adolescent affected by depression, however, recognizes that his mood level has been lowered.

SELF-ESTEEM AND SELF-CONCEPT

The depressed adolescent often views himself as bad, unacceptable, or inadequate. What the observer is likely to see are the adolescent's emotional defenses against this bad self-image and lowered self-esteem-denial, reaction formation, and action equivalents (Krakowski 1970). Frequently the teenager defends himself against this emotional pain by setting up distancing defenses.

The class clown may be putting on a false facade of gaiety to cover over his emotional uncertainty and self-doubt. As the teenage clown sometimes admits, "It is easier to make a fool of yourself; then the other teenagers will not tease and make a fool of you!" The adolescent who feels incompetent may overemphasize to himself and to the world that he really is competent by his rebellious behavior and pseudomaturity. When the adolescent feels inwardly bad or worthless, he may act out his anguish in aggressive delinquency (Martimor 1966). Drugs can give relief from the pain of depressive self-doubt or self-contempt. Marijuana may give a brief peace. Amphetamines will raise the mood temporarily. Heroin and cocaine can provide a short-lived euphoria. The depressed teenage girl who believes that she is unloved and unlovable can find a few moments of consolation in the arms of a male, and the next and the next, but the promiscuity that relieves her loneliness temporarily may do so only at the price of increasing self-contempt.

Unfortunately these emotional defenses often lead to alienation of the adolescent from sympathetic people, make it more difficult for the teenager to obtain the intimacy and support he needs, and frequently provoke punitive environmental responses (Cytryn and McKnew 1972).

PSYCHOMOTOR EFFECTS

As in adult depression, in adolescent depression drive is reduced and energy lowered. The quiet teenager, the model student, may in reality be the depressed adolescent. "It is so nice that she has settled down"—but she may be depressed. The depressed teenager finds it more difficult to concentrate. School or job failures may indicate that the adolescent is suffering from an underlying depression. Lack of energy is manifested outwardly by boredom, restlessness, and the inability to settle down (Toolan 1962). Intellectual and emotional growth-slowing often leads to further self-depreciation and perpetuates the cycle of depression (Torre and Rovera 1969, Hollon 1970). When the teenager recovers from an initial depressive episode, he may find himself so far behind his peers socially and intellectually that he becomes depressed anew.

SOMATIC MANIFESTATIONS OF DEPRESSION

As in adult depressed patients, frequently the reduced available energy and the bad self-image of the depressed adolescent are manifested outwardly in somatic symptoms.

Pain. When the depressed teenager feels continual emotional pain, this discomfort may be expressed in any form of somatic pain or ache. Headache, stomach ache, and dysmenorrhea may all be outward signs that the teenager is hurting psychologically. A pain that is unexplained, unduly prolonged, or not responsive to minor treatment procedures should be suspected as indicating depression.

Energy level. The reduced level of energy available to the depressed adolescent may manifest itself as constant tiredness. The depressed teenager "just lies around." The depressed adolescent girl may watch television all day. The youngster is feeling "the blahs." Life is dull and flat. Why bother? What's the use?

Eating variations. A depressed teenager can show appetite loss or even weight reduction. These symptoms may be a manifestation of a profound, pervasive, chronic depression. Since the adolescent may be normally a voracious eater, the depressed youngster may appear to be eating very well to adult eyes even though his appetite is reduced. Most often the depressed adolescent does not lose significant weight, but excessive weight loss is an ominous sign of severe depression. Some teenagers overeat during periods of depression: their resultant obesity may accentuate their feelings of ugliness and self-hatred and perpetuate their depression.

Sleeping. Sleep disturbance is a common sign of adolescent depression, but sleeping may be increased or decreased. Owing to his lack of energy, enthusiasm, and low self-esteem, the depressed adolescent often sleeps more and does less. It is more comfortable in bed. "There is nothing to get up for." "It is just another day."

Other depressed adolescents sleep less than normal but this reduction in sleeping time may go unrecognized. While parents are often upset when their adolescent boy or girl sits up at night listening to records or to television, they are usually much happier if the same teenager spends the late night hours reading. In truth, both the loud entertainment and the quiet reading may be outward signs that a depressed teenager cannot sleep and is filling the night hours.

Other somatic manifestations. In adolescence, elimination difficulties are usually late symptoms of severe depression. Encopresis even more than enuresis seems to be associated with depression in childhood or adolescence (Frommer 1968). Impotence also occurs as a manifestation of adolescent depression, but this is a very private symptom, rarely revealed and usually difficult to evaluate. Some adolescents say that it is possible to recognize a depressed adolescent by the condition of the teenager's skin— the dull sheen of the complexion, the worsening of the acne.

Social Manifestations of Depression

While many depressed adolescents tend to withdraw socially and to keep to themselves, others may gravitate towards peer groups of depressed teenagers. Depressed adolescents who feel bad, lonely, and inadequate can always find other teenagers who feel equally worthless. In a high school or college setting, it is sometimes possible to diagnose that a teenager has become depressed because he has started to associate with other teenagers who have already been recognized as feeling depressed, inadequate, or inferior. Sometimes the depressed adolescent acts out his inner pain by becoming part of an acting out peer group. He can join with other self-despising adolescents, and they can try to show that they are not really inadequate, inferior, or unmanly. The loners and the lost can together show the world. The pain of teenage depression can be acted out in group rebellion and destructiveness or manifested in shared drug-taking. As with any social group where the main relationship bond is pain, inadequacy, or maladaptation, such depressive peer groups tend to bind each other emotionally, to limit health-producing growth, and to perpetuate a depressive way of life (Chwast 1967).

Depressive Syndromes in Adolescence

Normal depressive-like states in adolescence recur as part of the normal teenage adjustment to physical and emotional growth. These depressive states are usually brief, do not interfere with the adolescent's overall development, or lead to emotional and intellectual stunting or distortion. The phase specific depressive-like states lack the full range of emotional and physical symptomatology seen in pathological depressions. During these temporary dysphoric episodes, the teenager does not experience a bad self-image or severely lowered self-esteem; in some instances the adolescent's self-image is enhanced even though he has other depressive symptoms.

The pathological adolescent depressive states tend to be longer lasting, chronic, or recurrent. These depressions produce slowed, distorted, or stopped emotional and intellectual growth. The depressed adolescent usually shows the physical and emotional manifestations of depression and typically maintains a bad self-image.

Normal Depressive States

EMANCIPATION MOURNING

Each developmental advance inevitably means something is left behind. Every new relationship widens the adolescent's intellectual and emotional horizon and, simultaneously, forces him to relinquish some relationships and the experiences formerly cherished (Lorand 1967). Now, there is no tooth fairy, no Easter bunny, and no Santa Claus, and all these were very warm and gratifying experiences. No longer can the teenage girl sit on Daddy's lap, because she is "too big"; Daddy and she used to have so much fun together and now it has changed. Growing teenagers mourn as their childhood leaves them with appropriate sadness, anger, and anxiety about the future.

In adolescence, the growing teenager must face and come to accept his self-reality. The physical reality—too tall, too short, too fat, or too thin—will not change very much and the teenager must live with it. The adolescent may have dreamt of being a movie star but now must accept the truth that the mirror shows. Is the nose too long and the hair too straight? Will those teeth never grow together and will they always protrude? The physical body takes its final adult shape; the teenager must accept this reality and mourn for what will never be.

During childhood, the growing youngster may have hoped for some cherished career, but adolescence may blight these hopes as the teenager comes to terms with the intelligence level at which he functions. The dreams, hopes, fantasies, and fears all meet reality during the adolescent years and for many adolescents this reality normally and naturally brings a time of sadness and mourning (Unwin 1970).

Over the years, many authors have commented about this period of mourning which occurs as the teenager integrates and adapts his ego ideals with the realities of his young adult self. This mourning process is usually very private and rarely shared, even with the peer group. In boys the emancipation mourning seems to occur primarily in the twelve- to fifteen-year period and somewhat earlier for girls. By mid-adolescence, the normal teenager should have worked through most of the adolescent maturation mourning and should have more comfortably accepted himself and his world.

In considering adolescent growth, usually the main family focus of emancipation is on the teenager's moving away from the parents. In reality, the parents often emancipate themselves from the adolescent rather than the adolescent from the parents. The adolescent may find himself pushed out of the family nest as father and mother begin to live their own lives. Many parents state openly, "We were glad to see the children grown up." Sometimes the parents withdraw from the growing teenager before the child is fully prepared emotionally for independence. This parental emancipation may leave the adolescent feeling lost and abandoned and may make the normal emancipation mourning more acute and temporarily more disabling.

NORMAL ENDOGENOUS DEPRESSIVE-LIKE STATES

Moodiness is a quality often attributed to the adolescent years. "It is just one of her days." "He woke up grouchy this morning." "She is feeling low." "He has the blues."

This moodiness of the teenage years seems to be most marked in early and mid-adolescence during the period of maximum physical growth and greatest hormonal readjustment—and of major separation and emancipation. These depressed and irritable moods are usually recognized by the teenager and those around him as transient emotions. Parents and teachers accept much of this moodiness as normal. Often it is stated—and quite correctly—"she will grow out of it, it is just a phase," but, as parents and teenagers will admit, teenage moodiness does make life more difficult for everyone.

The normal age-specific moodiness has many of the features of clinical depression. The adolescent feels emotionally sad and low, sometimes even to the point of weepiness. The moody adolescent is tired, listless, and unusually irritable. Sleep may be disturbed and early morning awakening is common. The adolescent girl who feels blue may stop eating; the moody, grouchy teenage boy may find it difficult to concentrate on his studies. For most teenagers, this moodiness, this normal, endogenous, depressive-like state clears spontaneously. Teachers do not refer these moody students for evaluation or treatment because they have seen many similar adolescents in high school. Since other adolescents know that "everyone goes through it," they are usually understanding and supportive until the teenager's moodiness clears. A typical episode of this normal moodiness lasts only for a few hours or days but, during this time, the teenager feels emotional pain and discomfort, and those around have to be tolerant and understanding.

Pathological Depression in Adolescence

ENDOGENOUS DEPRESSION

Moodiness is normal during the teenage years but sometimes a teenager's mood swings down and stays down so that the adolescent is emotionally and intellectually incapacitated by persistent depression. In pathological endogenous depression, the adolescent has recurrent depressive episodes during which the dysphoric mood may last for weeks or even months. These depressive swings may be demonstrably cyclic, unipolar or bipolar, and may appear and clear without obvious cause. The depressed adolescent usually does not seek help during the teenage years because he often considers these more pronounced mood swings as part of normal adolescence. The teenager knows that if he swings down, eventually he swings up. Often these teenagers attempt to relieve their nagging depression and, in these endogenous depressive states more than in other depressive syndromes, the adolescent is liable to self-medicate. When a teenager is feeling chronically low, he is apt to take a euphoria-producing drug. When the effect of these drugs wears off, the adolescent is liable to feel even more depressed and is more prone to take drugs again. In this way a drug-taking cycle is perpetuated and depressive symptoms are accentuated and sometimes made chronic.

Even though teenagers with persistent pathological endogenous depression often accept this depression as a normal part of their adolescence, these youngsters are likely to have friends or family members who are concerned and feel the adolescent should be helped (Olsen 1961, Berg et al. 1974). Classmates worry because a teenage friend is always "down in the dumps." Teachers note the adolescent's chronic tiredness and lack of appetite. The family physician treats the recurrent headaches and the dysmenorrhea symptomatically and is concerned about unexplained underlying factors. However, it is rare for a pathological endogenous depression to be recognized clinically or treated effectively in adolescence: this illness is usually diagnosed only in retrospect when these symptoms recur in adult life (de Ajuriaguerra 1970).

REACTIVE DEPRESSION

A reactive depression, at every stage of life, occurs as a pathological emotional response to loss. It is important to recognize that this is a psychological reaction to what the subject feels to be a loss, not merely to what people around see as a loss. In adolescence, each emancipation step inevitably brings emotional loss. Each growth toward new friends and new experiences usually means that some former relationships end. Every added responsibility and opportunity brings a new anxiety and a new loneliness.

It is easily recognized that an adolescent may develop a reactive depression following the loss of a meaningful or gratifying relationship. When the boyfriend is no longer interested, the neglected teenage girl is almost expected to become depressed. If the other adolescents do not want him on the team, the adolescent boy will disappoint his peers if he does not show sadness, anger, and some depression. A teenager frequently becomes depressed not because of the loss of existing reality, but due to the loss of a fantasy. When the hopes of the growing adolescent are dashed, sometimes the teenager becomes reactively depressed. He hoped to try out for the football squad, but the coach did not want him. She dreamed of being a cheerleader, but they did no even propose her name for the vote. He secretly wanted to become a radio engineer, but his grades were not good enough for technical school. Belittling adults, sometimes more than they appreciate, may undermine or destroy adolescent hopes and precipitate a reactive depression (Brandes 1970).

In the industrial nations, family mobility is an increasing part of life. Parental occupations and ambition necessitate frequent moves. When the family moves, the adolescent leaves behind a familiar home, a comfortable bedroom, established friends, and a predictable school environment. With the move, the teenager loses much that was familiar, warm, and comfortable, and after this move, he may become reactively and understandably depressed.

Handicapped adolescents seem to be more vulnerable to a disabling reactive depression because they have a special problem in accepting themselves. The retarded child will have had additional growth burdens during the preadolescent years, but the intellectually handicapped teenager must face the full, final meaning of his retardation (Glaser 1967). Parents and teachers cannot now protect the retarded adolescent who has to come to a personal and emotional acceptance of his own self-reality and unique self-potential. The sadness and the mourning of these handicapped adolescents may be more acute and severe than the nonhandicapped teenager and may persist in a disabling reactive depression, handicapping their growth and adaptation even further.

The epileptic teenager, the diabetic adolescent, and other growing youngsters with chronic illnesses must accept their illness as they plan their independent role in society. The chronically ill teenager often has to work through a period of bitterness and self-recrimination as he struggles over his continued need to take pills or have injections. Because of a chronic illness, the adolescent may be unable to participate in social and athletic activities in school. The epileptic teenager may have to face the fact that he cannot get a driver's license. The adolescent with a heart defect is often forbidden to participate in sports. The rage, the bitterness, the sadness, and the mourning that the chronically ill teenager has to face and work through can lead to a reactive depression with a wide range of depressive symptoms that further complicate the management of his physical illness. Chronically ill adolescents may also have to face the fact that they are very successful invalids, but rather inadequate in other social roles. Invalidism or persistent depression may be an easier life style that could persist to become a pattern of adult character.

As the adolescent matures, parents are also getting older and sometimes die. If a father or mother dies during the emancipation struggle between the teenager and the parent, the adolescent will be left with a great deal of unresolved guilt. Adolescents want parents to provide the continued stability and security of a home during the teenage years. When adolescents become adults, parents should then be their closest friends and companions. Teenagers need parents to give that final appreciation. When parents die, adolescent children usually feel a profound loss and deprivation and may become severely reactively depressed.

When an adolescent's emotional loss is recognized by others, the teenager's depression is more likely to be recognized also. However, it must be emphasized that a reactive depression develops as a pathological response to what is felt by the adolescent as a loss. Since the loss is frequently private and very personal, the adolescent may have to live through a persistent, unrecognized, but disabling reactive depression until, by his own strength and the passage of time, the symptoms are relieved.

ANHEDONIC OR PLEASURELESS DEPRESSIONS

"I have nothing to live for."

There are adolescents emancipated enough to be emotionally independent but who, when they observe themselves and evaluate their life situation realistically, decide they have nothing to live for. After logical, sensible consideration, these teenagers recognize that there is little pleasure for them in continuing to live. When they ask themselves, "What is the use?" of their existence, they can honestly find no purpose (Walters 1970, Pokorny, Kaplan, and Tsai 1975). These adolescents are sufficiently emancipated to be sure of their independence, but they recognize that their existence is emotionally sterile, that their family relationships are shallow and unrewarding, and that they themselves are emotionally and intellectually inadequate. To the honest unbiased observer, these adolescents may be absolutely correct in their self-evaluation (Hendin 1975).

With adolescent emancipation, these teenagers may be forced to recognize realities denied or hidden during their childhood. Parental unavailability or malevolence becomes more obvious. Parents who have been severely traumatized themselves may have found it difficult to trust and be trusted: they have been emotionally unavailable to their growing children who, then, in adolescence must face the meagerness of their own self-trust and the lack of emotional nourishment in their attenuated family relationships. With emancipation, the adolescent has to face persistent and unchangeable personal inadequacies. Social and academic deprivations and handicaps may be insurmountable (Masterson 1970).

When an adolescent emancipates emotionally to face this kind of cheerless reality, he may decide, with resignation and with minimal or no anxiety, that life is indeed not worth living. The suicidal potential of these anhedonic teenagers is very high, even though their depressive symptoms may be minimal. Their internal and external emotional barriers to suicide are lacking. In a very deliberate fashion, pleasureless teenagers can plan to end their ungratifying and hopeless existence.

Since adolescents in an anhedonic state may show few or no outward signs of depression, the first indication of their pleasureless existence may be an attempted or successful suicide.

Pat, a sixteen-year-old boy, was admitted to a general hospital in a deeply comatose state. When he was twelve years old, after two seizures, he was diagnosed as having grand mal epilepsy and, at that time, he was started on anticonvulsant medication. He had been the outstanding athlete in his school class, but he was forbidden to participate in athletics by his physician and this prohibition was maintained, even though he had no further seizures. Pat had an average intelligence level but, with hard work, he had maintained "A" and "B" rankings in his school subjects, much to the pleasure of his mother. By eleventh grade, however, he was finding the school work more difficult and, in the year prior to his suicide attempt, his school grades had slipped to the "C" or "D" level.

Pat's father had always been emotionally distant and was usually away from home, working on some business project. His mother, a chronically ineffective woman, was easily moved to tears and tore her clothes when she was upset. Just two weeks prior to the patient's suicide attempt, his brother had left home to join the Navy; Pat had no other siblings. This sixteen-year-old teenager swallowed anticonvulsant medication that he had collected over several months, and his suicide attempt would have been successful without very intensive treatment measures. When he recovered consciousness, the adolescent still stated, without obvious anxiety, "I have nothing to live for. Why did you not let me die?"

ANACLITIC DEPRESSION IN ADOLESCENCE

When an individual, child, adolescent, or adult, loses a relationship that provides both essential emotional gratification and necessary external support, an anaclitic depression is likely to occur. In an anaclitic depression, there are symptoms both of loss reaction and of personality

268

overload. Owing to the loss of an important gratification, there is a profound mourning reaction or a reactive depression, and since the lost relationship also provided support necessary for decision-making and for direction, the subject is unable to cope and is emotionally overwhelmed. The younger and less mature a child is, the more prone is the youngster to develop an anaclitic depression due to relationship loss. Spitz (1946) first described anaclitic depressions in infants separated from the mothering adult. Pediatricians are likely to see anaclitically depressed patients in the young preschool children who are hospitalized in an emergency crisis. However, anaclitic depression can occur at every stage throughout life where there is a loss of a relationship that is both gratifying and supportive (Blatt 1974).

Many of the symptoms of the anaclitic depressive syndrome occur briefly and to a minor degree during normal adolescent emancipation. The adolescent's awareness of his own inadequacies and of his need for other people pushes him to grow emotionally and to reach out to others. Sometimes, due to internal or external pressures, adolescents emancipate too early and give up relationships necessary for gratification, decision-making, and direction. Parents may emancipate from the teenager and leave the youngster before he is able to cope or make the necessary substitute friends.

Where a preadolescent has been unusually protected or gratified emotionally, the youngster may have never developed the necessary emotional strengths for emancipation: such a child may be emotionally unable "to go it alone." The "special" child may have had the most gratifying relationships during the first decade of life, but this gratification and this additional external support may have led to emotional dependence rather than independence.

Anaclitic depression, at any age, is a syndrome combining the reactions of inability and of loss. Usually the symptoms of emotional overload are more obvious. The teenager experiencing an anaclitic depressive reaction acutely feels an inability to cope. His anxiety mounts swiftly and rises into panic and, if the panic is not relieved, the youngster becomes emotionally overwhelmed and decompensates. In addition to this overload reaction, the anaclitically depressed adolescent is responding also to a loss of gratification with mourning, sadness, and, in some cases, deep pervasive depression. Usually these depressive symptoms are less obvious than the more prominent signs of personality overload but, once the adolescent is given enough support to reintegrate emotionally, the loss reaction may then become more apparent and the teenager will become sad, weepy, depressed, and complaining of physical discomforts.

John was a sixteen-year-old boy who had spent all of his life on a small family farm in rural Appalachia. He attended the local school and had never been more than twenty miles away from home. He was a bright adolescent with a fine command of words and, much to his parents' pride and his own satisfaction, he won a state essay competition. As part of the essay prize, he was invited to spend one week at the state university, where he would join with other prize winners in visiting university facilities, participating in group discussions, and in seeing the entertainment of the big city.

So, early in the summer, the young man found himself lodged in the university dormitory. Since it was the academic vacation, there were few people around and he had a room all to himself. No one noted anything amiss but, two days after his arrival, John was found curled up on his bed, crying quietly and refusing to talk. Initially it was thought that he had suffered a stroke. In reality he was showing the symptoms of an acute anaclitic depression.

John had never been away from home. He was totally unprepared for these sudden new demands placed on him. He missed his family and his friends, and he did not know how to relate to these outwardly sophisticated teenagers he was meeting. He was homesick, lost, unable to cope, and was overwhelmed eventually. When the patient's anaclitic depression was recognized, his family was invited to join him and, twenty-four hours after their arrival, he was recovered sufficiently to participate, albeit somewhat awkwardly, in the remaining activities.

Adolescents emancipating into a new culture or unfamiliar social environment are especially vulnerable to the development of an anaclitic depressive reaction. Youngsters bussed to schools in different neighborhoods may temporarily find themselves without a rewarding identity in their new society or without readily available gratification or rewards when they have left their familiar childhood surroundings. Since these youngsters have often greater than normal adolescent pride and are unwilling to admit defeat, they may mature to more absolute emancipation and self-sufficiency at the risk of increasing emotional isolation and personality overload—which can lead to anaclitic depression.

WILLIAM M. EASSON

Symptomatic Depression

DEPRESSIVE SYMPTOMS OCCURRING IN THE COURSE OF OTHER EMOTIONAL DISORDERS

In schizophrenia, depression may be a prominent symptom at the onset of the psychosis. Where disturbing thoughts are intruding and emotional control is loosening, a frightened, despairing teenage patient may become profoundly reactively depressed. As the psychosis develops, primitive angers and uncontrolled self-hate can intrude into awareness, leading to a pervasive, depressive state. As part of an established schizophrenic illness, a psychotic adolescent may have obvious depressive symptoms.

Not infrequently, depression may occur during the recovery phases from a schizophrenic episode (Hoedemaker 1970, McGlashan and Carpenter 1976). As the psychotic adolescent develops better reality contact, he is obliged to face his emotional awkwardness, his social isolation, and the residual handicaps of the psychotic illness. The schizophrenic youngster has to mourn the fact that he will never completely make up for those teenage experiences he missed during the time of his psychosis. Sometimes a depressive reaction is the first major sign that an adolescent is recovering from a schizophrenic illness and is now beginning to face a sad, bitter depressing reality.

DRUG INDUCED OR DRUG RELEASED DEPRESSION

Many chronic adolescent drug abusers use drugs to turn themselves on and off emotionally. After months or years of drug usage, the teenager loses the normal adolescent ability to feel awe and ecstasy without drugs. The chronic drug user may give up drugs only to find that his emotional existence is bland and barren. Frequently, these former drug users seem emotionally shallow. They do not have the natural vitality or enthusiasm of young adults, they have become emotionally stunted, and they no longer can generate excitement from within themselves. When an adolescent realizes that he has lost the ability to "turn on" normally and has only himself to blame, his flattened affect may become more depressed.

DEPRESSIVE MANIFESTATIONS OF PHYSICAL ILLNESS

Depression may be a reaction to the emotional stress of a physical illness or a specific manifestation of that illness (King 1972). Viral illnesses,

271

especially, seem to produce depressive symptoms that often last months after the physical manifestations of the illness have cleared. The teenager convalescing from infectious mononucleosis, hepatitis, or other viral infections may find himself unusually low emotionally, weepy, unable to concentrate and tired beyond what would be expected due to the physical illness itself.

Treatment

Depression in adolescence is frequently caused by many interacting factors. Depressive syndromes overlap and change from one type to another. A reactive depression in adolescence often has major anaclitic aspects or may be superimposed on an endogenous depression. Treatment must be directed toward the causative factors and must be modified as these change during the treatment process.

A therapeutic program should be directed especially toward those aspects of the teenager's illness that are disabling or handicapping his growth. Many adolescents will only accept or tolerate treatment for problems that are causing them pain. Though the clinician may feel that other aspects of the teenager's depression are more critical, the adolescent may be unwilling to participate more fully in the suggested treatment program. As with any adolescent illness, the physician treats what can be treated, whatever the adolescent allows.

In America and the Western European countries, antidepressants are most likely to be used with depressed teenagers where the endogenous or constitutional factors are prominent in the depressive syndrome. In Eastern European countries and the Soviet Union, antidepressants are used much more extensively and for a wider range of depressive syndromes. In most countries, the tricyclic antidepressants would be the drugs of choice in treating teenagers. While manifestations of adolescent depression seem similar in adolescents around the world, treatment centers place different emphasis on diagnostic and treatment criteria. Thus it is often difficult to judge how effective different procedures are in the management of teenage depression.

With depressed adult patients, it is sometimes unclear whether the symptomatic relief of depression is due to natural improvement or to the medication. In the adolescent years, it is even more difficult to gauge the therapeutic effect of medication, but it does seem that tranquilizing and sedative drugs are likely to deepen or perpetuate the depressive mood. Psychotherapy is beneficial in all depressive syndromes, but seems to be most beneficial where reactive or environmental factors are prominent

(Feinstein 1975). Where the teenager's depression is primarily anaclitic in nature, treatment must be planned to give a combination of strong support and supportive psychotherapy. Without adequate emotional support, the anaclitically depressed patient is liable to continue so disabled by anxiety that the concomitant depression cannot be treated.

The treatment for an anhedonic depression in adolescence and, at any stage of life, is simply to help the patient to get something, someone, anything that makes life worth living. If the teenage patient does not find some purpose in his existence, the anhedonic state will continue and the possibility of suicide will be always present. Where depression is symptomatic of other physical or emotional illnesses, it is essential, first of all, to treat the underlying illness. Frequently, this treatment will result in the alleviation of the depressive symptoms but, if these symptoms continue, specific antidepressant or psychotherapeutic treatment should be prescribed.

NATURAL CURE

With the normally high teenage energy and the usual adolescent emotional flexibility, there is a strong potential for natural cure in most teenage emotional disorders (Unwin 1970). The clinician must be very careful that he does not unnecessarily make an adolescent into a patient. Anthony (1970) points out the adolescent's increased ability for self-therapy. The normal adolescent growth process may produce a cure for teenage depression, especially if external demands and stresses can be reduced. In the management of adolescent depressive syndromes, often the most important aspect of treatment is the lowering of external stresses. With no further specific treatment, the normal teenage growth drive sometimes allows the adolescent to develop additionally adequate emotional strengths and sufficient capacity to deal with depression, both endogenous and exogenous in origin.

Conclusions

Depression, a very common symptom during adolescence, may be a manifestation of age-appropriate adjustment, or an indication of disabling psychiatric illness. Severe adolescent depression is frequently undiagnosed or is often considered to be merely a temporary phase-specific reaction. Pathological depression can severely incapacitate a teenager and lead to adolescent suicide or may cause residual life-long psychological stunting or maladaptation. Normal depressive-like states and pathological depressive syndromes in adolescence are described and the appropriate treatment is discussed.

REFERENCES

Anthony, E. J. (1970). Two contrasting types of adolescent depression and their treatment. *Journal of the American Psychoanalytic Association* 18:841-859.

———— (1970). Self-therapy in adolescence. *This Annual* 3: 6-24.

Berg, I., Hullin, R., Allsopp, M., O'Brien, P., and MacDonald, R. (1974). Bipolar manic-depressive psychosis in early adolescence: a case report. *British Journal of Psychiatry* 125: 416-417.

Blatt, S. J. (1974). Levels of object representation in anaclitic and introjective depression. *Psychoanalytic Study of the Child* 29: 107-157.

Brandes, N. S. (1970). A discussion of depression in children and adolescents. *Clinical Pediatrics* 10: 470-475.

Chwast, J. (1967). Depressive reactions as manifested among adolescent delinquents. *American Journal of Psychotherapy* 21: 575-584.

Cytryn, L., and McKnew, D. H. (1972). Proposed classification of childhood depression. *American Journal of Psychiatry* 129: 149-155.

de Ajuriaguerra, J. (1970). La psychose maniaco-depressive. In *Psychiatrie de l'Enfant*. Paris: Masson et Cie.

Feinstein, S. (1975). Adolescent depression. E. J. Anthony and T. Benedek, eds., *Depression and Human Existence*. Boston: Little, Brown.

Frommer, E. A. (1968). Depressive illness in childhood. A. Coppen and A. Walk, eds., *Recent Developments in Affective Disorders*, Chapter X, pp. 117-136. *British Journal of Psychiatry*: Special Publication II.

Gallemore, J. L., and Wilson, W. P. (1972). Adolescent maladjustment or affective disorder? *American Journal of Psychiatry* 129: 608-612.

Glaser, K. (1967). Masked depression in children and adolescents. *American Journal of Psychotherapy* 21: 565-574.

Hendin, H. (1975). Growing up dead: student suicide. *American Journal of Psychotherapy* 29: 327-338.

Hoedemaker, F. S. (1970). Psychotic episodes and postpsychotic depression in young adults. *American Journal of Psychiatry* 127: 606-610.

Hollon, T. H. (1970). Poor school performance as a symptom of masked depression in children and adolescents. *American Journal of Psychotherapy* 25: 258-263.

King, L. J. (1972). Affective syndromes in normal young people. *Diseases of the Nervous System* 33: 736-741.

Krakoswski, A. J. (1970). Depressive reactions of childhood and adolescence. *Psychosomatics* 11: 429-433.

Lorand, S. (1967). Adolescent depression. *International Journal of Psychoanalysis* 48: 53-60.

McGlashan, T. H., and Carpenter, W. T. (1976). An investigation of the postpsychotic depressive syndrome. *American Journal of Psychiatry* 133: 14-19.

Malmquist, C. P. (1971). Depressions in childhood and adolescence. *New England Journal of Medicine* 284: 887-893, 955-961.

Martimor, E. (1966). Contribution a l'etude medico-psychologique du vol; les etats depressifs. *Annals Medico-Psychology* 2: 635-643.

Masterson, J. F. (1967). *The Psychiatric Dilemma of Adolescence*. Boston: Little, Brown.

—— (1970). Depression in the adolescent character disorder. *Proceedings of the American Psychopathological Association* 59: 242-257.

Olsen, T. (1961). Follow-up study of manic-depressive patients whose first attack occurred before the age of 19. *Acta Psychologica Scandanavia* 37: 45-52.

Pokorny, A. D., Kaplan, H. B., and Tsai, S. Y. (1975). Hopelessness and attempted suicide: a reconsideration. *American Journal of Psychiatry* 132: 954-956.

Poluan, O., and Cebiroglu, R. (1972). Treatment with psychopharmacologic agents in childhood depression. A. A. Annell, ed., *Depressive States in Childhood and Adolescence*. Stockholm, Sweden: Almquist and Wiksell.

Schacheter, M. (1971). Etude des depressions et des episodes depressifs chez l'enfant et l'adolescent. *Acta Paedopsychiatrica* 38: 191-201.

Spitz, R. (1946). Anaclitic depression. *Psychoanalytic Study of the Child* 2: 313-342.

Teicher, J. D. (1973). A solution to the chronic problem of living: adolescent attempted suicide. J. C. Schoolar, ed., *Current Issues in Adolescent Psychiatry*. New York: Brunner/Mazel.

Toolan, J., (1962). Depression in children and adolescents. *American Journal of Orthopsychiatry* 32: 404-415.

Torre, M., and Rovera, G. G. (1969). Aspects de l'insuffisance scolaire dans les etats depressifs de la preadolescence. *Acta Paedopsychiatrica* 36: 346-351.

Unwin, J. R. (1970). Depression in alienated youth. *Canadian Psychiatric Journal* 15: 83-86.

Walters, P. A. (1970). Depression. *International Psychiatric Clinics* 7: 169-179.

17] SCHIZOPHRENIA IN ADOLESCENCE

PHILIP S. HOLZMAN AND ROY R. GRINKER, Sr.

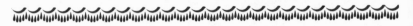

Most investigators agree that seventeen is the high-risk age for the onset of schizophrenic psychoses. Although occurring among younger children, it is the adult form that is the most prevalent. Moreover, it is striking that the age of visible onset varies very little across national boundaries. Middle and late adolescence seem to coincide with a marked increase in the incidence of schizophrenic psychoses, at least as measured by the number of first admissions per year to mental hospitals (Mayer-Gross, Slater, and Roth 1969). We are making here a clear distinction between schizophrenia on the one hand, and schizophrenic psychosis or overt schizophrenia on the other hand. The former describes a long-standing pattern of withdrawal, general apathy, poor object-relationship, and peculiar and even disorganized thinking, with occasional impulsive, antisocial acts but without hallucinations or delusions. The latter denotes a severance of reality constraints with many secondary features of psychosis, such as delusions and hallucinations in a setting that is otherwise schizophrenic and of neither organic nor cyclic-affective etiology. Statistical data from both the United States and the United Kingdom, as Table 1 shows, indicate that at the younger ages more males than females enter hospitals with schizophrenic psychosis, and it is only after age thirty-five that the ratio shifts. The age-specific rate rises from about 1 per 100,000 under fifteen years to about 25 per 100,000 between ages fifteen and twenty-four. Table 2, which shows the cross-national relative rates of first admissions, dramatically underscores the constancy of the picture internationally.

Reprinted from the *Journal of Youth and Adolescence,* Volume 3 Number 4, 1974. Copyright 1974, Plenum Press.

TABLE 1

**Admission Rate for Schizophrenia in England and
Wales in 1960 (from Mayer-Gross, Slater, and Roth 1969, p. 239)**

Age Group	Annual Admission Rate Per Million		Sex Ratio M/F
	M	F	
10 to	11	13	0.87
15 to	247	224	1.18
20 to	348	283	1.46
25 to	403	350	1.15
35 to	254	275	0.95
45 to	119	195	0.58
55 to	70	139	0.48
65 to	30	84	0.42
75 plus	23	68	0.38

TABLE 2

**Relative Rates of First Admissions for Schizophrenia to Mental Hospitals by Age:
United States (1964), England and Wales (1960), Czechoslovakia (1963), Denmark
(1961), Victoria, Australia (1962). (From Yolles and Kramer 1969).**

Age	United States	England & Wales	Czechoslovakia	Denmark	Victoria, Australia
15	8	3	7	2	3
15-24	148	171	156	137	108
25-34	217	216	189	208	187
35-44	171	152	180	137	193
45-54	103	01	102	112	126
55-64	55	61	60	104	67
65 & Over	12	34	28	67	73

What factors can account for the clear emergence of overt schizophrenic illness during adolescence? Are adolescence and schizophrenia unrelated to each other, and is their coincidence therefore attributable to chance factors? Is schizophrenia a disorder that, like Huntington's chorea, occurs at a particular age because of the time necessary for its inexorable "incubation"? Is adolescence a pathogenic agent—an intrinsic factor—which potentiates or triggers schizophrenia? Or do the social demands of adolescence—extrinsic factors—precipitate schizophrenia in a person who is vulnerable to that disorder? Will a vulnerable person manifest symptoms because social demands have begun to intrude significantly on the growing adolescent?

This chapter examines these possibilities and draws upon data from an ongoing study[1] of young adult schizophrenic patients to attempt, after first considering the nature of adolescence and schizophrenia, a resolution of these questions. We believe that our data support the hypothesis that adolescence imposes severe demands for social, interpersonal, and intrapersonal competence on the biologically and psychologically vulnerable adolescent. These demands seriously challenge him, thus precipitating retreat from the development of competence into psychopathology.

The Nature of Adolescence

Although there is a tendency in common usage to elide the two, it is helpful to distinguish puberty from adolescence. Puberty is a biologically unfolding maturational phase of development that consists in hormonal shifts and results in the appearance and development of secondary sex characteristics. The age of onset varies from one geographic region to another, but generally in girls puberty begins at about ten to twelve years with the onset of breast growth, appearance of pubic hair, and the beginning of menstruation; in boys puberty begins at about eleven to fourteen years, with the enlargement of the penis and testicles, growth of pubic hair, and the occurrence of ejaculation. These changes bring with them psychological adaptations principally in awareness of sexual and sensual feelings within one's own body, an awareness of one's changed physical appearance, an awkwardness felt in the new bodily changes, feelings of shame, guilt, and concern over measuring up to cultural ideals of appearance and behavior.

Adolescence, on the other hand, may be viewed as a culturally defined stage of transition in roles from childhood to adulthood. The age of onset, as with puberty, varies from culture to culture, but in the case of adolescence, it is initiated by cultural rather than biological events. The principal characteristic of adolescence is a shift from childhood dependence to adult independence, from demanding of others to being demanded of, from being provided for to providing for. This transition involves a movement from the nuclear family to a new and different primary group. Ties with one's own family must be severed as the fledgling adult begins to develop skills in working and loving. Attention turns from caring for oneself to caring for one's mate, one's offspring, and one's social and cultural milieu. The onset of adolescence is more or less indicated by the already developed biological markers of puberty. The end of adolescence which merges into young adulthood is even more highly individual and indefinite. It has no specific age, no biological marker, and may continue far into what, chronologically, we call adulthood.

Cultures differ in the demands they place upon young adults as well as in the degree to which they ease the young into adult roles. Thus, the behavioral manifestations of adolescence vary from one culture to another. That which seems to be constant, however, is the fact of resistance to or ambivalence over changing roles, a resistance that may be experienced more or less consciously, depending upon the sanctions of the society and of the times. In contemporary Western culture, adolescents express their ambivalence over assuming new adult roles by rebelliousness, sullen negativism, zealous compliance, asceticism, overintellectuality, regressive passivity, and others. Society, in its demands for a new generation to assume early responsibilities, has disrupted the adaptations of childhood and strained those aspects of psychological organization that must now be mobilized.

Most adolescents manage to endure the bodily changes of puberty. They grow psychologically into their new bodies; mental maturity gradually becomes congruent with sexual maturity; acne clears; and awkwardness gives way to modicum of grace. But the social and psychological demands of adolescence place a different quality of strain upon the youth. These behavioral demands occur several years after the onset of puberty, generally in the first post-high school year. It is then, particularly in the middle classes, that the youth begins to separate himself from his nuclear family, leaves home either for work or higher education, begins to form his own family, and incurs the myriad expectations that society requires one to fulfill. This phase of development is not without its psychological consequences, and few young people leave it without experiencing forms of loneliness, anxiety, fear, challenge, elation, or thrust. Responses of clinical anxiety, despair, and depression are not infrequent.

As Erikson (1974) formulated it:

279

In youth you find out what you *care to do* and who you *care to be*—even in changing roles. In young adulthood you learn whom you *care to be with*—at work and in private life, not only exchanging intimacies, but sharing intimacy. In adulthood, however, you learn to know what and whom you can *take care of.*

Psychoanalytic observers have typically regarded adolescence as, intrinsically, a time of turmoil and imbalance, a developmental period which occasions the revival of earlier conflicts that reproduce oedipal struggles, and oral and anal concerns. It is the revival of these conflicts in sufficient strength that leads to their resolution by disengagement from the nuclear family. The adolescent struggles against accepting the support his family offers while feeling that he needs that support. His increased fantasying activity includes an exaggeration of his own capacities. This grandiosity can be both a source of comfort and of disillusionment when reality probes the unrealistic aspects of the fantasy. The adolescent finds additional comfort and solace in temporary identifications of himself with figures outside the home, some of which are congruent with his own and his family's previous ideals and some of which are polar opposites. Psychoanalytic investigators, moreover, have shown that the psychological nature of these struggles tends to become concretized. Fantasies of engagement and disengagement with people are regarded as real, to be acquired, exploded, or hoarded. Feelings for others can be pierced, or they may be engulfed, poisoned, or paralyzed by them. Although these are metaphoric ways of speaking about internal mental states, they are also feelings in the adolescent who must contend with such issues.

But psychoanalytic insights have been based on studies of adolescents who experience intense conflict and whose pain has motivated them to seek professional help. Some others have sought help because of a prolongation of adolescent struggles and because they required more time and additional help in maturing to adult responsibilities. Is the intensity of the struggles of these young people representative of that of the entire population of adolescents? Although the indepth scrutiny made possible by the unique psychoanalytic interview is not available for general populations surveys, several studies of normal adolescents—of those who have not sought clinical help—emphasize the continuity between childhood and adulthood. They suggest that the disruptive and disjunctive patterns of disturbed adolescents may not be at all typical, and that the pathological degrees of anxiety, negativism, rebelliousness, isolation, asceticism, may not be inevitable in adolescence but rather predictable from the quality of earlier patterns of coping with adversity, stress, and challenge. The family, regarded by many adolescents-in-turmoil and by some of their healers as noxious, may actually provide a supportive relationship to the adolescent, representing a positive factor. Studies of normal development to which we refer are the Berkeley (Block 1971), Cambridge (Vaillant 1971), Haverford (Heath 1965), and Chicago (Grinker, Grinker, and Timberlake 1962, Offer and Offer 1973) studies.

In the Berkeley study, Block evaluated longitudinal data on 171 subjects. The data included school grades, teachers' reports, interviews, ratings of social behavior, and many psychological test scores. Results show that a number of subjects remained relatively stable while others changed a good deal between their high school years and adulthood. Yet even in the most extreme changers, continuity is evident. Male "nonchangers" seemed to be self-confident, quick, resourceful, and vigorous in contrast to the male "changers" who seemed to be dependent, unsure of themselves, tense, and guarded. For females, however, the "changers" seemed to be the ones who were assertive, competent, and eager to chart their own independent destinies. Incidence of psychopathology in this group of 171 was extraordinarily small.

At Haverford, Heath studied a number of "mature" and "immature" students and did longitudinal assessments of them for several years. Although most students showed periods of disorganization and instability when first confronted with the novelty of college life, most settled into a stable and autonomous life. Although the majority of the young people in Heath's sample experienced regressive periods of disorganization, most of them emerged without permanent psychopathological handicaps.

Vaillant studied 240 persons by interview and questionnaire methods at two-year intervals over a period of thirty years. The subjects, chosen in 1940 while they were college sophomores, were presumed psychologically and physically healthy, to be more intelligent, more verbal, in better physical health, and better motivated for achievement than the average college student. Continuity of defensive behavior was the principal focus. Vaillant's periodic interviews may be compared with time lapse photography, as they present in a short interval the major shifts in style of defense which took place over thirty years.

The conceptual scheme in which Vaillant's group viewed defense takes the form of a hierarchy. The first level, containing psychotic denial, distortion, and delusion, he labeled *narcissistic*. These defenses are discernible in healthy persons prior to the age of five, and in adults they continue to appear in primary-process formations such as dreams and fantasies, functioning to alter an unbearable reality. The second level, called *immature defenses* and containing projection, schizoid fantasying, hypochondriasis, acting out, and passive-aggressive behavior, appears in healthy persons from age thirteen to late adolescence, functioning to alter distressing affects that attend threats of object loss. The third level, or *neurotic defenses*, contains intellectualization and related mechanisms of repression, displacement, reaction formation, and dissociation or neurotic denial. These seem characteristic of healthy people from the age of three through life, functioning to alter "private feelings or instinctual expression." The highest level, labeled *mature defenses*, are common in healthy persons from puberty through life. These defenses—altruism, humor, suppression, sublimation, and anticipation—are based on mature cognitive functions and include sophisticated identifications with appropriate objects.

The long follow-up period made it possible to discern continuity and structure in behavior. Data on thirty subjects suggest that whether a person employs immature or mature defenses separates the subjects into poor and good life adjustment groups, although all subjects showed liberal use of neurotic defenses. Continuity could be discerned in a reliance on mature and immature defenses. Severe psychopathology did not contravene in a setting of mature adaptation. The intervention of severe life stresses, however, could force a reliance on progressively less adaptive defensive patterns from which recovery was probable with an abatement of the stress.

In the Chicago project, Grinker et al. studied eighty male students (and later a second group of fifty-four of a small midwestern college. They determined that these young men of average intelligence and lower middle-class origins reported little adolescent turbulence, although there was some increase in conflict with their parents during adolescence. They called this group of subjects *homoclites* in order to characterize their general conformity. Only six of the eighty showed some mildly deviant characteristics in the form of tendencies to act out and mild bitterness of outlook or shyness. Generally, however, these men experienced their adolescent transitions as smooth. They displayed good physical health from childhood on. Birth and pregnancy complications were minimal or absent. They reported positive, affectionate, and warm relationships with both parents, and experienced continual communication with them. Sociability, general contentment in a setting of striking conventionality were typical. A follow-up of these subjects fifteen years later shows that none had experienced psychological disorganization serious enough to warrant hospitalization or a visit to a mental health worker (Grinker and Werble 1974). The rather good adjustment, absence of psychopathology, freedom from serious social and work failures that characterized the "homoclites" in 1958 remain typical of them fifteen years later.

These qualities of normal adolescents were also described by Offer and Offer (1973) who studied eighty-four high school students over several years. Less than fifteen percent of the group dropped out of college, but half of these returned to school after working for one year. The Offers described three "routes" through adolescence: (1) Continuous growth. Those in this group—about 23 percent of the total population—seemed to be the steadiest, most adaptable of the subjects. (2) Surgent growth. These subjects showed some significant incidence of crises, with a slight tendency to react with mild depression. Yet these subjects never lost sight of their long-range goals. About 35 percent of the total group showed this quality of growth. (3) Tumultuous growth. The adolescents in this group were those who reacted to external trauma as if it were "a major tragic event." Separation from the family was an important issue and self-confidence was not well established. About 21 percent of the total group were so classified. The Offers' conclusions emphasized that turmoil and pathology do not define the adolescent period, although periods of disruptive behavior do occur.

These studies suggest that adolescence is not an intrinsically pathogenic period. Although some turmoil is discernible, there is no indication of major disruptions in young persons whose earlier behavior was not deviant. All of these studies of normal adolescence emphasized that there are many styles of adaptation and only a small number of these predict later psychopathology. The emphasis, however, is on the fact that the tasks of adolescence demand social and interpersonal, motor and intellectual competence. They do not demand high degrees of skill in any particular area, but they do require a nidus of competence in most of these areas, for genuine emancipation from one's nuclear family is built upon revision, modulation, flexible acceptance of adversity, and a mastery of opportunities. Just as adolescence does not produce pathology, it does not produce competence. But given a previously competent child, the tasks of adolescence will be mastered well, even though temporary regressions will be encountered.

Some Aspects of the Schizophrenias

Since 1970 we have studied young adults who have suffered a psychotic episode diagnosed as schizophrenic. In an earlier report (Grinker and Holzman 1973), we detailed one aspect of our studies and focused on the clinical examination, via a semistructured interview. From the tape recordings of these interviews our research team rated a number of aspects of the patient's functioning. Five features of these young adult schizophrenic patients emerged with some prominence. The first was their striking difficulty in maintaining what we called "organizational coherence," or an inability to keep percepts and ideas from disorder, fluidity, and disorganization. Even in periods of remission this quality of organizational instability was noteworthy. The second was the patient's prominent pleasureless demeanor, a quality of affect referred to by Rado (1956) as "anhedonia." The third feature was an excessive dependency of these patients on their families, hospital staff, and therapists. The fourth feature was the absence of definitive evidence of general competence; patients achieved less in school, jobs, and social life than one would have expected solely on the basis of intellectual levels. A fifth feature was that the precipitating circumstances surrounding the need for hospitalization depressed their self-esteem, highlighting an exquisitely vulnerable sense of self-regard.

Of particular significance for our present inquiry into the relationship between adolescence and schizophrenia is the appearance of evidence of poor competence in our group of young schizophrenic patients. The strain experienced by the typically maturing schizophrenic underscores issues of competence in already vulnerable people. Whether the vulnerability specifically implicates schizophrenia or represents a general vulnerability to psychopathology was not answered by our initial inquiry. It thus becomes important to compare the premorbid histories of schizophrenic and nonschizophrenic psychiatric patients and of nonpatient normals for evidence of poor competence in premorbid adjustment.

In this data sample we looked at forty-nine schizophrenic patients, eighteen nonschizophrenic patients (manic-depressive and personality disorders), and thirty-seven normals. In our study, age, socioeconomic status, and intelligence level have been matched, eliminating the possibility of a confounding of these variables with the evidence of premorbid histories involving school, occupation, and social difficulties. Table 3 shows the distribution of these subjects. The comparison shows dramatically that the two patient groups did not differ from each other in any of the principal variables tapping competence: social and work adjustment prior to hospitalization, runaway history, school performance, dropping out of school, experimenting with street drugs, and an inner experience of themselves as lonely individuals. The normal subjects on the other hand showed no incidence of running away from home, poor social and work adjustment, troublesome school records or substantial drug-taking.

TABLE 3

Percentage of Subjects in Each Group of Young Adult Patients (Ages 17-24) Who Manifested Evidence of Poor Competence and Premorbid Ineffectiveness.

	Schizophrenic Patients (N = 49)	Non-Schizophrenic Patients (N = 18)
Rate of Onset:		
Unknown	2	6
Sudden	20	33
Gradual	78	61
Adjustment Prior to Onset:		
Unknown	9	
Good	10	33
Fair	51	50
Poor	38	16
Antecedent Stress:		
Unknown	59	50
External Stress	12	11
Developmental Stress	10	5
External and Developmental Stress	14	11
Other	4	22
Runaway History:		
Unknown	2	0
Present	69	77
Absent	29	22
School Performance:		
Unknown	4	11
Excellent	10	27
Good	18	11
Fair	28	11
Poor	39	39
School Dropout:		
Unknown	2	5
No	31	33
Yes	67	61

TABLE 3 (Cont'd)

	Schizophrenic Patients (N = 49)	Non-Schizophrenic Patients (N = 18)
Drug-taking:		
No	39	44
Yes	61	56
Lonely:		
Unknown	2	44
No	31	5
Yes	67	50
Prominent Dependency:		
Unknown	0	0
No	24	33
Yes	76	67
Little Affection:		
Unknown	4	0
No	24	44
Yes	71	56

With respect to general competence, young adult schizophrenics do not differ from other young adults who have had behavioral and interpersonal difficulties severe enough to warrant hospitalization. Both groups, however, are significantly different from the nonpathological group. Lack of competence in adolescence does relate to later psychopathology, whatever its form, though this does not imply that all disturbances of adolescence that differ from disturbances in the nonpathological group constitute aspects of a "schizophrenic spectrum" (Kety, Rosenthal, Wender, and Schulsinger 1968). The later behaviors, difficulties, and varieties of disorganizations indicate that the nonspecific matrix of pathology in adolescence includes all those who are destined to become severely disturbed, including those who become overtly schizophrenic. Other investigators such as Bromet, Harrow, and Kasl (1974) contend that certain specific premorbid factors can predict a future "process" schizophrenia. We believe, however, on the basis of our data, that these premorbid disturbances are quite nonspecific with respect to the future form of psychopathology.

Our findings are not unique; other investigators have reported similar patterns. Rodnick and Goldstein (1972) studied interactions in families of adolescents at risk for serious psychopathology, reporting a range of intrafamilial conflicts, significant frequency of withdrawal behavior, excessive dependency on parents, isolated social behavior, and antisocial behavior. Holmes and Barthell (1968) reported that school performance of later schizophrenic patients showed poor academic and social achievement. Watt, Stolorowrd-Lubensky, and McClelland (1970) report similar data, with boys and girls showing deficits in competency in specific areas. Watt (1972) further noted that about 50 percent of schizophrenic patients showed deviant social behavior by early adolescence, a statistic in substantial agreement with ours. Robins' study (1966) of the precursors of psychopathology reported that children who later became schizophrenic differed in significant ways from those who remained free of major psychopathology. Those who became schizophrenic had more infectious illnessess in early childhood, more physical handicaps, a greater number of eating and sleeping disturbances, and antisocial behavior. Antisocial behavior was a particularly striking symptom, with 50 percent of those children having had an incident of physical aggression and incorrigibility.

Nameche and Ricks (1966) reported a slower motor development and inferior coordination among schizophrenics as children than any comparison group. Delayed development of speech, unclear speech, and social isolation were striking. These data are congruent with those reported by Bender and Freedman (1952) and Fish and Hagin (1972).

Are these patterns of maladaptation and inferior competence to be regarded as precursors of early manifestations of later serious psychopathological symptoms, as prodromal symptoms of the disorder? Are they the preconditions for the development of major psychopathology? Are they artifacts of the method of retrospective recall, a method notoriously subject to contextual distortion (Haggard, Brekstad, and Skard 1960, Hilles 1967)? It would seem that the follow-back methods used by Watt and Robins established that these data are not artifacts of the recall by distraught parents; these investigators organized data that had been recorded many years before major mental illness had been diagnosed. Garmezy (1974) has suggested that, perhaps, these indications of behavior difficulties in childhood are themselves the manifestation of the disorder that later established itself. This is a reasonable view and one that implies that the schizophrenic psychosis is merely a phase in an evolving pathological process, a phase marked by serious disorganization and loss of allegiance to reality.

It appears to us that the schizophrenias refer to a dysorganization of

287

adaptive and defensive functions which in turn reflect more fundamental dysfunctions of basic physiological and psychological processes. By fundamental we mean early in time—perhaps prenatally; and we mean genotypic. The particular derailments in development are too heterogeneous to reflect specific pathologies of specific organ structures. The persistent and ubiquitous disturbances in a variety of areas of functioning are sufficiently nonspecific to suggest that the pathology is to be characterized in terms of degrees of failure of developmental differentiation. Such failures may be more or less observable, depending upon the psychological, social, or physical tasks required of the person. In early childhood, strains on psychological resources are for the most part considerably less than they would be in later life. School and parental demands for conformity or for achievement may represent serious strains to some particularly vulnerable children. These children are probably those who show behavior deviations noted in the Robins' (1966) study.

But adolescence, with its insistent demands for separation and individuation, for taking a role in society and for perceiving it with competence, imposes inescapable burdens on a vulnerable organism. Response can be weak, ineffective, desperate, eccentric, or complaint-at-great-cost.

It is understandable then that statistics regarding first hospitalizations for schizophrenic patients show that young males outnumber young females until the fourth decade of life, when females are in the majority. Task demands on young adult males are vastly greater than those on young females. Requirements for competence in the social, occupational, and sexual realms are also greater on males. The young male must, in most cultures, establish himself in an occupation, become sexually aggressive enough to court and marry a woman, and to maintain sexual, social, and occupational potency. Thus, in men, limitations in competence become apparent early, and task demands impose heavy challenges. For young women in our culture, on the other hand, the requirements for independence and initiative are less than they are for young men. Thus the appearance of overt disorganization—the psychotic phase of the disorder—is less apparent. During the fourth decade of life, however, when child-rearing activities are less insistent, families will more readily extrude a schizophrenic female as now expendable. Hence, the higher hospitalization rates for women than men after age thirty-five.

In our view, then, the relationship between adolescence and schizophrenia is that of a catalyst to a biological reaction. The potential for disorganization is characteristic of the person. The social tasks of adolescence, however, place powerful strains on a vulnerable youth, and such a person must draw upon limited resources in response to these task requirements. Responses expose deficits, and the strain of the requirement to become competent can potentiate disorganization. The consequences of such failures to the adolescent's sense of worth, self-esteem, and pride are great; they add finite burdens to failures already sensed throughout the preceding years.

NOTE

1. This study, supported in part by Public Health Service grants MH-05519, MH-18999, and MH-19477, is part of a program investigating schizophrenia which is being conducted jointly by the Psychosomatic and Psychiatric Institute of Michael Reese Hospital, the Department of Psychiatry, Pritzker School of Medicine, University of Chicago, and the Illinois State Psychiatric Institute

Dr. Holzman is a recipient of a Career Scientist Award from NIMH (MH-70900).

REFERENCES

Bender, L., and Freedman, A. M. (1952). A study of the first three years of maturation of schizophrenic children. *Quarterly Journal of Child Behavior* 1:245-272.

Block, J. (1971). *Lives Through Time*. Berkeley: Bancroft.

Bromet, E., Harrow, M., and Kasl, S. (1974). Premorbid functioning in outcome in schizophrenics and non-schizophrenics. *Archives of General Psychiatry* 30:203-207.

Erikson, E. H. (1974). *Dimensions of a New Identity*. New York: W. W. Norton.

Fish, B., and Hagin, R. (1972). Visual-motor disorders in infants at risk for schizophrenia. *Archives of General Psychiatry* 27:594-598.

Grinker, R. R., Sr., Grinker, R. R., Jr., and Timberlake, I. (1962). "Mentally healthy" young males: homoclites. *Archives of General Psychiatry* 6:405-453. (Also in *This Annual* 1:176-255).

————, and Holzman, P. S. (1973). Schizophrenic pathology in young adults: a clinical study. *Archives of General Psychiatry* 28:168-175.

————, and Werble, B. (1974). Mentally healthy young men (homoclites): fourteen years later. *Archives of General Psychiatry* 30:701-704.

Haggard, E. A., Brekstad, A., and Skard, A. G. (1960). On the reliability of the anamnestic interview. *Journal of Abnormal and Social Psychology* 61:311-318.

Heath, D. (1965). *Explorations in Maturity.* New York: Appleton-Century-Crofts.

Hilles, L. (1967). The realiability of anamnestic data. *Bulletin of the Menninger Clinic* 31:219-228.

Holmes, D., and Barthell, C. (1968). High school yearbooks: a nonreactive measure of social isolation in graduates who later become schizophrenic. *Journal of Abnormal Psychology* 73:313-316.

Kety, S. S., Rosenthal, D., Wender, P. H., and Schulsinger, F. (1968). The types and prevalence of mental illness in the biological and adoptive families of adopted schizophrenics. D. Rosenthal and S. S. Kety, eds., *The Transmission of Schizophrenia.* Oxford: Pergamon Press.

Mayer-Gross, W., Slater, E., and Roth, M. (1969). *Clinical Psychiatry.* 3rd ed. Baltimore: Williams and Wilkins.

Nameche, G. H., and Ricks, D. F. (1966). Life patterns of children who become adult schizophrenics. Presented at the Annual Meeting of the American Orthopsychiatry Association, San Francisco, Calif., April 16, 1966.

Offer, D., and Offer, J. (1973). Normal adolescence in perspective. J. C. Schoolar, ed., *Current Issues in Adolescent Psychiatry.* New York: Brunner/Mazel.

Rado, S. (1956). *Psychoanalysis of Behavior: Collected Papers.* New York: Grune and Stratton.

Robins, N. (1966). *Deviant Children Grown Up.* Baltimore: Williams and Wilkins.

Rodnick, E. H., and Goldstein, M. J. (1972). A research strategy for studying risks for schizophrenia during adolescent and early childhood. Paper presented at Conference on Risk Research, Dorado Beach, Puerto Rico, October 1972.

Vaillant, G. E. (1971). Theoretical hierarchy of adaptive ego mechanisms. *Archives of General Psychiatry* 24: 107-118.

Watt, N. F. (1972). Longitudinal changes in the social behavior of children hospitalized for schizophrenia as adults. *Journal of Nervous and Mental Diseases* 155: 42-54.

Watt, N. F., Stolorowrd-Lubensky, A. W., and McClelland, D. C. (1970). Social adjustment and behavior of children hospitalized for schizophrenia as adults. *American Journal of Orthopsychiatry* 40: 637-657.

Yolles, S. F., and Kramer, M. (1969). Vital statistics in the schizophrenic syndrome. L. Bellak and L. Loeb, eds., *The Schizophrenic Syndrome.* New York: Grune and Stratton.

VARIOUS PERSPECTIVES
ON
ANOREXIA NERVOSA

HILDE BRUCH

Anorexia nervosa used to be extremely rare and few clinicians could study more than an occasional case. In the last decades there has been a considerable increase in its occurrence, so much so that probably every physician dealing with adolescents will sooner or later be confronted with an anorectic youngster. This increase has been reported not only from different parts of the United States, but also from many other Western countries.

Anorexia nervosa is the diagnostic label for a state of pitiful emaciation which is observed mainly in young women and which is the result of self-inflicted starvation. However, there is no true loss of appetite and the term *anorexia nervosa* is a misnomer for the condition to which it refers. Instead of lethargy and exhaustion, commonly associated with severe malnutrition, a marked drive for activity persists, and even extreme thinness is defiantly defended as justified, the only protection against the dreaded fate of being fat (Bruch 1973).

Initial reports about anorexia nervosa as a distinct syndrome appeared simultaneously in England and France about a century ago. Various efforts to explain it in psychological terms led to much controversy, until the whole issue was thrown into a new direction when in 1914 pathological lesions were described in the pituitary gland of a cachectic woman. For several decades the search for some endocrine deficiency persisted, with increasing vagueness in what was diagnosed as anorexia nervosa. At present there is renewed interest in possible endocrine and neurophysiological factors which are carried out with greatly refined laboratory techniques, though it is not yet possible to establish whether the described or postulated deviations are the cause or the result of severe malnutrition

(Boyar et al. 1974, Garfinkel et al. 1975). During the 1930s a psychological syndrome of anorexia nervosa was distinguished from the "Simmonds disease." Psychoanalytic investigations played an important role in this clarification. The focus was on exploring the disturbed eating, the oral component, in the hope of explaining the entire complex through one specific psychodynamic formulation (Waller, Kaufman, and Deutsch 1940). Unconscious pregnancy fantasies were assumed to be the basic dynamic issue; even today, fear of impregnation is still looked for as a causal factor.

Reports on larger patient groups which have appeared since 1960 reflect a definite change in this approach. It is now generally accepted that there is a true or primary anorexia nervosa syndrome which represents a separate nosological entity, with pursuit of thinness as the leading symptom and from which an unspecific weight loss, which occurs in various psychiatric conditions, needs to be differentiated. The somatic pictures in both forms look deceptively alike; amenorrhea is associated with severe weight loss and various signs of malnutrition. Primary anorexia nervosa is characterized by an intense interest in food and extreme hyperactivity, whereas in the atypical form loss of appetite and fatigue and indolence are common.

Primary Anorexia Nervosa

In true anorexia nervosa, the form that occurs with increasing frequency, the basic psychological issue is a frantic effort to establish a sense of control and identity (Bruch 1973). It occurs mainly in girls following menarche, though it may develop either in prepuberty or later in adolescence or young adulthood, usually at the time of decision-making or changes in the family or environment. Few conditions arouse as much bewilderment, compassion, and frustration as the spectacle of a young person pursuing a course of self-starvation, with conflicts about eating dominating the surface picture. Analysis of the interactional patterns preceding the manifest illness reveals forces that have resulted in deficiencies in conceptual and perceptual awareness of bodily needs.

The true syndrome is amazingly uniform, and disordered psychological functioning can be identified in three areas: (1) a disturbance in body image and body concept of delusional proportions, (2) inaccurate and confused perception and cognitive interpretation of stimuli arising in the body, with inaccurate hunger awareness as the most pronounced deficiency, and (3) a paralyzing sense of ineffectiveness which pervades all thinking and activities.

BODY IMAGE DISTURBANCES

True anorectics are identified by their emaciated and gruesome appearance. However, they deny any abnormality and actively maintain their emaciation. Excess weight precedes the illness in only about 15 to 20 percent. Prior to onset most were of normal weight and a few on the thin side, but they start dieting because they feel they are "too fat." Many patients will regain weight for a variety of reasons, but without correction of the body image disturbance, relapses are common. Even with treatment, many express for quite some time bewilderment about their inability to see themselves realistically, or they will confess that they had felt that by starving themselves they were hurting their parents, gaining satisfaction from the concern of others, but unaware that they themselves were undergoing the ordeal of starvation, as if their body was not their own. During the illness the body is experienced as extraneous, as separated from the self. Lasting recovery involves the development of an active and positive acceptance of one's own body and concern for its health.

MISPERCEPTION OF BODILY FUNCTIONS

Anorectics' refusal to eat is the symptom that arouses most concern, anxiety, frustration, and rage. Though there is no true loss of appetite, awareness of hunger in the ordinary sense seems to be absent. They are frantically preoccupied with food and develop unusual, even bizarre eating habits which, like dawdling over food, are similar to those of victims of famine. Anorectics will complain about feeling full after a few bites. Some patients even report this after watching others eat; this seems to be a phantom phenomenon.

In about 25 percent of the cases, food refusal alternates with uncontrollable eating binges (bulimia) which are experienced as loss of control, a submission to something they do not want to do. Anorectics are terrified by this and try to remove the unwanted food through self-induced vomiting, laxatives, enemas, and diuretics. These practices may result in serious disturbances in the electrolyte balance, at times with fatal outcomes (Bruch 1971).

Another characteristic manifestation of falsified body awareness is the absence of fatigue in spite of constant hyperactivity, such as walking, swimming, or doing calisthenics by the hour. The absence of sexual feelings, failure of sexual functioning, and amenorrhea may also be considered in this context. Other sensations, such as temperature awareness or sensitivity to pain, are also incorrectly perceived or responded to. This has been interpreted as indicating hypothalamic dysfunction (Mecklenburg et al. 1974). Anorectics are also deficient in identifying emotional states, and even severe depressive feelings may remain masked.

INEFFECTIVENESS

Underneath their spirited facade anorectics suffer from a deep sense of ineffectiveness—a conviction of acting not on their own initiative, but only in response to demands coming from others. Their early development is described as having been free from difficulties and problems to an unusual degree, the later anorectic child having been the parents' pride and joy, of whom great things were expected. Such perfect and overconforming behavior is a camouflage for serious underlying self-doubt, of not feeling in control of one's own life, and of lacking in self-directed identity. The extreme control over the body provides a sense of accomplishment; even a slight gain in weight is apt to precipitate depression and self-hatred.

FAMILY TRANSACTIONS

Most families are socially ambitious, financially successful, and present themselves as happy. They appear to be stable on superficial impression, with few broken marriages. They are of small size with a conspicuously greater number of daughters than sons. Intimate contact reveals that underlying the apparent marital harmony are serious and concealed problems. In their dissatisfaction with each other, each parent seeks affection and confirmation from the perfect child who feels obligated to fulfill their demands (Selvini 1974). The illness represents an effort to establish a sense of independent selfhood and an escape from this overdemanding role. In these success and achievement oriented homes, which offer many privileges and much cultural stimulation, these youngsters make pleasing compliance a way of life until the new tasks of adolescence demand self-directed behavior and regulation of goals.

To visualize the development of such a failure in acquiring a sense of adequacy and effectiveness, I have constructed a simplified model of personality development (Bruch 1973). Behavior from birth on requires differentiation into two forms, that initiated in the individual and that in response to external stimuli. For normal development, for all areas of development, appropriate responses to clues originating in the child are as essential as stimulation from the environment. How it operates can be observed in the feeding situation where a mother, who is sensitively attuned to her child's expressions, offers food only for nutritional needs. Thus the child learns to recognize hunger as a distinct sensation. If a mother's reactions are inappropriate or contradictory, be it neglectful, oversolicitous, or inhibiting, the child will not learn to differentiate between being hungry or other sources of discomfort and will grow up without a discriminating and regulatory awareness of his bodily sensations. Without the conviction of living his own life, he will feel helpless under the influence of internal urges and external demands.

Atypical Anorexia Nervosa

No general picture can be drawn for the atypical group where weight loss is incidental to a variety of psychiatric problems, is frequently complained of, or is valued only secondarily for its coercive effect. In hysterics, the morbid rejection of food may follow some frightening or disgusting sexual experience. Here, the unconscious fear of impregnation, the traditional psychoanalytic explanation for all cases, may be a relevant issue. Schizoid patients with their disturbed sense of reality misinterpret the whole eating function and may refuse food for feeling unworthy, or suffer delusional fear of swallowing. Characteristically they are apathetic, indolent, and indifferent about the emaciation. Depressive feelings are common in anorexia nervosa. Occasionally severe depression and social withdrawal, traceable to repeated early experiences of separation or desertion, precede the onset of anorectic behavior which may represent an effort to fight the depression. Absent, in these cases, are hyperactivity, perfectionism, and the defiant pride in being thin.

Anorexia Nervosa in the Male

Anorexia nervosa occurs conspicuously less often in males than in females. Both the primary and atypical syndrome have been described (Bruch 1973). As in females, pursuit of thinness is the leading motive in the primary picture with a similar family constellation, overcompliance, and exceptional performance during childhood. The illness becomes manifest when the assured status of superiority is threatened by new demands or changes in the environment. Rigid self-starvation, often with eating binges followed by self-induced vomiting, bring about severe weight loss. Hyperactivity and drive for achievement persist, often with remarkable athletic accomplishments, in spite of the severe emaciation. In contrast to females, primary anorexia nervosa in boys occurs nearly exclusively during prepuberty. It may well be that pubertal development, with the outpouring of male sex hormones and powerful new sensations, protects against its occurrence later on.

The atypical picture may occur in adults who become anorectic, with true loss of appetite and exhaustion, in response to stressful life situations. Anorexia occurs also in pubertal boys where it may serve various symbolic meanings, such as atonement for sins. Such boys are generally apathetic, indifferent, and will cease attending school.

Treatment

Treatment involves two distinct tasks that require integration: restitution of normal nutrition and resolution of the underlying psychological problems, including the disturbed patterns of family interaction. Anorexia nervosa has always been considered a condition that offers difficult and frustrating treatment problems. Death or continued invalidism are not infrequent results. Recently, a whole series of optimistic reports have appeared speaking of nearly invariable success with gain in weight. By whatever method this is achieved, weight gain alone is an unreliable sign of rehabilitation. Relapses are frequent and the histories of those with fatal outcome illustrate the fallacy of considering restitution of weight alone a cure (Bruch 1971).

Such claims have been made in the past for the greatest variety of methods ranging from implantation of the pituitary gland, insulin injections, and electro-convulsive shock therapy to psychotropic drugs. The latest claim of invariable success with rapid weight gain is being made for treatment with behavior modification (Agras et al. 1974, Blinder, Freeman, and Stunkard 1970). Unfortunately, such claims are being made without the benefit of information on long range results. From numerous requests for consultation on unsuccessfully treated patients it appears that many forms of behavior treatment are utilized. Freely chosen activities may be used as a reward for gaining weight, or making conditions extremely uncomfortable, such as withholding all desirable activities, granting various privileges only as reward for weight gain. With this method substantial weight increases are achieved which, however, often are short-lived. Follow-up findings dramatically illustrate that the weight gain in itself is not a cure for anorexia nervosa and that enforcing it this way may be damaging. Proponents of the method do not seem to be unaware of the possible dangers. A dramatic example was given in the case of a young woman who had gained satisfactorily while hospitalized but who committed suicide after discharge (Blinder et al. 1970). The patients I have seen in consultation, after they had been exposed to this method, had experienced the program as brutal coercion. Some had become depressed, even suicidal, and the family interactions, social relations, and eating patterns had deteriorated (Bruch 1974). It seems to undermine the last vestiges of self-esteem and to destroy the crucial hope of ever achieving autonomy and self-determination. Such serious symptoms follow so often that this method must be considered dangerous. Even Wolpe (1975) admits that behavior therapy is often carried out by poor and inadequately trained practitioners.

I do not wish to imply by these critical comments that improvement of nutrition is not often a matter of great urgency; the very survival of a youngster may be at stake. There have been continuous debates on how to accomplish the seemingly impossible task of getting food into a patient who is stubbornly determined to starve. Under emergency conditions intravenous hyperalimentation may offer the solution. This method avoids the patient's being forced to take food by mouth and, if necessary, by tube feeding. Impressive weight gains are achieved without the traumatic struggle over eating.

A certain degree of nutritional restitution is a prerequisite for effective psychotherapy. The course of the illness may be unnecessarily prolonged when a therapist indulges in the unrealistic expectation that the weight will correct itself once the unconscious meaning of the food refusal and the underlying conflicts are made conscious. This approach overlooks that one cannot do meaningful therapeutic work with a starving patient. Much anorectic behavior is a direct expression of starvation, which has such a distorting effect on all psychic functioning that no true picture of the psychological problems can be formulated until the worst malnutrition is corrected. The same applies to the handling of binge eating and vomiting which may have become habitual by the time a psychiatrist is consulted. A passive attitude on the part of the therapist implies that he condones the abnormal behavior, and the problems which are camouflaged by it do not become accessible to therapeutic investigation.

Equally enthusiastic are the claims made for family therapy whereby family conflicts are supposedly resolved during a few dramatic sessions after which the patient resumes eating (Barcai 1971, Liebman, Minuchin, and Baker 1974). This seems to be an effective approach for young patients soon after the onset of the condition, but less so for those with serious psychiatric problems and after the illness has existed for any length of time. In these cases, too, disengagement and redirection of the malfunctioning forces in the family is essential. The deficits in the psychic development require individual psychotherapeutic help. Here the results are closely linked to the percentage of the psychodynamic understanding, and are excellent when meaningful treatment goals are pursued (Bruch 1973, Selvini 1971).

The theoretical considerations which I have offered here are closely related to the therapeutic approach which I have developed from traditional psychoanalytic technique. It was recognized that the classic psychoanalytic setting, with the analyst interpreting the unconscious meaning of the patient's free associations, contains elements that represent for the patient the painful repetition of old patterns, namely of being told by someone else what to feel and think, with the implication of being incapable of knowing his own mind. The life long profound sense of ineffectiveness is thus confirmed and reinforced.

In the new approach the focus is on the patient's failure in self experience, on the defective tools and concepts for organizing and expressing needs, and on the bewilderment when dealing with others. One aspect of therapy is the effort to repair conceptual defects and distortions, and to recognize the roots for the deep seated dissatisfaction and sense of isolation. This is accomplished by assisting patients to develop awareness of their capabilities and potentials so that they become capable of handling their own problems in more competent ways. These modifications are in good agreement with modern concepts of psychotherapy for schizophrenia, borderline states, and narcissistic character disorders.

The therapist's task is to be alert and consistent in recognizing any self-initiated behavior and expressions by the patient. He must pay minute attention to the discrepancies in a patient's recall of the past, to the way current events are misperceived or misinterpreted. He must be honest in confirming or correcting what the patient communicates. These patients suffer from an abiding sense of loneliness, often feeling that they are not respected by others. They may feel insulted and abused though the realistic situation does not contain these elements. The anticipation or recall of a real or imagined insult may lead to withdrawal from the actual situation and to flight into an eating binge, vomiting, or to more rigid starvation. Exploration of the dynamic aspects of these experiences and examination of alternatives in such situations eventually helps a patient to experience himself as not utterly helpless. He can then begin to feel competent to approach problems realistically.

Conclusions

Through such active participation in the treatment process, patients will learn to recognize impulses, feelings, and inner needs in areas where they had been deprived of adequate early learning. They become capable of living as self-directed, authentic individuals, enjoying what life has to offer. Using this approach, even patients who had been unsuccessfully in treatment for several years, and who were filled to the brim with useless, though not necessarily incorrect, knowledge of their psychodynamics, will begin to change and then relinquish their self-punishing rituals. Examining their own development in realistic terms, with emphasis on their own contributions, serves as an important stimulus for acquiring thus far deficient mental tools.

In spite of an overt negativistic attitude, these patients are unusually alert to what is going on. Indications of some change may become apparent in the first few sessions, when they recognize that what they have to say is regarded as important. Instead of focusing on the motives underlying the disturbed eating, I find it useful to inquire about their general development and about their feelings of self-confidence and satisfaction with themselves. Most will reply that they never had confidence in themselves, that they had lived by doing only what was expected of them. Some will name some definite event which made them aware that something was wrong with this way of life.

What a patient offers as vital issues varies, of course, from case to case. It is important to recognize that seemingly ordinary, even silly memories are taken seriously as contributing to a meaningful explanation of the illness. Having never trusted themselves to acknowledge their own needs, therapy must help them discover that they have the right to express and pursue their own wants and wishes.

Once patients feel understood and respected in their deepest concerns and recognize that the therapist follows their lead in clarifying important issues, they are more apt to listen to his explanations that meaningful psychotherapy is not possible as long as they are in a state of acute starvation which, in itself, provokes abnormal psychological reactions. The cadaverous appearance interferes with all human relationships since it arouses strong reactions. It also keeps the therapist anxious and concerned, and this may hinder the progress of treatment. The problems that precipitated the whole illness will remain inaccessible to clarification as long as the nutrition is abnormally low. When rapport has been established on this level, patients will permit the weight to rise without experiencing a loss of self-esteem and pride. Better physical health contributes to their becoming capable to face problems of increasing independence, autonomy, and maturity, and they no longer need to manipulate the body and its functions in this bizarre way.

Though early institution of a comprehensive therapeutic program improves the chances of recovery, long standing illness does not preclude good treatment results. Evaluation of the long range outcome led to the conclusion that not any one factor is predictive of success or failure, but that results are directly related to the relevance of the therapeutic intervention with development of autonomy as its primary focus.

REFERENCES

Agras, W. S., Barlow, D. H., Abel, G. G., and Leitenberg, H. (1974). Behavior modification of anorexia nervosa. *Archives of General Psychiatry* 30: 279-286.

Barcai, A. (1971). Family therapy in the treatment of anorexia nervosa. *American Journal of Psychiatry* 128: 286-290.

Blinder, B. J., Freeman, D. M. A., and Stunkard, A. J. (1970). Behavior therapy of anorexia nervosa: effectiveness of activity as a reinforcer of weight gain. *American Journal of Psychiatry* 126: 77-82.

Boyar, R. M., Katz, J., Finkelstein, J. W., Kapen, S., Weiner, H., Weitzman, E. D., and Hellman, L. (1974). Immaturity of the 24-hour luteinizing hormone secretory pattern. *New England Journal of Medicine* 291: 861-865.

Bruch, H. (1971). Death in anorexia nervosa. *Psychosomatic Medicine* 33: 135-144.

——— (1973). *Eating Disorders: Obesity, Anorexia Nervosa and the Person Within*. New York: Basic Books.

——— (1974). Perils of behavior modification in treatment of anorexia nervosa. *Journal of the American Medical Association* 230: 1419-1422.

Garfinkel, P. E., Brown, G. M., Stancer, H. C., and Moldofsky, H. (1975). Hypothalamic-pituitary function in anorexia nervosa. *Archives of General Psychiatry* 32: 739-744.

Liebman, R., Minuchin, S., and Baker, L. (1974). An integrated treatment program for anorexia nervosa. *American Journal of Psychiatry* 131: 432-436.

Mecklenburg, R. S., Loriaux, D. L., Thompson, R. H., Andersen, A. E., and Lipsett, M. B. (1974). Hypothalamic dysfunction in patients with anorexia nervosa. *Medicine* 53: 147-159.

Selvini, M. P. (1971). Anorexia nervosa. S. Arieti, ed., *The World of Psychiatry and Psychotherapy*. New York: Basic Books.

——— (1974). *Self-Starvation: From the Intrapsychic to the Transpersonal Approach to Anorexia Nervosa*. London: Chaucer.

Waller, J. V., Kaufman, M. R., and Deutsch, F. (1940). Anorexia nervosa: a psychosomatic entity. *Psychosomatic Medicine* 2: 3-16.

Wolpe, J. (1975). Letter: behavior therapy in anorexia nervosa. *Journal of the American Medical Association* 223: 317-318.

19] NARCISSISTIC DISTURBANCES IN ANOREXIA NERVOSA

ALAN GOODSITT

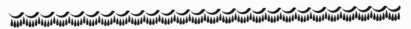

Anorexia nervosa, a syndrome most frequently affecting adolescent girls, but also occurring in males, is characterized by the initiation of restrictive dieting. Anorectics are obsessed with an unreasonable fear of becoming fat, even while enduring emaciation. Despite massive weight loss they delusionally insist their weight and bodily shape are normal. Accompanying these symptoms one typically finds a maniclike hyperactivity and amenorrhea (in girls). Mortality rates of seven to fifteen percent have been reported (Sours 1969).

Anorexia nervosa is a symptom complex that can occur with any variety of ego pathology, but Bruch (1973) has identified a core group of anorectics that she signifies as "primary anorectics." They manifest severe body-image distortions and a marked disturbance in their awareness of inner feelings and bodily sensations. Primary anorectics claim to be unaware of sensations of hunger, sexual impulses, and feelings. They become frightened when asked to talk about themselves, their feelings, and their reactions since they are incapable of answering questions about inner perceptions, frequently responding with a blank stare or an, "I don't know." One anorectic, when asked about her feelings, referred me to her mother for an answer.

The problem does not seem to be simply a matter of lack of self-observation, nor is it primarily defensiveness against sharing feelings, but rather an impaired capacity to live within their bodies and to experience their internal conditions. When anorectics refer to their bodily state, they reveal gross inaccuracies in their self-perceptions. A severely emaciated anorectic will insist the shape of the body and weight are perfectly normal,

304

a distortion Crisp (1974) has demonstrated experimentally. Delusions about body size and image, and disturbances of internal experiences are not consistent with a diagnosis of neurosis. Bruch suggests a core schizophrenia. It is my impression that a diagnosis of borderline psychosis fits many or most of these primary anorectics that are the subject of this chapter.

A review of the literature reveals few attempts at integrating recent psychoanalytic discoveries with anorexia nervosa. The early literature favored explanations in terms of conflicting drives. The cessation of eating was considered a defense against fantasies of oral impregnation. These formulations left unexplained the peculiar body delusion, the impairment of body self-experience, as well as the hyperactivity, which is a striking component of the syndrome. More recent publications have emphasized the symbiotic-like attachments anorectics form with their parents, the incompleteness of the separation-individuation process, and the anorectic's sense of unpreparedness for growing and assuming an adult, heterosexual identity.

The patient who asked me to consult her mother when asked how she, the patient, felt is a good example of someone who has not differentiated herself and her inner processes from others (Goodsitt 1969). Bruch has emphasized these patient's lack of identity or individuation and their severe sense of helplessness and ineffectiveness, but the concept of identity in reference to these patients requires further clarification in terms of psychic structure. I propose to examine those deficits which give rise to the lack of identity and necessitate symbiotic mergers, and explain the psychic meaning and function of the characteristic hyperactivity of anorectics.

Bruch (1973) describes the distorted body-image and severely impaired awareness of internal feelings and sensations of anorectics as manifestations of a perceptual disorder. What is disturbed, in my opinion, are not all perceptions, but primarily perceptions of the self which include the body. Bodily sensations are the nucleus around which the sense of self is organized. Freud's (1923) assertion that "the ego is first and foremost a bodily ego" applies to the sense of self. Typically, when a cohesive sense of self becomes unstable, bodily symptoms (hypochondriasis) result. Since disturbances in bodily experience often reflect interior disturbances, the study of a syndrome with prominent bodily delusions is useful in understanding self-pathology.

Kohut's (1971) concept of the cohesive self refers to an experience of oneself which remains stable and continuous in time and space. This self-constancy is comparable to object-constancy and both are probably established in normal development at about the same age. Initially, this sense of cohesiveness is dependent upon a symbioticlike relationship with a parental figure, who provides mental functions which the child has yet to acquire. The infant and young children without the parent's provision of security, judgment, and empathy are vulnerable to overstimulation both from external and internal sources, to severe fluctuations in self-esteem, and to disruption or fragmentation of the sense of cohesion.

How the child feels about himself is very much dependent upon the reliability of supporting external objects. Prior to the child's internalizing the regulating functions of the need-satisfying object, external factors loom large in the child's maintenance of narcissistic equilibrium. When there is a disruption in the dependent relationship with a nurturing object the child or adult, arrested at this level of development, is liable to feel helpless, ineffective, overwhelmed, unworthy, unreal, incomplete, or empty. One of Bruch's anorectic patients described such a state when she said, "I am like a balloon with hot air on the inside and just some skin on the outside." Activities are perceived as boring, mechanical, and routine; life is passively experienced. Regulation of tension, narcissistic equilibrium, and self-cohesion are specific functions provided by an external object.

Again, it was Bruch who found that an overwhelming sense of helplessness, ineffectiveness, and passivity is a cardinal feature of anorexia. It is my thesis that this helplessness reflects the anorectic's deficiency in self-regulating psychic structure which allows vulnerability to external contingencies. Anorectics complain of being easily exploited and excessively influenced. This is vividly depicted by one anorectic in her description of what happens when she eats. She experiences the food remaining in her stomach undigested—in the same form as prior to ingestion. Similarly, another anorectic believed that if she ate chicken breast, it would give her breasts. They experience eating as being occupied by a foreign substance. What is missing is the conviction that their bodies are active agents which metabolize the food, break it down into component parts, and transform it into a part of their own bodies. In their conception of the relationship between their bodies and food, their bodies are strangely passive, insignificant, and unable to regulate metabolic activities.

It is only after one has achieved a stable, cohesive sense of self that one can process external stimuli, be it food or information, and maintain a sense of wholeness and integrity. Further it permits one to confront external influences, digest or process them, convert them into self, or reject them with equanimity. It is a well-integrated self that allows one to feel in control and not just an empty receptable subject to foreign occupation. The anorectic's experience of bodily helplessness indexes a lack of integrity of the sense of self.

Anorectics frequently complain that if they take one bite of food, they will not be able to stop; if they eat a full meal, they will gain weight at once. Again, this directs our attention to the profound sense of helplessness, lack of control, and ultimately a lack of a self-regulating psychic apparatus. Anorectics feel inordinately influenced by external events, and deal with this by a characteristic rigidity and defensiveness in controlling their environment. We observe an obsessive preoccupation with counting calories, rigidly monitoring caloric intake, and attempting to exercise strict control over their peers, families, and therapists to the degree that these people feel tyrannized. Furthermore, anorectics compulsively schedule their daily routine and react with profound tension, extreme vacillations in mood, and disturbances in their sense of self when their environmental control is undermined. One anorectic described feeling "in pieces" during the daily staff changes on the hospital ward. The concern here is not simply one of identity, in the sense of "who am I and what is my role?" but rather one of being threatened with fragmentation of the self. Faced with the threat of fragmentation, the anorectic's efforts to maintain external control are understandable.

Self-starvation is frequently precipitated by some event which signifies a loss of control such as being forced to go to a school not of his choosing, the onset of menstruation, or an undesired chubbiness. The anorectic then decides that there is only one thing that he can exert the control over, and that is his body—its shape and weight, intake, and output. The body's allegiance cannot be to anyone or anything outside oneself. In its total control the anorectic can again feel omnipotent. The demand for constancy so futilely asked of the environment is now directed to the body. One observes in the anorectic a hypochondriacal preoccupation with his body and little else (although the efforts to control the environment are never abandoned). I believe this focus on the body serves for self-definition and stimulation, and is directed against a sense of fragmentation.

The anorectic denies his parents their former role in choosing a menu and regulating the quality and quantity of food intake. His eating habits become bizarre, with an insistence on fad diets. One such patient told me that when she ate and saw others happy that she was eating, she could no longer eat because she did not know whether she was eating for herself or for them. These patients struggle against the feeling that eating and control over the body does not belong to them. Who owns their bodies is a matter of contention and not something taken for granted. An anorectic when told of dangerous ischemic changes in her heart, secondary to malnutrition, remained unperturbed. She said, "That is my doctor's problem, not mine," and she continued her strenuous physical activity as if her heart's precarious condition was truly not her problem. Feeling states and bodily experiences are not integrated into a defined, stable sense of self. The refusal of the parent's food seems to be a desperate attempt to extract an autonomous self out of a confused undifferentiated relationship.

Although these patients may perceive and understand their precarious condition, they deny its significance because it conflicts with their megalomanic belief in self-perfection. Thus the anorectic feels that he need not eat, and can delusionally proclaim that his emaciated condition is perfectly normal. Further testimony regarding this phenomenon is provided by one of Bruch's patients who said, "I don't know why I feel food is unnecessary," and, "I still don't see why I should eat." Another reports, "My body could do anything—it could walk forever and ever and not get tired." My patient, disregarding the precarious condition of her heart, said that if God had intended her to die, she would have before now, and she continued her dangerous starvation.

The following case material illustrates some of these formulations and will be utilized to examine the meaning and function of the anorectic's hyperactivity and compulsivity.

Cindy was sixteen when she sought treatment. She had been amenorrheic for two years and during that time weighed between fifty-six and ninety pounds. She was five feet two inches tall. She had a miserable first year in high school. Her parents had overcome her objections and persuaded her to attend a parochial school, thereby separating her from her friends who continued in public school. Cindy then formed an inseparable relationship with a new girlfriend, and they decided to diet together. Weight loss became a test of self-discipline and effectiveness; she wanted to see just how much she could lose. Losing weight was a "conquest"— meaning that she was master in her own house, in her life, and in herself. Cindy had been a shy girl. Although she had friends, she felt herself on the social periphery. She wanted to be somebody. Weight loss, now, made her different in a way that "stood out." She complained to me that her father was preoccupied with his work and that for him she did not exist, but she admired her athletic brother.

Cindy had always been active, but now she was driven to activity. She could not sit still. Her daily routine was completely planned and she could not deviate from her schedule without feeling desperate. She told me about taking the "round about way home," watching television for fifteen minutes, biking for half an hour, cleaning up and doing homework, walking for half an hour, dinner, biking again for half an hour, going to the park for half an hour, etc. She described the activities as "just having something to do, anything to relieve feelings." She didn't want to be "lazy" which she defined as a terrible sense of boredom. She hated her compulsive routine and bemoaned that every day was just like the others. She complained about going through the motions of life, about life passing her by, and about feeling prematurely aged. Cindy could see that others got up and went to school just as she did, but she knew that something was missing in her experience of it. There was little that was interesting or that provoked enthusiasm. When she was not busy, she would begin to think and feel bad. She described her future as going into empty space. Cindy felt some direction and reason for her existence only when she had something planned or scheduled. Her artificially contrived *raison d'etre* for any one day would be to make it to her late night treat of ice cream or a candy bar. If she tried to do without her treat, she felt that she had no purpose, nothing to look forward to. Cindy had difficulty settling down at night and would occupy her mind during these anxious hours by repeatedly reviewing her next day's schedule. She bought several diet books, memorized the caloric value of food, counted her calories, and knew exactly what her caloric intake was at any given moment. She insisted on strange diets—for example, fish every night or no meats—which she referred to as "wild kicks." Eventually she complained that she felt like two people—one inside and one outside, with the former telling her not to eat. As she lost weight, she couldn't think clearly; she would "feel a fog in my mind."

Cindy left no room in her life just to be with herself and her inner feelings, because these were unbearable feelings of emptiness, dullness, and aimlessness. They had to be drowned out with constant activity which only provided a semblance of a life truly lived. She seemed to have no sense of true self-participation in her own activities; they were devices to fill up empty space and time. Strenuous physical exertion, in particular, was not simply aimed at losing weight, but was an attempt at stimulation in order to feel alive.

Cindy's anorexia also strives toward establishing an identity and being noticed even if she were perceived as a "skin and bones kid." She could no longer be treated with indifference. Her illness screamed out at her family, and they had to take notice of her. Her family had to defer to her by making changes in their living and dining arrangements. This is not the identity seeking of an adolescent who has come to the point in her life when she has to make final role choices (Erikson 1959). The question is not what will I do with a self whose existence is taken for granted, but rather how can I feel myself as present, whole, and alive. Her activities are not the outward manifestations of an inner self with specific goals and values; she requires props which give the illusion of being somebody at least for the time being.

The exhibitionistic aspect of an anorectic's demanding, dramatic behavior implores an environment to react and confirm a sense of self. Noneating puts the anorectic into abrasive conflict with the family, and this allows him to feel, through the impact he has made on them, that he exists. When anorexia becomes episodic, it can often be correlated with disruptions in narcissistically sustaining object relationships. The patient then feels depleted and is unable to cathect sufficiently those parts of the self that would impel him to eat.

Patients suffering from anorexia nervosa frequently find eating conflictful because of its various meanings and functions. Eating reduces a tension which protects many anorectics from fragmentation. Food however is also experienced as an intrusion into the tenuous sense of self, as a foreign occupation, thereby intensifying fragmentation. Thus we see the well-known anorectic pattern of compulsive, tension-reducing eating, followed by self-induced vomiting to counteract the fear of fragmentation.

Anorectics generally reach adolescence before their disturbances are apparent. Their lack of individuation has not been problematic. They are known as good, compliant children who are somewhat robotlike. The onset of puberty and adolescence poses a special threat to these children who have not internalized self-regulating psychic structure. The task of separating from the parent is not the same as that of a child who has achieved self and object constancy along with a stable self-object differentiation. For the child who has internalized the parental functions of tension neutralization, self-esteem regulation, and maintenance of self-cohesion, the process can be accomplished with minimal difficulties. Still, even for the normal child, self-cohesiveness is tested during adolescence (Gradolph 1976). The adolescent fluctuates from being full to being empty of himself. For the anorectic, deficient in internal psychic apparatus, decathexis of the parental imago threatens a disintegration of the self which can result in hypochondriacal preoccupations and bodily delusions.

One way of dealing with internal psychic disorganization is to exert rigid environmental control. A stable, controlled environment provides, of course, a sense of stability. Yet, if there is anything constant about adolescence, it is change itself—both internal and external. For example, parents have to adjust to the newly pubescent child and the child, in turn, makes adjustments to changes in the parents. The pubescent child also needs to integrate his bodily changes into a new body-self concept which includes these changes. For the anorectic with poor self-constancy, these demands on the ego's synthetic function are extraordinary. Pubescence with its associated sexuality is dangerous to these psychically impoverished children not because of threatened superego retaliation, but because it disturbs the previous relationships required for self-cohesion.

What does it mean to treat the anorectic with behavior modification programs which aim at weight gain by means of reward or punishment, and that carefully monitor and control behavior in order to eliminate resistance? Often, psychological issues are ignored or deemphasized while the therapists concentrate on the primary goal of weight production (Maxmen, Silberfarb, and Ferrell 1974). The negativism of the patient is considered a peripheral issue, and he is treated with tranquilizers.

Behavioral modification therapy, in my opinion, duplicates the same conditions that probably produced the illness in the first place. The potential for individuation is not only ignored, but forced further underground as the anorectic learns to exclude his inner being, and to conform to a totally controlling environment. There is no possibility of understanding the disorder, integrating the various conscious and unconscious aspects of the personality, and releasing the potential for growth previously constricted. The body-self split is intensified as the anorectic is forced to surrender control of his body to the therapist. Gaining weight is accomplished at the cost of further fragmentation of the body-self, and this, I submit, is the central pathology. What one now obtains is a person who suffers as before, but looks normal—an anorectic clothed in weight.

Conclusions

The therapy of a patient with anorexia nervosa is difficult. The core pathology is an aborted development of a cohesive self, and conditions have to be established to allow resumption of the growth process. The two primary goals are establishing a better narcissistic equilibrium and maintaining life. If, in addition, an early goal is weight gain, one may jeopardize the chance of forming a workable therapeutic alliance by provoking a negative transference. One must not take the symptom for the illness. Treating the symptom—attempting to put on weight—interferes with the other goal of correcting the psychic pathology.

The therapist allows the patient to reestablish a symbiotic transference in which the patient feels comfortable enough to utilize him to perform functions he is incapable of. He wishes to convey to the patient his understanding of the desperate sense of helplessness and ineffectiveness.

He acknowledges that the patient may have found it necessary to take emergency measures such as hyperactivity and noneating to deal with these painful states, but that when the patient is more comfortable with himself, he will be able to give up these inadequate and unsuccessful solutions. The therapist serves as an auxiliary ego for him; narcissistic injuries are minimized and a new, more stable equilibrium is achieved.

Long term hospitalization is frequently necessary. The therapist must accept that the patient might kill himself or cause damage to vital organs through malnutrition. The patient's capacity for realistic judgment and self-regulation is defective, and the therapist must direct these functions. When tube feeding or other coercive means of food intake become necessary, the therapist must stress that this is an emergency measure to maintain life and not an intrinsic psychotherapeutic maneuver. This is in contrast to coercive measures forcing the patient to eat so that he will gain weight and look normal. When the patient is ready to gain weight, he will do so because he is ready to accept the added portion to his body as part of himself and not as something grafted onto him.

REFERENCES

Bruch, H. (1973). *Eating Disorders: Obesity, Anorexia and the Person Within*. New York: Basic Books.

Crisp, A. H., and Kalucy, R. S. (1974). Aspects of the perceptual disorder in anorexia nervosa. *British Journal of Medical Psychology* 47: 349-361.

Erikson, E. (1959). The problem of ego identity. *Psychological Issues: Identity and the Life Cycle* 1: 101-164. New York: International Universities Press.

Freud, S. (1923). The ego and the id. *Standard Edition* 19: 3-68. London: Hogarth, 1961.

Goodsitt, A. (1969). Anorexia nervosa. *British Journal of Medical Psychology* 42: 109-118.

Gradolph, P. (1976). From panel discussion: individual psychotherapy of the severely disturbed adolescent. The 11th Annual Weekend Meeting of the Chicago Society for Adolescent Psychiatry, March 1976.

Kohut, H. (1971). *The Analysis of the Self*. New York: International Universities Press.

Maxmen, J. S., Silberfarb, P. M., and Ferrell, R. B. (1974). Anorexia nervosa. *Journal of the American Medical Association* 229: 801-804.

Sours, J. (1969). Anorexia nervosa: nosology, diagnosis, developmental patterns and power-control dynamics. *Adolescence: Psychosocial Perspectives*. New York: Basic Books.

20] INPUT AND OUTCOME OF FAMILY THERAPY IN ANOREXIA NERVOSA

BERNICE L. ROSMAN, SALVADOR MINUCHIN,
RONALD LIEBMAN, AND LESTER BAKER

This chapter is an account of the development of a family therapy model for the treatment of anorexia nervosa, a behavioral disorder of self-starvation, in children. While the work to be described has always been characterized by a family in contrast to an individual approach, the conceptual framework and the strategies of treatment have undergone a differentiation and development of their own. This is due to our increasing experience with this at one time esoteric but recently more common symptom, and our ongoing efforts to evaluate and reevaluate the effectiveness of the psychotherapeutic techniques.

Minuchin (1970) first discussed the application of structural family therapy in anorexia nervosa, the use of an ecological framework in the treatment of a child, to the case of a fifteen-year-old boy who refused to eat. He contrasted more traditional child psychiatric approaches which localize the psychological disorder within the individual with that of the ecologically minded therapist who is concerned with the child in significant contexts, most typically the family, and whose interventions are directed toward those contexts.

The treatment described in that case exemplifies some of the key aspects of the structural family approach:

1. The therapist focused on the family system, that is, on the family member's characteristic ways of relating to each other, rather than on the individual child. The "crazy" symptom of not eating exhibited by the patient was redefined as an interpersonal problem. Family members were seen as mutually regulating each other's behavior. While this required a more complex approach by the therapist, who had to consider the multiple

impact of his interventions, it also offered more opportunities for introducing change.

2. The family system was not conceived of merely as a system of interchangeable parts, but rather as internally structured; hence the term structural family therapy. Family members have individual characteristics and identities; simultaneously they are members of subsystems within the larger system, that is, spouse subsystem, parental subsystem, sibling subsystem, etc. These subsystems are functionally related in ways that are culturally, but also idiosyncratically defined. The structural therapist addresses himself to the dysfunctional relationships within and between the systems. His efforts at changing or restructuring dysfunctional patterns in this case were directed toward increasing the unity and executive effectiveness of the parental subsystem and diminishing a coalition of mother and patient against the father. The results were quite different than if the interventions had been made because the boy was too close to his mother or was rejected by his father.

3. The therapist essentially worked with the ways in which the family dealt with each other at the present time. Little or no time was spent on historical reconstruction of the development of the family's problem, the patient's problem, or the reason for (the intrapsychic meaning of) the anorexia symptom. Diagnostic efforts were directed toward examining the current dysfunctional patterns of relationships, with particular emphasis on transactional sequences, and the way in which the family organized itself around the illness.

4. Therapeutic interventions consisted of arranging experiences for the family members which would enable them to perceive each other and interact in new ways. This was done by strategic redefining of behaviors (not interpretations of inner thoughts and feelings) and through the assignment of interaction tasks to be done at home. While this approach is similar, in some ways, to family behavior modification (Eisler 1973), it differs in that the modifications were planned according to an overall view of the family system and the requirements of restructuring the internal organization.

Many of these points are generally applicable to family work with childhood disorders (Minuchin 1974). After this beginning, more cases of anorexia were treated, and a larger research into the familial context of psychosomatic illness in children was begun. In particular, children with psychosomatic asthma and with superlabile or "brittle" diabetes were being treated with family therapy in much the same way (Minuchin, Baker, Rosman, Liebman, Milman, and Todd 1975). In the course of this study, it was noted, with some excitement and interest, that while the identified symptoms of the children were all quite different, the family patterns of functioning were similar, with the symptomatic child playing a similar role in the dysfunctional family system. The formulation of a conceptual model of psychosomatic illness in children which outlined specific and treatable characteristics of their family's functioning was a great step forward in differentiating our approach to anorexia nervosa.

According to this model of the psychosomatic family, four general characteristics were identified and a fifth specified which had to do with the involvement of the symptomatic child.

First, psychosomatic families were found to be highly enmeshed, or overinvolved. While in all families individual members are regulated by the family system while functioning also in individually differentiated ways, in enmeshed families the individual becomes submerged in the system. Interpersonal differentiation is poor and family members may be seen to intrude into each other's thoughts and feelings to a great extent. It is often difficult to tell where one person's business leaves off and the other's begins. Another aspect of enmeshment is the poor differentiation of subsystems. This may result in inadequate performance of functions associated with a given subsystem—that is, ineffective parental control—or in the crossing over of boundaries so that children are inappropriately parental to their parents or siblings. Subsystem boundaries may also be impaired due to frequent coalition formation which occurs in these families as a way of maintaining stability, for example when a child or children may join one spouse against the other in conflict or decisionmaking.

Second, these families were found to be very overprotective not only to the symptomatic child, but as a way of family life. Overprotection often extended beyond physical care or concern over illness into other areas of life, and frequently hampered the development of autonomy and interests or activities outside of the safe family.

Third, the families were resistant to change, and denied having any problems other than their sick child. These families are particularly vulnerable to pressure for changes in family organization coming from within, such as a child reaching adolescence, or from without, such as changes in occupation or geographic relocation.

Fourth, the families had a very low tolerance for conflict and inadequately developed techniques of conflict resolution. In some cases families bickered or complained a lot, while others totally avoided disagreement. However, inability to confront differences to the point of negotiating a resolution was characteristic of all the families. As a result, most of the families lived in a state of constant tension.

315

Within this type of family context, the symptomatic child was involved in parental conflict in particular ways. Parents unable to deal with each other directly might unite in protective concern over their sick child. A marital conflict might be transformed into a parental conflict over the patient. The child might be recruited into taking sides by the parents, or might intrude herself as a mediator or helper. The value of the symptom in regulating the internal stability of the family seemed to reinforce both the continuation of the symptom and the peculiar aspects of the family organization in which it emerged.

The development of this conceptual framework greatly facilitated the therapists' work with the anorectic patients and their families. Each family had its own particular style of interaction, its own set of conflictual issues and stresses to which it was responding; nevertheless, awareness of the underlying similarities in family organization enabled the therapists to focus more quickly on the problems and to develop a systematic program of therapy. In presenting an outline here of this program, its goals, and overall strategy, we will not do justice to many ingenious interventions and family tasks devised by therapists to accommodate the individual styles and needs of families. Some of these have been described elsewhere (Minuchin 1974, Liebman, Minuchin, and Baker 1974a, 1974b, Combrinck-Graham 1974, Rosman, Minuchin, and Liebman 1975). However, we believe that the overall effectiveness of the treatment, carried out to date by sixteen different therapists, comes from the development of a general strategy based on this conceptual schema.

The first step in the treatment of this illness is to eliminate the symptom of not eating. This may seem to be a rather paradoxical statement because after all everybody, using any form of treatment, wants or expects to cure the symptom. Usually, however, this is considered to be the ultimate goal, with earlier stages of treatment devoted to uncovering causes, resolving conflicts, rewarding improved behavior, and so forth. However, it is our view that while the underlying problems may take a while to clear up, the symptom must be dealt with at the beginning. First, anorexia is a destructive and potentially fatal illness. The therapist must reverse this process as rapidly as possible. Secondly, the emotional charge of this behavior keeps the family strongly organized around the identified patient and around issues of health and food, thus inhibiting a broader exploration of the family relationships which are contributing to the illness. Finally, when the symptom is no longer available, submerged conflicts and other dysfunctional patterns which have been circumvented and avoided will emerge to be dealt with in treatment.

A variety of strategies are employed to accomplish symptom remission. Slightly more than half of our patients were admitted to a pediatric medical unit for a brief period of from one to four weeks. This is usually done for medical evaluation, to restore some of the more physically debilitated patients, and to determine if a brief period of disengagement from the family scene, coupled with an exposure to a behavioral paradigm, in which participation in activities is made contingent on weight gain, will reverse the eating behavior. Other patients were treated completely on an out-patient basis. Family therapy begins, in almost all cases, with a session in which the therapist meets with the patient and family around the lunch table. This practice derives from the ecological schema mentioned earlier according to which the wise therapist looks at the problem in its context. The ensuing family encounters at the lunch sessions are programmed by the therapist in a variety of ways (Rosman, Minuchin, and Liebman 1975) so as to accomplish three goals: (1) To change the family's perceptions of the patient as helpless, sick, or crazy and to broaden the therapeutic focus to include the rest of the family, relieving the patient of the need to carry the burden for others. (2) To redefine the eating problem as an interpersonal problem. This permits changing the arena of conflict so that the fight may be carried on more directly with less harm to the patient. (3) To block the parents from using the child's deviant behavior for conflict detouring, thus removing the motive force for the maintenance of the symptom.

Changes in the family organization which have been initiated in the therapy sessions are reinforced by family interaction tasks to be carried out at home. When these interventions are successful, and we have some good evidence that they most usually are, a rather rapid remission of the symptom will be achieved.

The therapist who from the first has had to deal with overprotectiveness, enmeshment, rigidity, and poor conflict resolution around the eating issue now moves into other areas of life where these patterns pervade. As the symptoms of anorexia diminish, other family problems emerge, sometimes revealed in the most trivial events of daily life, which can then be explored in therapy. For example, the six members of one family all had the same kinds of socks, which they washed together, and then had unresolvable arguments about how to tell whose was whose. The opening and shutting of doors and the maintenance of privacy (Aponte and Hoffman 1973), the distribution of responsibility for household chores, conflicts over discipline, all provide content for the therapist to deal with in his work with the family. Goals for this middle period of therapy are clarification of boundaries, developing problem and conflict solving strategies, and increasing the life space of family members. This can be achieved only when the family and parents are less preoccupied with the medical problems of the patient.

In the final stage of treatment, when the eating problems are more remote and family members are functioning at a more differentiated level, the therapist is able to deal with some of the specific and more long standing problems coming from within the subsystems. Marital problems of the spouses and sibling and peer relations of the children can be treated in separate sessions where required. It is very important these issues be dealt with to avoid a recurrence of the illness or of other symptoms in the patient, or in other family members, and to enhance the individual development of family members.

Now, within this overview of the structural family approach to anorexia nervosa, we must go to one further level of differentiation. On the basis of a survey of the work of the sixteen therapists with all of the fifty-three patients, it appears that while the general schema applies to the treatment of all the families, specific goals of family restructuring vary systematically with the age of the child and the developmental stage of family. The therapists have been very sensitive to these differences and have modified the treatment accordingly.

First let us consider the youngest group, the preadolescents, ranging in age from nine to twelve. Fourteen of the patients or 25 percent of the group treated fell in this range. In these families, therapists almost universally stated as their primary goal: increasing parental effectiveness and parental control, and strengthening the parental coalition especially around executive functioning. To begin this process, some of the parents in the lunch sessions were encouraged to work together to force their child to eat, particularly when the child was most defiant and resistant. Other parents were instructed to maintain a behavioral paradigm at home, similar to that used at the hospital. Parents were helped to become effective at controlling their children's behavior and in setting limits. This strategy not only served to diminish the symptom, but reinforced the boundaries between subsystems, increased the distance between parents and children, and minimized the child's involvement in parental conflict. While these tactics seemed to reduce the autonomy of the patient, the reverse actually proved to be the case. The child, while anorectic, was trapped in the conflict with and between the parents. Freed from this position, the child was able to return to the normal tasks of developing competencies at home, in school, and in social life which had been neglected during the illness. Positive effects of this strategy on the patient could be seen not only in symptom remission, but in a more relaxed and cheerful affect state, the giving up of babyish behaviors, and better relations with siblings. When working with this age group, therapists used family sessions initially, shifting to parent sessions in the latter phases. Preadolescent patients were not seen individually.

The adolescent group of patients were the most numerous in the sample treated; thirty-one patients, or 60 percent of the group, were between thirteen and sixteen years of age when first seen. Therapists' aspirations for children in this age group were directed towards development of autonomy and increasing independence. Parents and children, in some cases, were disengaged around the issue of eating and redirected toward negotiating more typical adolescent conflicts. In other cases, children were encouraged to become more self-sufficient in monitoring their own diets, but with the parents supervising the weight gain and behavioral regime. Therapists aimed at reduction in parental overprotectiveness and fostered increased assignment of responsibilities for the child in the home as well as for the self.

It is interesting to compare our work with this age group with that of Bruch (1973). This author has suggested that the central issue for anorexia nervosa patients is the conflict around autonomy and control. She proposed that, as a result of an intrusive and domineering early mother-child relationship, the patient has not developed feelings of mastery and ownership of her own body. The illness is seen as a distorted but heroic effort on the part of the patient to regain control of her body and to assert autonomy. Her therapeutic work with patients is directed toward a more constructive resolution of this problem. While we would agree that our adolescent patients do engage in this kind of struggle, we submit that this is only a partial picture. The anorectic patient while struggling to free herself of the constricting control of the enmeshed family is herself controlling, manipulative, and intrusive into the domains of her parents and siblings as are all the members of her family toward her and toward each other. To work alone with the adolescent patient to disengage her from this involvement is to make the therapeutic task more difficult. Only by submitting the mutually restrictive involvement of parents and child to the therapeutic process, and clarifying which parts of the struggle belong truly to the patient and which parts belong to others, can autonomy and independence be accomplished. To facilitate this process, the therapists push the children into increased peer and sibling group participation. In working with adolescents, therapists will see the sibling subsystem and occasionally the individual patient in addition to family and marital sessions.

319

Progressing into late adolescence and early adulthood, eight patients, 15 percent of the sample, were seen who were between the ages of seventeen and twenty-one. This was the period in which separation from the family was impending or had actually been attempted. Anorexia at this age seemed to reflect inability of patient and family to negotiate a successful launching of the child into independence. Therapists worked only initially in family sessions, moving quickly to separate the patient into individual sessions to foster disengagement and self-confidence, and to work with parents in marital sessions to reduce their need for and pull on the patient. Subsequently, patients were able to begin or return to college, get a job, rent an apartment, acquire a boyfriend, and successfully lead an independent life.

We have elaborated on these points to emphasize that commitment to an overall approach, which is highly structured and programmatic, need not inhibit flexibility in the use of different therapeutic techniques to adapt the overall strategy for the particular characteristics of the family and patient. Individual therapy sessions with the patients or the parents, in addition to occasional family sessions, are most important in the late adolescent and young adult group to underline and reinforce the disengagement and individuation processes vital to successful recuperation. Behavioral modification techniques may also be incorporated.

Conclusions

The characteristics of the fifty-three patients whose outcomes are reported here are typical for this diagnostic group as described in psychiatric literature. Patients came from a variety of middle and upper middle-class backgrounds; all were white. Six of the patients (11 percent of the group) were male. Their cases and course of treatment were similar to those of the girls. Patients were diagnosed as anorectic on the basis of a weight loss of 20 percent or more body weight not due to any organic cause as determined by pediatricians. In our sample, the range of weight loss went from 20 percent to 50 percent, with a median of 30 percent. In their behavior and verbalizations, patients exhibited pathognomic signs of anorexia nervosa: denial of hunger, delusional body image, and fear of fatness. Forty percent of the patients had been treated prior to referral to us, usually with some form of individual treatment; almost 20 percent had been previously hospitalized. The interval between onset and referral to us ranged from one month to three years; median time was six months; the median course of treatment was six months long. These figures do not include three cases who dropped treatment after two or three sessions, (attrition of 6 percent).

Therapeutic outcome was evaluated in two areas: degree of remission of the anorexia symptoms, and a clinical assessment of psychosocial functioning in relation to home, school, and social adjustment.

Patients were scored as recovered from anorexia when eating patterns returned to normal and body weight stabilized within normal limits for height and age. If patients improved, gained weight, but still showed some effects of the illness, such as a borderline body weight, obesity, problems around eating such as occasional vomiting, a score of fair was given. Patients who did not respond to treatment were rated as unimproved.

In the clinical assessment similarly, a patient's status was scored as good if adjustment in the family situation, participation in academic and extracurricular activities at school or work, and involvement with peers were judged satisfactory. A rating of fair was given when adjustment in one or another of these areas was unsatisfactory. Patients were judged unimproved if they were unable to function even at borderline levels and continued to show disturbances of behavior, thought, and affect.

Evaluations were based not only on the patient's condition at termination of therapy, but also on information obtained through follow-up contacts with patients, families, and pediatricians. Follow-up intervals range from three months to four years, with a median follow-up time of one year, and 25 percent have been followed for at least two years.

Of the fifty patients who continued treatment, forty-three made complete recoveries from the anorexia, four were judged to be only in fair condition, and three were unimproved, and were transferred elsewhere for treatment with some success. Within the recovered group, two of the children relapsed, were treated again, and have remained in recovered condition for six months or more. If we count only the absolute recoveries, we can say we have achieved an 86 percent successful outcome. Since most published samples of this size report success rates more closely approaching a 30 percent improvement rate on follow-up, we consider our findings to be substantial evidence of effective psychotherapy.

Results of the clinical assessment have been similarly gratifying. Forty-four of the patients were rated as making a good adjustment, three as only fair, and three unimproved. Counting only the satisfactory adjustments, the outcome is 88 percent effective.

It is of some interest that four of the patients were reported returning at a later date for some brief individual counseling. In these cases, the problem or issues did not concern eating, but were related appropriately to a later stage of psychosocial development. The purpose of these additional visits was to, as one patient so nicely put it, "work out normal problems."

321

In conclusion, we have reviewed the development and increasing differentiation of a model for effective treatment of a difficult and threatening psychosomatic illness. We believe that the increasing specificity of the concepts and the development of therapeutic strategies closely tied to our theory have enabled sixteen different therapists to carry out an effective, systematic approach to treatment which is economical and transmissable to other workers in the field.

REFERENCES

Aponte, H., and Hoffman, L. (1973). The open door: a structural approach to a family with an anorectic child. *Family Process* 12: 1:1-44.

Bruch, H. (1973). *Eating Disorders*. New York: Basic Books.

Combrinck-Graham, L. (1974). Structural family therapy in psychosomatic illness; treatment of anorexia nervosa and asthma. *Clinical Pediatrics* 13: 10:827-833.

Eisler, R., and Hersen, M. (1973). Behavioral techniques in family-oriented crisis intervention. *Archives of General Psychiatry* 28: 1:111-116.

Liebman, R., Minuchin, S., and Baker, L. (1974a). The role of the family in the treatment of anorexia nervosa. *Journal of the Academy of Child Psychiatry* 13: 2:263-274.

——— (1974b). An integrated treatment program for anorexia nervosa. *American Journal of Psychiatry* 131:4:432-436.

Minuchin, S. (1970). The use of an ecological framework in the treatment of a child. E. Anthony and C. Koupernick, eds., *The Child in His Family*. New York: Wiley.

——— (1974). *Families and Family Therapy*. Cambridge, Mass.: Harvard University Press.

———, Baker, L., Rosman, B., Liebman, R., Milman, L., and Todd, T. (1975). A conceptual model of psychosomatic illness in children: family organization and family therapy. *Archives of General Psychiatry* 32: 8: 1031-1038.

Rosman, B., Minuchin, S., and Liebman, R. (1975). Family lunch session: an introduction to family therapy in anorexia nervosa. *American Journal of Orthopsychiatry* 45: 5: 846-853.

21] BEHAVIOR THERAPY
IN ANOREXIA NERVOSA

KATHERINE A. HALMI AND LINDA LARSON

Recent controversies over behavior therapy in anorexia nervosa (Bruch 1974) give the impression that the use of behavioral contingencies is a new treatment modality. This is not so. Sixteen years ago, while Dally and Sargant (1960) were announcing chlorpromazine as a new treatment for anorexia nervosa they were concurrently employing behavioral contingencies. Their patients were put to bed at the start of treatment and not allowed up until they regained near normal weight. Again, this powerful reinforcer was used with chlorpromazine and psychotherapy in twenty-one patients by Crisp (1965) who also reported follow-up information. Russell (1973) mentioned a restriction regimen which is progressively relaxed through a series of rewards as the patient cooperates and gains weight. Behavior conditioning has been used along with family therapy (Liebman, Minuchin, and Baker 1974) and promoted as a "practical initial management in a general hospital" (Maxmen, Silberfarb, and Fenel 1974). The usefulness of behavioral contingencies in conjunction with other therapies in treating anorexia nervosa has become widely recognized.

The rational for using behavioral techniques derived from learning theory was stated by Brady (1972), "The anorectics behave as though they suffer from an eating phobia—eating generates anxiety and their failure to eat represents avoidance." Cessation of eating after ingesting a very small portion of a meal (or removing it from the body by self-induced vomiting) is reinforced by anxiety reduction. From such an analysis two treatment procedures suggest themselves; deconditioning the anxiety associated with eating or shaping eating behavior (and hence weight gain) by making access to powerful reinforcers contingent on eating. The former procedure has never been reported as the sole treatment. Hallsten (1965) treated a twelve-year-old anorectic girl using Wolpe's systematic desensitization by pairing Jacobsonian relaxation with a hierarchy of anxiety producing eating and weight gaining scenes. However, he used this reciprocal inhibition technique concurrently with the powerful reinforcer of making visits by relatives contingent on weight gain. The patient gained weight and was regarded as having a satisfactory adjustment after a five month absence. Leitenberg, Agras, and Thompson (1968) using operant conditioning strategy with selective positive reinforcers based on "the assumption that each behavioral step forward will reduce anxiety," showed this technique effective in inducing weight gain in two anorexia nervosa patients. Using the patients as their own controls, they showed "the effects of reinforcement were isolated from effects of separation from home, expectations of therapeutic success imported by physician's instructions, and noncontingent therapist attention."

Blinder, Freeman, and Stunkard (1970) using a daily reinforcement of access to physical activity contingent upon one-half pound weight gain were able to induce a rapid weight gain in three anorectic patients. Brady and Rieger (1972) using a similar program reported a follow-up on thirteen patients plus three patients treated by Blinder. This follow-up ranging from four to fifty-nine months after hospital discharge reported two deaths (13 percent) and three patients (21 percent) with a poor adjustment.

Elkin, Hersen, Eisler, and Williams (1973) in a sequential single-case design showed that combinations of increasing the amount of food plus providing feedback on weight and positive reinforcement resulted in a greater caloric intake than any of the three methods used alone. Bhanji and Thompson (1972) reported weight gain in ten of eleven anorexia nervosa patients with operant conditioning using individualized reinforcers. A follow-up (two to seventy-two months) on seven of these patients showed on a global rating only one had a good outcome, three had some continuing problems, and three had a poor outcome.

Agras, Barlow, Chapin, Abel, and Leitenberg (1974) in five single-case experiments with anorectics demonstrated: (1) hospitalization has a negative reinforcing effect of inducing weight gain, (2) knowledge of weight gain is necessary for positive reinforcers to be maximally effective, and (3) the larger the amount of food served to anorectics the more is eaten.

Halmi, Powers, and Cunningham (1975) reported the effectiveness of an operant-conditioning program using formula feeding initially in eight anorexia nervosa patients. No ataractic drugs were given concurrently. All patients gained during hospitalization and at follow-up (two to thirteen months after discharge) all had continued to gain as outpatients on individualized positive reinforcers. Only one patient had major adjustment problems.

From a review of literature it is apparent that controlled studies on the behavioral treatment of anorexia nervosa both during hospitalization and post-hospitalization are necessary. No long term posthospitalization open study using behavioral techniques has been reported. Thus we thought it worthwhile to design and conduct controlled treatment studies comparing an operant conditioning paradigm with a psychotherapy and family therapy program containing virtually no behavioral contingencies related to weight gain.

Table 1

Criteria for Anorexia Nervosa

1. Onset between ages ten and thirty years.

2. Weight loss of at least 25 percent of original body weight. Patient must be at least 15 percent below normal weight for age and height. (Normal weights will be obtained from the Metropolitan Life Insurance Company Scales and the Iowa Growth Charts for Children.)

3. A distorted, implacable attitude and behavior toward eating, food, or weight that overrides hunger, admonitions, reassurance, and threats—for example:
   a. Denial of illness, with a failure to recognize nutritional needs.
   b. Apparent enjoyment in losing weight, with overt manifestation that food refusal is pleasurable indulgence.
   c. A desired body image of extreme thinness, with overt evidence that it is rewarding to the patient to achieve and maintain this state.
   d. Unusual hoarding or handling of food.

4. At least one of the following manifestations:
   a. Lanugo (persistence of downy pelage)
   b. Bradycardia (persistent resting pulse of 60 or less)
   c. Periods of overactivity
   d. Episodes of bulimia (compulsive overeating)
   e. Vomiting (may be self-induced)

5. Amenorrhea of at least three months duration, unless illness occurs before onset of menses.

6. No known medical illness that could account for the anorexia and weight loss.

7. No other known psychiatric disorder, with particular reference to primary affective disorders, schizophrenia, obsessive-compulsive and phobic neuroses (it is assumed that even though it may appear phobic or obsessional, food refusal alone is not sufficient to qualify for obsessive-compulsive or phobic disease). Other psychiatric disorders are excluded according to the criteria of Feighner et al. If during the course of the present illness, the patient meets concurrently criteria 1-6 and that of depression or obsessive-compulsive neurosis, she will be considered to have anorexia nervosa.

Methodology

In order to be admitted to the study, all seemingly eligible female patients between ages ten and forty must meet the criteria of Table 1 with two psychiatric interviewers. They are then admitted to the Clinical Research Center at the University of Iowa Hospital where, during a seven-day adjustment pretreatment period, a complete medical evaluation is done and two pretreatment behavioral evaluation are made using a battery of assessments both self and observer rating for mood, typical anorectic behavior and attitudes, and interpersonal behavior. On the seventh day the patients are randomly assigned to behavioral therapy or no behavioral therapy. A structured social and psychiatric history is obtained by a social worker from the patients and family. On admission, all patients are given a target weight, the lowest weight in a normal weight range of their age and height according to the Metropolitan Life Insurance height-weight norms and the *Girls Growth Chart* from the Iowa Child Welfare Research Station. The patients are told this is the lowest medically acceptable weight for them. Throughout their hospitalizations all patients are weighed at 7:00 A.M. daily and are informed of their weight. Daily caloric counts are done by a dietician blind to the treatment program. The daily caloric intake necessary to maintain the patient's weight on the seventh pretreatment day is calculated to be 125 percent of basal requirements as determined by a nomogram. All patients receive Sustagen, diluted to 1 kcal/cc and given in six equal feedings, as their only source of nutrient for the first fifteen days of treatment. For the first five days the patients receive the caloric level estimated to maintain body weight (baseline calories). The second five days they are offered 150 percent of baseline calories and the third five day period they receive 200 percent of baseline calories. Following this, the patients have three meals of a regular diet including a morning, afternoon, and evening snack. The meals are taken in the unit dining room, where the patient is given one-half hour to complete each meal. The amount of calories offered to the patient per day is increased by 50 percent each five-day period.

All patients receive three hours per week of individual therapy sessions with a psychiatric social worker who focuses on the patient's relationship with other family members and with her peers. The family, parents, siblings, or spouse are seen in therapy regularly and separately from the patient during most of the latter's hospitalization. These sessions emphasize interpersonal relationships in the family. The patient is seen with her family in one or two therapy sessions before her discharge from the hospital.

Behavior therapy is essentially that of operant conditioning with positive reinforcements of social activities, increased physical activities, and visiting privileges contingent upon weight gains. Although the patient will be weighed every morning and informed of her weight, weight gain will be evaluated at the end of five-day periods. In order to earn increased privileges, the patient must gain 0.5 kg per five-day period. An exception is the first five days, when she will be required only to maintain her weight. If the patient does not gain weight at the end of five days, she receives no advanced privileges. Later, if she has lost weight at the end of a five-day period, privileges will be withdrawn.

The first day of the behavior therapy program the patient will be isolated and restricted to her room. For five days she will receive no visitors, no phone calls, and no mail. She will drink her formula in her room and only hospital staff will enter her room. A radio, but no T.V., is allowed in the room. If the patient maintains her weight, on the sixth day or the beginning day of the next five-day period, she is allowed to make one phone call, receive her mail, have one visitor for one hour, and be out of her room one hour every day for the next five days. The end of the next and each succeeding five-day period, the patient is required to gain 0.5 kg and then 1 kg when she is on the regular diet in order to have an additional visitor or the same number of visitors for an additional hour, to receive her mail, to make additional phone calls, and to be out of her room each day for an additional hour. Phone calls, visitors, and mail can be received only on the

327

TABLE 2

Characteristics of Adolescent Anorexia Nervosa
Patients During Hospitalization
Behavior Therapy Program

11 Cases	Admission Age	Height cm.	Pre-Treatment Weight kg.	Percent Standard Weight	Hospital Discharge Weight kg.	Percent Standard Weight
1	16	161	32.9	68	40.4	84
2	15	164	41.4	80	51.4	99
3	15	157	34.6	76	45.3	100
4	17	160	44.3	85	48.4	93
5	14	158	33	69	41.8	88
6	16	162	30.8	59	39.7	76
7	15	162.6	36.6	73	42.6	85
8	17	158	33.1	69	42	87
9	14	163	35.4	67	51.5	97
10	14	149	27.3	65	42.0	100
11	14	157	28.1	61	43.8	95
Mean	15	159	34.3	70	44.4	91

TABLE 3

Characteristics of Adolescent Anorexia Nervosa
Patients During Hospitalizations

No Behavioral Contingencies

9 Cases	Admission Age	Height cm.	Pre-Treatment Weight kg.	Percent Standard Weight	Hospital Discharge Weight kg.	Percent Standard Weight
12	15	167.5	36.1	69	41.4	79
13	16	170.8	43.1	79	49.3	90
14	16	170	38.9	71	47.0	86
15	16	162	38.4	80	46.3	96
16	17	162.5	37.0	74	44.0	88
17	14	164	39.9	77	47.7	92
18	12	150.5	35.5	78	41.8	92
19	12	161	36.5	72	47.6	93
			38.4	75	46.7	92
Mean	15	163	38.2	75	45.7	89.8

TABLE 4

**Characteristics of Adult Anorexia Nervosa
Patients During Hospitalization
Behavior Therapy Program**

18 Cases	Admission Age	Height cm.	Pre-Treatment Weight kg.	Percent Standard Weight	Hospital Discharge Weight kg.	Percent Standard Weight
21	26	156	31.4	69	40.3	89
22	20	158	28.7	62	36.9	80
23	22	168	40.2	80	45.9	92
24	23	162	37.0	77	42.1	88
25	20	163	42.8	84	48	94
26	18	151	33.6	76	40.2	91
27	19	157	38.2	83	45.2	98
28	20	184	38.1	57	67.6	101
29	20	159	33.2	72	40.1	87
30	19	160	35.8	75	46.9	98
31	26	166	35.4	66	47	87
32	54	161	30	59	41.3	81
33	21	165	45.6	82	52	94
34	23	157.5	31.2	62	40	80
35	29	166	33	65	44.4	87
36	20	160	34.4	70	45.6	93
37	19	155	37.7	78	47.6	99
38	22	163	24.8	55	43.9	97
Mean	23	162	35	70.7	45.3	91

day privileges are earned. During the time earned out of the room, the patient may participate in any ward activity she wishes. She may choose which hours in the day she spends out of her room. While in her room the patient may engage in any crafts or reading of her choice.

After discharge from the hospital, the patients are placed on an outpatient behavior therapy program. Individualized positive reinforcements such as new clothes, special activities, etc. are given by the family for 0.5 kg weight gain per week until the patient reaches target weight. She is then expected to maintain her weight within 2 kg of her target weight. If at any follow-up visit the patient is below this 2 kg limit or has lost more than 1 kg on her way up to the target weight, she is rehospitalized. Initial weekly

TABLE 5

Characteristics of Adult Anorexia Nervosa
Patients During Hospitalizations
No Behavioral Contingencies

6 Cases	Admission Age	Height cm.	Pre-Treatment Weight kg.	Percent Standard Weight	Hospital Discharge Weight kg.	Percent Standard Weight
39	20	155	29.5	65	28.9	64
40	33	173	38.4	61	47.7	84
41	21	160	42.5	88	47.4	99
42	20	170.5	48.1	85	53.9	95
43	25	163	35.9	73	40	82
44	19	160	34.1	74	43.5	95
Mean	23	163.6	37.5	74	43.6	86.5

follow-up visits are gradually decreased to less frequent as the patient improves in weight maintenance and behavior. Whenever possible the patient is seen with her family in outpatient therapy sessions. Some parents are extremely resistant to becoming involved in therapy. However, most parents cooperate well with the outpatient operant conditioning paradigm.

Results

Adolescence has been arbitrarily defined to include patients between the ages of twelve and seventeen. Adult patients are those eighteen years and older. All consecutive anorexia nervosa admissions from 1972 until 1975 were treated with the behavioral therapy program described above. These patients, consisting of seven adolescents and eight adults, are included in this report. Since January, 1975, all consecutive anorectic admissions have been randomly assigned to behavior therapy or no behavior therapy and they complete this patient sample of forty-four.

Tables 2-5 summarize clinical characteristics of the four patient groups, adolescents and adults with and without behavior therapy, during hospitalization. A comparison of the percent of weight gain in these groups during hospitalizations is given in Table 6. The treatment program that included behavior therapy was more effective in inducing weight gain in both adolescents and adults. Since the results did not differ between these groups we felt justified in combining them. When this was done the difference in treatments become statistically significant ($p < .01$, simple *t* test).

TABLE 6

Percent Weight Gain In Hospital

	Adolescents			Adults	
	Behavior Therapy	No Behavior Therapy		Behavior Therapy	No Behavior Therapy
N	11	9		18	6
Mean	21.09	14.77		20.22	12.16
S.D.	8.73	3.23		9.32	7.70
	t = 1.9538			t = 1.8396	
	* P .05			* P .05	

	Combined Adolescents and Adults	
	Behavior Therapy	No Behavior Therapy
N	29	15
Mean	20.55	13.73
S.D.	8.96	5.38
	t = 2.70	
	P .01	

* directional t test

TABLE 7

Anorexia Nervosa Followup

Present Adjustment: (Key)

Good   The patient is maintaining weight and functioning well at home, school, work, and socially.

Adequate   The patient is maintaining weight, but having minor behavior problems.

Fair   The patient is maintaining weight, but is functioning marginally in one or more important life areas (given above).

Poor   The patient is not maintaining weight and is functioning marginally in important life areas.

TABLE 8

**Adolescent Anorexia Nervosa Patients
at Time of Followup**

Behavior Therapy Program

11 Cases	Months Since Hospital Discharge	Present Weight Kg.	Percent Standard Weight	Weight Change Since Discharge		Return of Menses Months After Discharge	Adjustment
				Kg.	% change		
1	13	62.7	131	+22.3	+47	none	poor
2	13	52	100	+0.6	+1	none	good
3	10	46.5	102	+1.2	+2	none	fair
4	7	51.1	102	+1.7	+2	1	good
5	34	52	100	+10.2	+12	NA	good
6	40	50	100	+10.3	+24	11	good
7	40	47	94	+4.4	+9	none	adequate
8	30	45	94	+3	+7	none	good
9	23	58	100	+6.5	+3	none	adequate
10	25	42.5	100	0	0	none	fair
11	18	45	98	+1.2	+3	none	fair

TABLE 9

**Adolescent Anorexia Nervosa Patients
at Time of Followup**

No Behavioral Contingencies

7 Cases	Months Since Hospital Discharge	Present Weight Kg.	Percent Standard Weight	Weight Change Since Discharge		Return of Menses Months After Discharge	Adjustment
				Kg.	% change		
12	18	52.8	100	+11.4	+21	4	good
13	17	51.8	95	+2.5	+5	none	fair
14	14	54.2	100	+7.2	+14	none	adequate
15	13	46.8	97	+0.5	+1	9	good
16	11	44.2	88	0	0	none	adequate
17	9	47.8	92	0	0	none	fair
18	6	37.7	83	-4.1	-9	none	poor
19	0	—	—	—	—	—	—
20	0	—	—	—	—	—	—
Mean	12.6		93.6	+2.5	+5		

TABLE 10

Adult Anorexia Nervosa
Patients at Followup
Behavior Therapy Program

8 Cases	Months Since Hospital Discharge	Present Weight Kg.	Percent Standard Weight	Weight Change Since Discharge		Return of Menses Months After Discharge	Adjustment
				Kg.	% change		
21	16	36.4	80	-3.9	-9	none	poor
22	14	35.5	77	-1.4	-3	none	poor
23	13	45.8	92	0	0	none	adequate
24	12	46.4	97	+4.3	+9	none	adequate
25	8	49.4	100	+1.4	+6	none	good
26	8	42.6	97	+2.7	+6	6	adequate
27	7	45	98	0	0	none	fair
28	1	63.2	94	-4.4	-7	none	poor
29	2	45.5	99	+5.9	+12	none	adequate
30	1	46.9	98	0	0	none	adequate
31	30	52	96	+5	+9	24	good
32	30	41.3	81	0	0	none	fair
33	23	54	98	+2	+4	18	adequate
34	29	49	96	+9	+16	none	good
35	26	49	90	+5	+3	none	adequate
36	25	51	104	+5.4	+11	6	good
37	19	50	104	+2.4	+5	none	good
38	16	43.9	97	0	0	none	adequate
Mean	15.8		94	+1.7	+3.4		

An operant conditioning paradigm (see methodology) was followed in the outpatient therapy program for all patients. A global adjustment (Table 7) was given to these patients by the social worker and psychiatrist at the time of a follow-up inquiry which was a personal or telephone interview. The raters were not blind to the hospital therapy program. The possibility of bias must be considered. However, the objective measure of weight can hardly be expected to be influenced by the therapist's knowledge of treatment. The weight change since the time of hospital discharge, the length of the follow-up, and adjustment ratings are given for each of the four patient groups in Tables 8-11.

Although the treatment differences in both adolescents and adults favor behavior therapy in the amount of weight change since hospital discharge,

TABLE 11

Adult Anorexia Nervosa
Patients at Followup

No Behavioral Contingencies

6 Cases	Months Since Hospital Discharge	Present Weight Kg.	Percent Standard Weight	Weight Change Since Discharge		Return of Menses Months After Discharge	Adjustment
				Kg.	% change		
39	11	26.6	59	-2.3	-5	none	poor
40	10	46	81	-1.7	-3	none	poor
41	9	50	104	+2.6	+5	none	good
42	6	57	100	+3.1	+5	none	good
43	2	34	68	-6	-14	none	poor
44	1	44.5	97	+1	+2	none	good
Mean	6.5		85	-.55	-1.7		

these differences do not reach statistical significance. This is due to the considerable variation within each group. The greatest difference occurred between the adolescents who received behavior therapy in the hospital and the adults who did not receive that program. Note that adolescents in both treatment programs gained more after hospital discharge than the adults. It is possible that with larger numbers this difference would become significant.

The length of follow-up from the time of hospital discharge ranged from one to forty months. It is commonly expected that shortly after hospitalization patients will continue to do well and thus a longer follow-up is needed for a more accurate assessment of treatment failures. In our follow-up sample of forty-two, seventeen patients were evaluated at less than one year and twenty-five patients received evaluations greater than one year from hospital discharge. Almost one-half of the patients who had follow-up ratings at less than one year were given a poor or fair adjustment. Whereas, only seven of the twenty-five patients followed greater than one year had poor or fair adjustment ratings.

Fewer patients who had behavior therapy while in the hospital had poor adjustment ratings (four of twenty-nine) than those without behavioral contingencies (four of thirteen). Only two of eighteen adolescents received poor adjustment ratings compared to six of twenty-four adults.

The strongest factor influencing outcome was a previous treatment failure. The latter was defined as a minimum hospitalization of one month specifically for treatment or a minimum of six months outpatient therapy during which time the patient remained the same weight or lost weight and made no improvement in her anorectic behavior.

All patients who had previous treatment failures received a poor or fair adjustment rating at follow-up (Table 12). Only five of thirty-one without previous treatment failures were given a poor or fair rating. Six of the eleven previous treatment failures were not maintaining their hospital discharge weight at follow-up, whereas only two of the thirty-one without prior therapy failure were losing weight (Table 12). Three of the previous treatment failures were adolescents and eight were adults. Of the nine patients referred from another state, eight had been previous treatment failures.

Of the eight patients who had a return of menses six had good adjustment ratings and two had adequate ratings. All eight were maintaining their weight between 96 percent and 104 percent of their target weights.

TABLE 12

**Adjustment at Followup
Compared with Previous Treatment Failures**

	Poor and Fair	Good and Adequate		Poor	Good, Adequate and Fair
Previous Treatment Failure	11	0		6	5
No Previous Treatment Failure	5	26		2	29

$X^2 = 20.79$, p .001 (Yates correction) $X^2 = 9.26$, p .005

Case Reports

CASE 3

This fifteen-year-old girl was admitted to the hospital weighing 35.9 kgs. Two months earlier she had weighed 45.3 kgs, her greatest weight, and a normal weight for her age and height. Her menses ceased one month prior to the time the patient started a voluntary diet. During a competitive swimming meet, one of the girls whom the patient admired remarked that the patient looked overweight. Shortly afterward, she started dieting by deleting from her meals high carbohydrate foods. She gradually eliminated more and more food items from her diet until she ate very little. She described bulimic episodes in which she would eat a large amount of ice cream or a dozen cookies. The patient denied ever abusing laxatives or self-inducing vomiting. She expressed a marked fear of gaining weight and stated that she was doing thirty situps twice a day to keep her stomach from sticking out. In the two months prior to admission she had been collecting recipes and doing much more cooking for the family than she had previously done. The patient would refuse to eat meals she prepared and hid candies and sweets about the house. She had the physical symptoms of bradycardia and hypothermia on admission.

Past history and family history. The patient was born in Cuba and moved here with her parents when only a few months old. She has one sibling, a younger sister, with whom there was extreme competition. When the patient was four years old her parents were divorced. During the next four years there was considerable dramatic fighting between the parent over the father's visiting rights. The mother was killed in a car accident when the patient was eight years old, and shortly after this, she and her younger sister came to live with their father. The father is a forty-six-year-old general surgeon who has diabetes and follows a special diet. He is anxious, controlling, overactive, and dramatic. He issues many rules and regulations for the household, but his daughters tend to compromise most of them. The father and daughters spend very little time together. The sisters are obviously envious of each other. The father had been dating casually until about two years ago and since then had consistently dated one person. About six months ago, the patient became very jealous over her father's dating and requested he stop dating entirely. He complied with her request. The patient was an excellent student and has been at the top of her class for several years.

Course in the hospital. The patient was treated with the behavior therapy program described earlier. She was dramatically superficial in her interactions with the staff and therapist. She constantly tested rules, exercised frequently, and would try to hoard food. She had a slow, steady weight gain while in the hospital and was discharged at 45.3 kgs.

Outpatient Course. Shortly after discharge the patient lost two kgs and maintained that weight for almost four months. In her weekly therapy sessions, she was resistive, and her housekeeper reported that she was again engaging in unusual food handling. This time after considerable effort the therapist was able to persuade the father, housekeeper, and sister to come in for family therapy sessions. When the patient lost another 2 kgs she was hospitalized for a week. She was initially tube fed until placed on a behavior therapy program which rapidly brought her back to target weight. The father was unable to follow through with any of the suggestions made during family therapy sessions. He continued to engage in a power struggle with the patient. Nine months after hospital discharge therapy was discontinued because the family moved to another state. Continued family therapy was recommended but thus far we have not been contacted for any information concerning this family.

CASE 4

This seventeen-year-old girl was admitted weighing 39 kgs. She was 55 kgs five months before when she started dieting. The patient started dieting shortly after her graduation from high school and after she left for Europe with her math teacher, ten years her senior. The patient described him as a compulsive and controlling man who frequently remarked that she was too fat. She gradually began to reduce her intake of high carbohydrate foods, and then deleted other food items from her diet so that intake, in the course of a day, was scant. Although she had originally planned to stay in Europe, she decided, after two months, to return. She returned with her companion, but then went to live at home and broke up with him. When she entered the hospital she was eating only vegetables and yogurt. She spent considerable time collecting recipes and cooking rolls and cookies which she could not eat. She stated she had a good appetite but was very afraid of losing control of it and becoming fat. She denied vomiting, bulimic episodes, or abuse of laxatives and these were not noted while in the hospital. Just before she left for Europe, the patient had started on birth control pills and still had sparse menstrual periods which stopped completely when taken off the pills. She exercised excessively, walking at least six miles per day and swimming one-third of a mile per day. She was not disturbed over her weight and in fact thought she was a bit fat. She complained of a sleep disturbance and had bradycardia and lanugo on physical examination. She came into the hospital wanting to escape considerable family tension and complete the separation from her boyfriend.

Past history and family history. Both parents were immigrants from Switzerland and were nonpracticing Catholics. The father, age forty-seven, was an industrial arts teacher at a school for handicapped children. The mother, age forty-nine, was a nurse who had just returned to work in the past year. An older married sister, who lived in town, was extremely dependent on the mother and her frequent return home caused a disruptive influence in the family. A younger sister, age fifteen, was also underweight (5' 7" tall and weighed 52 kgs). The younger sister had a problem with drug abuse; amphetamines, LSD, and mescaline. The mother prevailed on the patient to manage the behavior of her younger sister, and insisted on knowing every detail of her daughters' lives. While she tried to enforce excessively stringent laws concerning early curfews and attempted to make the girls report frequently as to their whereabouts, the mother also encouraged the patient's experimentation with sex and assisted her in getting birth control pills and in planning her trip to Europe with her teacher. The father was essentially uninvolved with the family. There was considerable tension between the mother and father, whose only interaction with each other was argument. They were in the process of discussing a separation when the patient was admitted to the hospital.

Course in the hospital. The patient was treated with the behavioral program. During treatment she gained from 43 kgs to 44.3 kgs. During the first ten days of treatment she lost 0.1 kg. The next ten days she went from 42.2 kgs to 45.3 kgs, gaining privileges. From then on, she continued to gain, obtaining greater privileges. She was discharged at 49.4 kgs, which was close to her target weight of 50 kgs. The patient was initially overactive, but cooperated well with the program. Her mother tried to bring her salt pills and a stool-softener. She responded well in her personal therapy sessions, and obtained excellent insight into family problems and of her own dependency in that regard. She decided to leave home and attend college despite the opposition from her parents. She was able to obtain a loan, allowing her to be financially independent of her parents.

Outpatient course. The patient went away to college for two quarters. She maintained her target weight for the first six months and by the end of the second six months had gained 4 kgs. While there, the patient got along well with her peer group and started to date. She had a job in the school cafeteria and became involved in social activities. Her menstrual periods returned four months after she had reached her target weight. The patient now has a summer job and is living at home, but is having minimal contact with the family. The parents were seen in separate sessions during the patient's hospitalization. They were extremely resistant to therapy and were reluctant to participate in outpatient therapy after the patient was discharged from the hospital.

CASE 15

This sixteen-year-old girl was admitted to the Clinical Research Center weighing 36.7 kgs. The patient's menses ceased ten months prior to her admission, and the parents stated they noted the onset of peculiar food handling nine months prior to her admission. The patient denied that she went on a voluntary diet but insisted she had no appetite and therefore could not eat. She had been giving away her school lunches and hiding food about the house. She was collecting recipes and cooking elaborate meals for the family. The patient did not engage in vomiting, but did abuse laxatives. She was exceedingly overactive, jogged several miles a day, rode her bicycle for long periods of time, and did ritualistic exercising. She enjoyed losing weight and did not feel she was ill or should be in the hospital. She had a fear of getting fat and felt her present shape was still too heavy. She had the physical symptom of bradycardia on admission.

Past history and family history. The patient was described by her parents as being outgoing and friendly, interested in sports, and performing well in school. She had many friends before the onset of her illness, who noted that the patient had to study very hard in order to get above-average grades. Since she had entered high school it had been very difficult for her to obtain above-average grades. The father, age forty-one, was a schoolteacher and the mother, age thirty-nine, worked as a nurse and was mildly obese. The patient had one sibling, a younger brother, who was described as having no problems, and who reciprocated in maintaining a good relationship. The parents were concerned that the patient was overly dependent on them.

Course in the hospital. This patient did not receive behavioral therapy and was treated with the family and psychotherapy program described above. During pretreatment the patient's weight changed from 37.2 kgs to 37.8 kgs. She continued to have a steady weight gain and at the time of discharge weighed 46.3 kgs; her target weight being 48.1 kgs during her hospitalization, the patient was cooperative with the staff. She needed, however, considerable support, encouragement, and reassurance. She came to acknowledge the fact that she did have an appetite and, in fact, felt hungry. She was able to discuss her dependent relationships with her parents and her fear of having to make plans for the future. Initially, the parents were seen separately in counseling sessions and then together with their daughter in family counseling sessions. The parents were able to express an understanding of their tendency to encourage superior performance in their children.

Outpatient course. The patient maintained her weight within 1.5 kgs of the target weight after she attained that weight about a month following hospital discharge. She had one drop in weight of 2 kgs but recovered within a week. Six months after discharge her menses returned but she is still having irregular cycles. The patient and her parents participated regularly in weekly outpatient therapy sessions for three months. They established an open and relaxed communication among themselves, and the patient became less dependent on her parents and more capable of making her own decisions. During her senior year in high school she again became active in social activities and started dating. She made a more realistic career goal for her abilities when she decided to go to a secretarial school instead of a prenursing college program. This summer she has a job and has made arrangements to go away to school next year.

CASE 17

This fourteen-year-old girl began dieting six months prior to hospital admission when she weighed 48 kgs. On admission she weighed 39.9 kgs, 24 percent below a normal weight for her age and height. Her last menstrual period was in the same month she began to diet. The patient admitted she began dieting because she felt overweight, associating that as a response to teasing by her younger brothers and sisters who thought she was getting plump. She began dieting by cutting out deserts and then starches and high fat foods. She could cut up her food in small pieces and dispose of it. Yet, she collected recipes and would cook dinners for her large family of eight siblings. She was constantly preoccupied with how she looked, and expressed an obvious fear of getting fat. She would look at herself in the mirror frequently throughout the day. She did not engage in vomiting or laxative abuse but did have ice cream bulimic episodes. She exercised regularly in order to lose weight. The patient had an early morning sleep disturbance and physical symptoms of bradycardia and hypothermia.

Past history and family history. The patient was the oldest in a Catholic family of eight children. Her father, a forty-one-year-old farmer, not only took care of his farm but in addition was employed at a farm implement dealer's store. He worked very hard and had little time to spend with his children. He was somewhat removed from his family, but it was only by his insistence that the patient was admitted to the hospital. The mother was a forty-one year old moderately obese housewife. It was obvious that she made most of the decisions in the family and took control of family affairs. She was defensive and hostile toward the therapist and the treatment program. The mother felt our target weight was too high for the patient and was unwilling to discuss any problems that might exist within the family or with the patient, essentially denying that a problem existed. The father felt that the patient had been doing well at home and at school until the onset of her illness. She then became concerned about getting excellent grades, although it was exceedingly difficult for her to do this. She spent considerable time studying to improve her grade average. Her illness brought attention from her father and the patient appreciated this.

Course in the hospital. The patient was on the treatment program that did not contain behavioral therapy (see methodology). She gained very slowly but steadily throughout her hospital course and at the time of discharge weighed 47.7 kgs—her target weight was 52 kgs. However, she did write to her parents complaining about her target weight and was able to solicit their support. Midway through the program she complained of flu symptoms, a stomach ache, and discomfort. She obtained some limited insight into the nature of her dependency on her mother, her fear of disagreeing, and being more assertive with her mother. She was able to discuss her angry feelings towards a younger sister who would successfully impose on the patient to do her chores. During the hospitalization the parents were seen separately in therapy on three occasions. The mother continued to make excuses as to why they could not meet the family therapy sessions. The mother felt that the patient should not return to school, since the program was perhaps too strenuous for her, and encouraged her to remain home for the rest of the school year. Excessive absences before the patient was admitted had caused the school to become very concerned about her health.

Outpatient course. The patient maintained her weight 0.5 kg below the discharge weight for six months. Then she lost 2 kgs because of the "flu." She has not regained that weight, is still excessively concerned with her appearance, and has made only a marginal adjustment at home. She states she has status because she is thin. The patient has difficulty with bulimic ice cream episodes. She has become more active in social activities with her peers, and was seen both separately and with her parents in outpatient therapy sessions. However the mother was resistive to the therapy and finally refused to come. The parents have arranged for their daughter to spend their summer away from the family with relatives.

CASE 26

This eighteen-year-old woman was admitted to the Clinical Research Center five months after she started dieting. Her greatest weight was 44 kgs and she had gone down to 32 kgs in the course of her dieting. She stopped menstruating during the first month of her diet. During her senior year in high school the patient decided to lose weight with several other girls. She gradually began to obtain a pleasure in how successful she was at losing weight and how much more effective she was than her peers in doing so. She indulged in ritualistic exercising and bike riding to lose weight. She became interested in cooking and started to collect recipes and cook gourmet meals for the family. She admitted to having bulimic episodes in which she would eat large amounts of cookies or rolls and then induce vomiting. This occurred about twice a week. She also abused laxatives. She described difficulty getting to sleep and waking up several times during the night. When she was admitted to the hospital she felt she was still too fat and had a fear of losing control of her appetite.

Past history and family history. Although the patient's father left her mother before she was born, the father still saw the patient at infrequent intervals. She expressed considerable hostility and bitterness toward the father. The patient had an older brother age twenty-nine and married sister age twenty-seven. Both had been away from the family for quite some time. Her mother remarried when the patient was thirteen. The patient spoke affectionately of her stepfather and described a close relationship with her mother, a very anxious and insecure person who stated she had always been overprotective of the patient. The mother felt ineffective in maintaining any kind of discipline and said she felt her daughter was always able to manipulate her. The mother and stepfather had a supportive and understanding relationship.

Course in the hospital. This patient was treated with behavioral therapy and gained slowly but steadily throughout her hospitalization. She was discharged weighing 39.9 kgs with a target weight of 43.5 kgs. The patient was hostile toward the entire staff whom she regarded as authority symbols. She was sarcastic and often pointed out mistakes that various staff members would make. She would try to pit one staff member against another. During her stay, she had many somatic complaints such as headaches, stomachaches, and backaches. She was compulsive about arranging her various arts and crafts activities and compulsive and ritualistic in her grooming and care of her hospital room. She was resistive in her personal therapy sessions and refused to talk about interactions with her mother, stepfather, and peer group. She stated she was in the hospital only at the insistence of the stepfather.

Outpatient course. The mother and stepfather were cooperative and attended all therapy sessions during the patient's hospitalization and all outpatient sessions. During the hospital course, the mother and stepfather were seen in separate sessions except for two family sessions before discharge. As an outpatient it has been very difficult for the patient to maintain target weight, but she has usually kept to within one kg of that weight. At first, the patient was very resistive to therapy and hostile. Her attitude seemed to change when the mother confronted her about her behavior. Her menses returned six months after hospital discharge when her weight was 42 kgs. A month after getting out of the hospital, she obtained a job but had difficulty getting along with her boss. Five months after discharge she moved out of the family house into an apartment with a friend, became more active socially, and is presently dating. Recently, she got another job which she enjoys and has also changed roommates. She has become much less dependent on her mother and has been more successful in working through her problems at work and with her roommates.

CASE 31

This twenty-four-year-old married woman was admitted to the Clinical Research Center weighing 34.7 kgs. She was 53 percent below a desirable weight for her age and height. During her sophomore year in high school the patient had been overweight, weighing 63 kgs. She had received teasing for being chubby from her peers and tried unsuccessfully to diet. During her senior year in high school she was successful in gradually losing weight and this continued throughout her first year of college. At the end of her first year of college the patient weighed 47.5 kgs, the time and weight at which she stopped menstruating. She continued to slowly but steadily lose weight over the following five years. On admission she stated she felt fat and would allow herself to eat only a small amount of vegetables. She stated she had a decreased sexual desire in the past several years, while admitting to having an appetite and to occasionally indulging in eating binges after which she felt very guilty. She was afraid that once she started gaining weight she would not be able to stop. She abused laxatives and tried to induce vomiting, but was unable to do this. She developed an interest in cooking, collected recipes, and would prepare gourmet meals for her husband. She complained of an initial and terminal sleep disturbance.

Past history and family history. The patient's menses began when she was eight years of age. She had an exploratory laporotomy at that time because cancer was suspected. Later, she was hospitalized at age fourteen for abdominal pains during a time when her parents were considering a divorce. She stated she then felt it was her responsibility to keep the

343

marriage together. The patient always did very well in school and graduated from college with an almost straight-A average and a B.A. in teaching. She was employed as a seamstress until her hospital admission because there were no teaching jobs available in the town where her husband was employed. She described herself as a perfectionist who lived by a rigid code of proper behavior. She stated she tried to accomplish everything perfectly and felt guilty when she was unable to do so.

The patient's father, a school administrator, had several job changes during the patient's childhood causing the family to move frequently. The patient worked very hard in school. She described her father as being a hard worker, conscientious, and a good provider for the family, but because of his scholastic endeavors (he had been throughout her whole life working toward his Ph.D. and did not obtain it until just this year) the family did not see much of him. The patient described her father as being anxious, aloof, critical, and unhappy. She described her mother as rarely expressing her feelings and trying to bind the children to her by indulging them with gifts. During the patient's adolescence, her parents threatened divorce many times, and she felt responsible to arbitrate. She stated the family felt her mother was stupid and of no value. The patient is the second of four children. An older and younger brother have left the family but another younger brother still lives at home and is rebelling against the parents.

The patient was married at age twenty-two when she weighed 41 kgs. She described her husband as a passive, indecisive man who was kind and understanding to her. She stated she never had an argument with him.

Course in the hospital. The patient was treated with the behavioral therapy program described above. She gained slowly and steadily throughout her hospital course and was discharged weighing 47 kgs—her target weight was 54 kgs. The patient was able to articulate in therapy excellent insight into the nature of her relationships with her parents and husband. She made it very clear she wanted to control her rate of weight gain and her final target weight. The behavior of other patients would frequently upset her, and she tended to become dramatic and to exaggerate minor incidents that happened on the ward.

Outpatient course. The patient maintained a weight of 50 kgs for one year after hospitalization. She returned with her husband for regular counseling sessions and was able to establish a satisfactory relationship with him. Three years after hospitalization she increased her weight to 54 kgs and began menstruating regularly. She described a very satisfactory sexual relationship with her husband and stated she worked on gaining weight because she and her husband wanted to have a child.

CASE 42

After fourteen months of dieting, during which her weight went from 70 kgs to 47 kgs, this nineteen-year-old was admitted to the Clinical Research Center for treatment. Her menses ceased five months after she started dieting, at which point she weighed 61 kgs. The patient started dieting during her sophomore year in college because she felt she was a little overweight and wanted to lose just a few pounds. She was very pleased at accomplishing her weight loss and continued to diet and lose weight, feeling that she was much larger than her actual size. The patient would run and exercise, and self-induced vomiting about once a month after a binge eating episode. She would hoard food and cook large dinners for her family on weekends, but not eat the food she prepared. She expressed a fear of losing control and eating until she became fat. Upon admission, she had the physical sign of bradycardia.

Past history and family history. The patient did well in school and had an active social life throughout her grade school and high school years. She is the second of five children and the oldest daughter. She had always been very close to her mother, but after the onset of her illness there had been considerable friction between the mother and the daughter because of a conflict over the patient's boyfriend. The mother was an overweight forty-six-year-old housewife who dominated the household. Her father, a forty-six-year-old factory worker, was passive and silent during most of the interview sessions. The patient described her father as being remote and distant from the family. The mother was defensive and hostile during the therapy sessions. She and her husband were seen in a few sessions separate from their daughter and then in some family therapy sessions.

Course in the hospital. This patient was treated with family therapy and psychotherapy without behavioral contingencies. She gained very slowly but progressively throughout her hospital stay. She was discharged weighing 53.9 kgs with a target weight of 57 kgs. The patient was cheerful and cooperative with the staff and enjoyed their encouragement and reassurance. She seemed to transfer her dependency on her mother to the staff and would frequently ask them to make decisions for her. She gained in therapy a good insight into the nature of her relationship with her mother and father, and was able to insist to the mother that she live in a dorm at college rather than live at home and live away from home during the summer while she worked. The mother was very opposed to this, but the patient was able to stand up to the mother and follow through with her plan.

Outpatient course. The patient attained her target weight two months after discharge and has since maintained it. She still occasionally expresses some fears about getting fat and eating compulsively. However, she has not done that. The mother has refused to come to any outpatient therapy sessions after the first few. She has also resented her daughter continuing in therapy alone. The father has been supportive of the patient, precipitating much tension between the mother and father. The patient has continued on in college in her major as a physical education student and is socializing well in group activities, although she is not dating. She is doing well academically and has a job for the summer away from home.

CASE 43

Two years before admission this twenty-five year old single woman began dieting. At that time she weighed 54.5 kgs. She steadily lost weight until she reached 34.6 kgs, her weight on admission to the Clinical Research Center. She stopped menstruating about six months after she started dieting. The patient stated she did not consciously go on a diet. During the time she started to lose weight, she became a vegetarian. She regularly self-induced vomiting, engaged in laxative abuse, and exercised to lose weight. She had carbohydrate eating binges after which she would self-induce vomiting. She was pleased with her thin body and enjoyed losing weight. She did not feel she was thin and expressed a fear of getting fat. On admission she was extremely emaciated with mottled skin, bradycardia, and hypothermia.

Past history and family history. The patient's parents were divorced when she was six years of age and since then she has lived with her mother. Her father is an alcoholic and she did not know him until she visited him about a year ago. She has two sisters, ages twenty-six and twenty-four, whom she describes as being mildly overweight. She also describes her mother as being mildly overweight. The patient attended college, receiving above average grades, and graduated with a degree in music. The first year after graduating she worked as a music teacher in a school for the retarded. She disliked that job intensely and after a year quit it and hitchhiked to Michigan. On route, she stated, she was raped while hitchhiking, which upset her a great deal. She states she hasn't been able to function well since. She worked as a waitress for six months in Michigan and then returned to North Dakota, her home state. She worked for a short time at an art gallery and then teaching in an elementary school, but was unable to continue this work and returned home to live with her mother. For the four months prior to hospitalization she had been living with her mother, teaching a few piano lessons, and working as a dietitian's assistant at a nursing home.

Course in the hospital. The patient refused to take any food or fluids while in the hospital. She repeatedly vomited and in the course of time developed a severe electrolyte disturbance requiring tube feeding. She was tube fed continuously for ten days during which time her weight increased from 36 kgs to 39 kgs. For the next seventeen days the patient was offered food and fluids and continued to exercise and vomit until her weight reached 35 kgs. She was on the treatment program without behavioral contingencies. When her weight went down to 35 kgs she also developed an electrolyte inbalance again requiring tube feeding. At this time she was regarded as a treatment failure and taken off the study. She was tube fed for the next six days continuously and discharged at a weight of 39.5 kgs. The patient passively agreed to the tube feeding and agreed to stay in the hospital until her fluids and electrolytes were back to normal. She insisted on leaving and returned to her home in North Dakota. The patient refused to participate in therapy sessions. She stated she was here at the desire of her mother and was not interested in therapy for her illness. She was quiet and most of the time refused to talk with the staff. Some telephone interviews were conducted with the mother who was unable to travel the distance for therapy sessions.

Outpatient course. Immediately after the patient returned home she was hospitalized for two weeks locally. There she was again tube fed and treated with Thorazine and Elavil. She had a 2 kgs weight gain before signing out of the hospital. She continued to live with her mother and obtained a part-time job, but soon developed another weight loss. At the present time she is participating in another research project for anorexia nervosa.

Conclusions

Many open studies have shown that behavior therapy can induce weight gain in anorexia nervosa. Only one randomly assigned, controlled treatment study has been conducted (Wulliemier, Rossell, Sinclair 1975) comparing the efficacy of an operant conditioning form of behavior therapy with a program of strict isolation, appetite stimulating drugs, and psychotherapy in anorexia nervosa patients. The latter program was not free of behavioral contingencies, as it contained the strong negative reinforcer of strict isolation. This study with a total of seventeen patients showed the rate of weight gain was three times as great for those patients receiving an operant conditioning program. Our study has shown the latter treatment is more efficacious in inducing weight gain than a therapy with no weight gain behavioral contingencies.

It is possible that considerable variation in the rate of weight gain can occur, depending on the reinforcement schedule within the operant conditioning paradigm. No controlled study has been done to show what interval of reinforcement is most effective in inducing weight gain. Comparison of two open studies, one with a five day reinforcer (Halmi, Powers, and Cunningham 1975) and one with daily reinforcements, (Brady and Reiger 1972) shows the latter produces a greater weekly weight gain (1.85 kgs vs. 1.4 kgs). Controlled studies are needed to determine the advantages and disadvantages of various reinforcement schedules.

Previous studies (Halmi 1973, Russell 1975) reported a favorable outcome associated with early age onset of anorexia nervosa. In this study the outcome variable of maintaining weight after hospitalization was accomplished by a greater percent of adolescents than adults (11 percent vs. 25 percent).

We recognize that weight is only one measure for the effectiveness of an anorexia nervosa treatment program. Therefore, each patient was evaluated for a general adjustment rating reflecting the patient's behavior and functioning at home, school, work, and socially. An analysis of these ratings at follow-up provides a method of examining the crucial question of whether the use of behavioral contingencies is harmful in the treatment of anorexia nervosa. If behavioral contingencies are harmful, then those patients exposed to them in both the hospitalization and outpatient therapy programs should have a greater number of poor adjustment ratings than those who had behavioral therapy only in the outpatient treatment. This was not the case. Only 14 percent of those who had behavior therapy during hospitalizations had poor ratings in contrast to 31 percent of those who had no behavioral contingencies while hospitalized.

In a recent follow-up study, Morgan and Russell (1975) showed that the closer the anorectic patient was able to maintain a normal weight the better were her scores on psychiatric, sexual, and socioeconomic adjustment scales. They also found that an early age onset was associated with a good prognosis. We found, in addition to better weight maintenance by adolescents than adults, an association between younger age and more favorable adjustment ratings. The average ages and standard deviations for each adjustment rating are as follows: poor = $21.5 < 6.46$, fair = $20.84 < 14.72$, adequate = $19.67 < 4.14$, and good = $18.53 < 3.29$.

Comparison of different treatments in various settings by evaluations made at long-term follow-up present some difficulties that should be mentioned. First, there could be a significant difference in the samples being treated and this in itself would affect outcome. Second, the criteria for satisfactory adjustment can vary considerably between investigators. Third, different standards of judgment can be applied to the same criteria.

The first example can be demonstrated by comparing this study's sample with the Morgan and Russell (1975) study sample. In our study eleven of forty-four (25 percent) patients were previous treatment failures. Whereas, in the Morgan and Russell sample nearly half (49 percent) of patients had previous treatment failures. In both studies it was independently determined that patients with previous therapy failures had a poor outcome. It is most likely that a sample containing twice as many poor risk patients as another will, on a follow-up evaluation, have more patients with a poor outcome irrespective of the type of treatment.

A psychoanalyst is undoubtedly going to have different criteria for satisfactory adjustment than a pediatrician. Likewise, if specific criteria were identified a psychoanalyst would use different standards of judgment for those criteria than a pediatrician. When all these factors are considered, it becomes exceedingly difficult to compare the various treatments reported for anorexia nervosa. Obviously, the most meaningful evaluation of treatments is done by randomly assigned controlled studies in the same setting.

In summary, this study demonstrates that behavioral contingencies can be used advantageously and not harmfully in the treatment of anorexia nervosa. At the follow-up evaluation thirty-four (80 percent) of our patients were maintaining their weight and of these fifteen (36 percent) were regarded as well adjusted.

NOTE

1. This research was supported by NIMH grant MH-26218 and Clinical Research Center grant RR-00059.

REFERENCES

Agras, W. S., Barlow, D. H., Chapin, H. N., Abel, G. G., and Leitenberg, H. (1974). Behavior modification of anorexia nervosa. *Archives of General Psychiatry* 30: 279-286.

Bhanji, S., and Thompson, J. (1972). Operant conditioning in the treatment of anorexia nervosa: a review and retrospective study of 11 cases. *British Journal of Psychiatry* 124: 166-172.

Blinder, B. J., Freeman, D. M. A., and Stunkard, A. J. (1970). Behavior therapy of anorexia nervosa; effectiveness of activity as a reinforcer of weight gain. *American Journal of Psychiatry* 126 (8): 1093-1098.

Brady, J. P., Rieger, W. (1972). Behavioral treatment of anorexia nervosa. *Proceedings of the International Symposium on Behavior Modification.* New York: Appleton-Century-Crofts.

Bruch, H. (1974). Perils of behavior modification in treatment of anorexia nervosa. *Journal of the American Medical Association* 230 (10): 1419-1422.

Crisp, A. H. (1965). A treatment regimen for anorexia nervosa. *British Journal of Psychiatry* 112: 505-512.

Dally, P. J., Sargant, W. (1960). A new treatment of anorexia nervosa. *British Medical Journal* 5187: 1770-1772.

Elkin, T. E., Hersen, M., Eisler, R. M., and Williams, J. B. (1973). Modification of caloric intake in anorexia nervosa: an experimental analysis. *Psychological Reports* 32: 75-78.

Feighner, J. P., Robins, E., and Guze, S. B. (1972). Diagnostic criteria for use in psychiatric research. *Archives of General Psychiatry* 26: 57-63.

Hallsten, E. A., Jr. (1965). Adolescent anorexia nervosa treated by desensitization. *Behaviour Research and Therapy* 3: 87-91.

Halmi, K. A., Brodland, G., and Loney, J. (1973). Prognosis in anorexia nervosa. *Annals of Internal Medicine* 78: 907-909.

Halmi, K. A., Powers, P., and Cunningham, S. (1975). Treatment of anorexia nervosa with behavior modification. *Archives of General Psychiatry* 32: 93-96.

Leitenberg, H., Agras, W. S., and Thomson, L. E. (1968). A sequential analysis of the effect of selective positive reinforcement in modifying anorexia nervosa. *Behaviour Research and Therapy* 6: 211-218.

Liebman, R., Minuchin, S., and Baker, L. (1974). An integrated treatment program for anorexia nervosa. *American Journal of Psychiatry* 131: 432-436.

Maxmen, J. S., Silberfarb, P. M., and Ferrell, R. B. (1974). Anorexia nervosa: practical initial management in a general hospital. *Journal of the American Medical Association* 229: 801-803.

Morgan, H. G., and Russell, G. F. M. (1975). Value of family background and clinical features as predictors of long-term outcome in anorexia nervosa: four-year follow-up study of 41 patients. *Psychological Medicine* 5: 355-371.

Russell, G. F. M. (1973). The management of anorexia nervosa. From

Symposium on Anorexia Nervosa and Obesity, Royal College of Physicians of Edinburgh, Publication No. 42:44-62.

Wulliemier, F., Rossell, F., and Sinclair, K. (1975). La therapie comportementale de l'anorexie nerveuse. *Journal of Psychosomatic Research* 19: 267-272.

22] THE SIGNIFICANCE OF THE THERAPIST'S FEELINGS IN THE TREATMENT OF ANOREXIA NERVOSA

BERTRAM J. COHLER

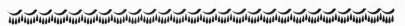

Anorexia nervosa refers to a syndrome characterized by a psychologically determined refusal of food. Not a specific nosological entity, and associated with a variety of both psychotic and nonpsychotic disorders, this disturbance occurs primarily in young women between the ages of twelve and thirty. While a loss of weight and emaciation are the most significant clinical symptoms, most female patients experience both amenorrhea and constipation, probably as a result of the nutritional deficit which accompanies loss of weight.

Recent reviews of the extensive literature arrive at several common conclusions (Nemiah 1958, Bliss and Branch 1960, Thoma 1967, Kaufman and Heiman 1964, Bruch 1965, 1966, 1970a, 1970b, 1973, Rowland 1970, Gifford, Murawski, and Pilot 1970, Goodsitt 1969, Thander 1970, Halmi 1974a, 1974b, Sours 1974): (1) Quite often, symptoms are directly connected with present interpersonal and intrapsychic conflicts; (2) anorexia nervosa symbolizes basic issues of feeding, orality, and nurturing care of the original mother-child relationship, and the expectation of care which is repeated anew in the transference; (3) about 10 percent of all anorectic patients die during treatment, a fatality rate relatively high for psychiatric illnesses. The possibility of fatality presents a particularly difficult problem for the therapist, who feels both personally and professionally threatened by the failure of his patient to thrive and respond to psychotherapy. The treatment of anorexia highlights transference and countertransference, providing greater understanding of these issues in psychiatric treatment.

The present chapter is concerned with certain problems in the psychotherapeutic treatment of anorectic patients, as illustrated by the detailed case of a late adolescent girl who, for the past five years, has been in a residential treatment center for children and adolescents. Through a discussion of this case, we will attempt to show that treatment of anorexia nervosa presents extreme difficulty. The very nature of the patient's transference disrupts the maintenance of a therapeutic perspective on the adaptive significance of the patient's symptoms (Eissler 1943, Berlin, Boatman, Sheimo, and Szurek 1951, Palazzoli 1971).

Countertransference in the Treatment of Anorexia Nervosa

Typically, a therapist is consulted when the patient's physical condition has seriously deteriorated, increasing the risk of fatality. The patient's disturbance is, of course, reflected in her emaciation. During periods of crisis in psychotherapy, however, weight gained is frequently lost, leading to increased criticism of treatment from both the patient's family and other mental health professionals. Such criticisms tend to make the therapist feel inadequate in providing good treatment, a feeling which is intensified by the patient's challenge that he (the therapist) cannot be of help and that she (the patient) will never get well. Additionally, the therapist is often faced with the prospect of treating a patient who does not believe that she is ill and who is terrified of the possibility that her therapist might control food intake and, therefore, her life.

Considering the intensity of anger and despair evoked in the therapist by prolonged psychotherapeutic contact with anorectic patients, it is little wonder that those who find themselves in the position of having to treat such patients often have recourse to behavioral manipulation and modification. Although such behavioral approaches do not appear to yield favorable results superior to those obtained with the best intensive psychotherapy (Bruch 1974), even psychodynamically oriented reports attempt to resolve problems resulting from the therapist's frustration by recommending manipulative procedures in the treatment of anorectic patients (Eissler 1943, Groen and Feldman-Toledano 1966, Bachrach, Erwin, and Mohr 1965, Lang 1965, Hallsten 1965, Leitenberg, Agras, and Thomoson 1968, Blinder, Freedman, and Stunkard 1970).[1]

Psychotherapy with anorectic patients leads to intense emotional reactions in the therapist; perhaps the most intense encountered in a therapeutic relationship. However, the capacity of the therapist to bear these feelings of anger, hopelessness, manipulation, and powerlessness is of the greatest importance for the treatment process. It is precisely when the patient can attribute these feelings to a therapist, who can accept and endure these feelings himself, that the patient is first able to achieve personality change and to experience a greater sense of intrapsychic integration.

Having attributed her distress to her therapist, the patient has successfully split off the hating and bad internal object from the loving and good internal object and, having excluded and regulated the bad object, she is able to perceive herself as a worthy person, in control of her own life. Only then is she able to relax her need for inner control which first motivated the development of anorectic symptoms (Sours 1969, Palazzoli 1970, 1971, 1974). The problem in psychotherapy with anorectic patients is not that of fostering such splitting of the ego, for the defense of splitting already exists as a characteristic of the patient's arrested emotional development (Freud 1938, Klein 1952, Winnicott 1950-1955). The problem is that of fostering the therapist's capacity to bear and sustain these painful feelings, and to accept the discomfort which develops as an inevitable concomitant to feeling so intensely the patient's pain and despair.

We believe that the therapist's feelings of anger and hopelessness in the treatment of anorectic patients is a genuine and intrinsic part of the treatment process and not, as often believed, an element of countertransference. The latter is typically regarded as the therapist's reactions to the patient, based on his earliest childhood experiences, which prevent him from being able to react to the patient as an individual. The concept of countertransference assumes that affective reactions to the patient interfere with the therapist's objectivity and, therefore, are harmful to treatment. Indeed, Freud (1912) recommends that the analyst adopt an attitude of emotional distance modeled after that of the surgeon. This recommendation must be integrated with his advice that the analyst use his unconscious as an instrument within analysis.

Two separate aspects of the psychotherapeutic process are often confused when defining the concept of countertransference: (1) feelings which are based on the therapist's own prior life history and relationships with significant figures in his own parental family and (2) feelings which arise from the therapist's sensitivity to the patient's self and to the patient's characteristic relations with others.

Feelings toward the patient based on the therapist's own prior life history and from the therapist's own unresolved intrapsychic conflicts, as determined by his entire life history, are those which are typically classified as countertransference. Typical of such countertransference reactions is that of the therapist who forgets an appointment with a patient who is, at that point in treatment, dealing with inner conflicts, the content of which are relevant to the therapist's own unresolved conflicts.

These countertransference feelings must be differentiated from another aspect of the therapist's reaction to his patient, based on his own empathic reaction to the patient's plight. For example, a therapist who feels overwhelmed and hopeless about how to reach a suicidal patient may be experiencing the patient's own affects empathically. This empathic response, described by Reik (1937) as a process in which the therapist shares the patient's experiences as if they were his own, has been termed recipathy by Murray (1938), trial or counter-identification by Fliess (1942, 1953), generative empathy by Schafer (1959), and empathy by Kohut (1959). It is widely recognized that we can only know the inner state of another through this process of empathic introspection in which the therapist gains increased understanding of the patient's feelings through awareness of his own affective responses, asking himself, "how does this patient make me feel?" It is less widely recognized that this empathic process is not only a means for coming to better understand the patient but also, in itself, an important part of the treatment process.

The patient experiences the therapist's efforts at empathic understanding as a sign of interest and concern. However, of even greater importance, particularly in work with seriously disturbed patients who split-off unacceptable or painful feelings (Freud 1938), as a result of this process of empathic response, the therapist becomes able to manage the responsibility of bearing painful feelings and unacceptable parts of the self, until such time as the patient is better able to "come to terms" with such disvalued aspects of self. This capacity for splitting represents an ego-adaptive achievement on the part of the patient which makes it possible to continue to function. Temporarily relieved of the burden of having to suffer such intense inner conflict, the patient is better able to begin the process of personality reconstruction.

In the case of the suicidal patient, the fact the therapist can feel overwhelmed and hopeless makes it possible for the patient to feel some hope; the therapist can be the bad or unacceptable aspect of the patient's self, while the patient becomes the benign or positive aspects of the self. The therapist empathizes with the patient's feelings and bears these feelings out of a sense of professional responsibility for the patient's welfare. Since he recognizes that these uncomfortable, painful, or even frightening feelings are an empathic, therapeutic response to the patient's distress, he feels little sense of danger or anxiety and little need for defense against them or for retaliation against the patient for precipitating distress. The therapist's empathic response is merely the complement of the patient's own feelings.

This use of the empathic process is described in greater detail by Flarsheim (1975) who, in discussing his treatment of a suicidal patient, observes his reaction to a wish that the patient not exist. He notes that this wish represented the complement of the patient's own wish for nonexistence. As he gradually came to assume this feeling of desperation for her, she felt his empathic response to her plight and could obtain relief not only from the fact that the therapist understood her problems (in itself a significant and hopeful act), but that her therapist could *be* her problems for her, bearing her suffering so that she would have less need for such suffering.

Early Childhood: Development of Symbiosis and Conflict Regarding Control

In a review of literature regarding the etiology of anorexia nervosa, two themes emerge: (1) conflict regarding the patient's capacity for individuation and for resolution of the mother-infant symbiosis (Mahler 1968, 1972a, 1972b, Goodsitt 1969), and (2) feelings of loss of control of her capacity to determine her own life (Sours 1969). All published reports considering the importance of family relationships in the development of this syndrome stress the significance of the mother's personality, life experiences, and relationship with her child from birth through adolescence as the most critical factor determining the development of anorexia (Cohler 1972). To summarize features observed repeatedly in these studies, we can describe a hypothetical paradigm: The mother of the typical anorectic patient is an emotionally immature woman who feels that she received poor maternal care. She was, and continues to be, dependent upon her own mother, a controlling woman who provides criticism but little support, and who feels an obligation to direct her daughter's life. This issue of control reaches a climax with the prospective patient's birth. At this time, grandmother attempts to run the family and to care for her daughter during the confinement and the immediate postpartum period while, at the same time, remaining aloof and critical of her daughter's childcare attitudes and practices.

The daughter feels unprepared to become a mother and resents having to care for another when she, herself, still wants to be cared for as an infant. She is uncertain of the meaning of the baby's cry or of the relationship between signs of the baby's distress, and inner needs such as hunger.

Feeling unfulfilled herself, she cannot understand her infant's needs as different from her own unmet needs. Since she could not understand the manner in which she might care for her own inner needs, she feels unprepared to care for her infant daughter. In addition, because the infant is a girl, self-object differentiation is even more difficult for the mother.

During childhood, the mother of the prospective patient controls her daughter's life just as her own mother had controlled her life. Unable to foster individuation, she remains tied to her daughter in special ways that are not true for other children in the family. Simultaneously, her daughter is willing to be compliant and is an especially helpful girl who enjoys emulating her own mother's life, particularly that part of her mother's life which focuses on food preparation. She also emulates her mother's concerns regarding eating, weight loss, and inner control, adopting her mother's regulatory mechanisms of control, and becoming domineering over herself.

During adolescence, experiencing renewed conflict regarding self-control, the prospective patient relies even more on the mechanism of strict self-control which she had learned from her own mother who was both controlling of her and controlled by grandmother. Simultaneously, the prospective patient experiences the demands of adolescence that she achieve greater psychological distance between herself and her own mother as a threat to this impulse control system founded upon emulation of her mother (Blos 1967). Unable to accept the extent to which she has been dependent upon her own mother for the maintenance of inner controls, and fearing both this dependence upon her mother, as well as the possible loss of this dependence, she begins to attack her mother's domineering and controlling behavior. Feeling defeated and controlled by her mother and, without recourse, she attempts to demonstrate inner control in terms of limiting her intake of food.

There are several reasons why food so often becomes the focus of this conflict regarding control. Initially, eating represents a highly cathected area of the patient's life in which conflict over control had already been experienced earlier in life both intrapersonally and interpersonally. This concern is heightened by the contemporary emphasis upon slimness in women (Palazzoli 1974). Renouncing food becomes a sign of will-power and of control over one's impulse to eat and realize immediate gratification. Control of food intake has fairly immediate and direct consequences. Changes in body proportions and loss of weight can be observed fairly clearly and directly, and can be clearly measured by such evidence as being able to wear smaller size clothes.[2] The ability to observe so directly this tangible evidence of inner control, as evidenced by the ability to refuse what is desired, becomes an important source of reassurance that other disturbing impulses may also be controlled, and that such control can come from within, rather than from without, in the person of the punishing and controlling mother.

Finally, it should be noted that dieting serves as a proof that the patient can control her own desire to swallow up other persons. As long as she is able to refuse food, and sees that she is becoming slimmer, she can be certain that she has not realized her own wish to perpetuate her symbiosis with her mother by having her mother live inside of her where she is always and immediately available.

What starts as an attempt to demonstrate the capacity for control of dangerous impulses becomes a process of emaciation which goes beyond what even the patient had expected to take place. Since hunger signals have been confused since earliest infancy, since it has always been difficult for the prospective patient to be certain when she was hungry, failure to eat at the usual times leads gradually to a loss of hunger signals and, over time, diminution of the desire to eat (Stunkard 1959). The patient is unaware of the extent to which her control of her eating threatens her very life, and cannot understand why it should be that her parents and others should become concerned about her weight loss. Of course, the daughter's refusal to eat and subsequent loss of interest in food lead her mother to become increasingly anxious about the quality of her own nurturant care; the ensuing guilt increases the mother's determination that her daughter should eat, and, in turn, this determination intensifies the daughter's determination not to eat and surrender her control to her mother's wishes by eating.

The conflict regarding control now becomes a real conflict in the mother-daughter relationship, and as long as the daughter can resist her mother's demands, she can assure herself that she has the necessary control to avoid impending inner chaos. As her mother becomes even more anxious and controlling in the attempt to make her daughter eat, her daughter becomes even more determined not to eat for she must be able to prove to herself her continuing capacity for control. As long as she does not give in to her mother she can both test and prove her capacity for inner control. For the daughter, although clearly not for her mother, the issue is primarily one of control rather than of survival. Of course, the longer conflict between mother and daughter continues, the more important it is to the daughter to refuse food. Feeling dominated by her mother, food refusal becomes her only means for obtaining control of her own life (Palazzoli 1974). It is usually at the time when the patient has lost more than a quarter of her original weight that the family first seeks psychiatric assistance.

Syndrome and Treatment: The Case of Rose

At the time of her enrollment in residential treatment, our patient, pseudonym Rose, was fifteen years old and had been cachectic for more than two years. A frail, beautiful girl, with long, dark brown hair, and intense, sad brown eyes, her emaciation only accentuated the delicacy of her appearance which, according to her mother, had been evident even in earliest infancy. Rose had always been a sad and frail child. Indeed, her mother notes that the first thing that she observed after Rose was born was how delicate she appeared to be.

Rose's intensity was keenly felt by other family members who regarded her as a distant, brooding, and somewhat menacing person. Her constant criticism of the apparent superficiality of other family members was particularly unusual in her family and neighborhood. Primarily Italian in ethnic background, most members of this lower class neighborhood in a large Midwestern city share a common outlook on the world which is cautious, conservative, and prosaic. Rose's devotion to the church was also unusual in its fervor, even in a culture in which women, in particular, are devout and dependent upon the church (Parsons 1969).

Catholicism has particular significance for Rose. As early in the morning as her father, a plumber, might arise in order to be at work by seven, Rose, his third child and eldest daughter, was always awake before him. At the age of thirteen, Rose regularly attended early morning Mass. She said that she enjoyed awakening early in the morning. At any rate, she had great difficulty sleeping, and she would arise frequently in the middle of the night to pace the floor. Often, she would encourage her mother to sleep while she fixed breakfast for her father, a task she particularly enjoyed.

Nowhere in the daily routine was Rose's personality so strongly felt as at mealtimes. Cooking was regarded as an important skill for a woman to have, and both Rose's mother and grandmother were superb cooks. Even Rose's grandmother, who criticized almost every other aspect of Mrs. M's life, admitted that she was a good cook.

After the onset of her illness, Rose continued to help her mother in the kitchen. She displayed grace as she served her parents, two older brothers, and younger brother. There was only one incongruous element: after serving her family, she did not eat what she had helped to cook, but retired to the kitchen where she nibbled at rare roast beef and red jello, which she insisted upon preparing by herself. Furthermore, she refused to sit with the rest of the family, explaining that "it made her sick" to watch other family members "stuff" themselves.

Everyone in her family and all her classmates in school knew that something profound was troubling Rose. When Rose walked into the room the girls in her classroom at the parochial school would cease their conversation in much the same way as when Sister came into the room. It was clear that she exercised the same influence over classmates that she exercised over her family. Her best friend at school, with whom she had grown up, said she was "mystified" about how best to help her. This capacity to mystify others is one of the most striking aspects of Rose's personality. She is both pleased and terrified of her capacity to baffle others, and even to baffle herself. In residential treatment, her continual question, which she poses to all who work with her, is whether they think they really understand what is "bothering" her and can help her to get well. She claims to feel a strange and powerful force within her, completely alien, which she cannot control, and which pushes her to be frantic.

Family Background and Early Childhood

Rose was born into a family in which there was considerable tension. The entire extended family was living together in one building. Mrs. M felt under great pressure to please her mother, a domineering and critical woman, who in Mrs. M's words, "can hurt an awful lot by what she says and what she does."

Mrs. M had considerable difficulty carrying pregnancies to term, and preceding each birth, she had several miscarriages. Indeed, over an eight-year period, Mrs. M was almost continually pregnant.

For Mrs. M, having a daughter was particularly difficult. Her difficulty in carrying to term had already led her to feel defective as a woman. As a child she had been envious of what she saw as her brother's relatively greater freedom, and the birth of her first daughter evoked conflicts regarding her own femininity that were not evoked by the birth of her two sons, who could provide her with the masculinity she envied.

The conflict between Mrs. M and her mother, and the impact of this conflict on her capacity to care for her baby, are consistent with the literature on the personality of mothers of anorectic patients. In the first place, as Rowland (1970) and Gifford, Murawski, and Pilot (1970) have observed, the mother of the anorectic patient is, herself, involved in a complex and symbiotic fashion with her own mother, and one in which the grandmother intrudes into the mother's relationship with her infant. Mrs. M's mother is quite obviously intrusive and controlling, and while Mrs. M resents her mother's involvement, she also seeks this involvement. She depends upon her mother's criticisms and advice and frequently calls or visits her several times a day. Unfortunately, these calls and visits provide little comfort or satisfaction. Mrs. M reports that she is quite tense all the time, but that on days when she has visited her mother, she feels especially upset. In view of the fact that her daughter developed an eating disorder, it is particularly significant to note that Mrs. M feels tension particularly in her abdomen. Finally, just about the same time that Rose became anorectic, Mrs. M developed a peptic ulcer for which she was hospitalized for several weeks. Following her doctor's suggestion, Mrs. M no longer eats with her mother, nor does she spend long periods of time with her.

From the outset, Rose was a difficult baby to care for. Jaundiced following birth, she was frail and her pediatrician became concerned that she might die if she became ill. Indeed, she developed febrile respiratory illness and was hospitalized for several days. Rose's feeding difficulty may have been due to her inability to suck adequately. Mrs. M complained that because Rose was so listless and difficult to care for, she was never certain when Rose was hungry.

Once more, we see a striking parallel between the literature on anorexia nervosa and Rose's early development. Bruch (1970d, 1971a) notes that the future anorectic patient is not taught in infancy that inner needs are related to satisfaction. Rose's mother could not read the cues which Rose provided.

Mrs. M reports that, as a young child, Rose showed relatively little feeling. Her mother remembers few times when she was either very happy or very sad. However, developmental milestones during early childhood were reached at the appropriate times, and Rose was able to sit up alone at five months, walked at about a year, and began talking in partial sentences by about the time she was a year-and-a-half old. There was little difficulty in toilet training. Mrs. M resolved, at about twenty months, that her daughter should be toilet trained and, within about a week, she was trained. Once she had established this control, Rose's control never again failed. In Mrs. M's description of how she toilet trained her daughter, we see the beginning of her determined control of her daughter's behavior which continued to the time of Rose's admission to residential treatment and which, together with the mother-daughter symbiosis, contributed so significantly to the development of Rose's later disturbance.

ILLNESS IN MOTHER AND DAUGHTER:
DIETING AS AN EXPRESSION OF THE SYMBIOSIS

Beginning with the sixth grade, Rose began to show violent rage when there was even the most minimal disturbance of order in the home. At about this same time, Mrs. M had become increasingly preoccupied with her relationship with her own mother. It was then that Mrs. M first complained of the pain in her abdomen, to be later diagnosed within the next months as an ulcer. At the same time, Mrs. M's doctor told her that she must begin to lose weight in order to control hypertension, which was also diagnosed.

In addition, Mrs. M began to experience menopause. This change, together with her illness and a subsequent hospitalization where she nearly died from internal bleeding associated with the recurrence of her ulcer, could not have come at a worse time for Rose. Just as she was beginning to notice changes in her own body, her mother became seriously ill, and just as she was beginning to menstruate, her mother was experiencing menopause. At a time when Rose's temper was becoming more difficult to control than before, as, indeed, was true for other aspects of her impulse life, her mother was hospitalized with a life-threatening illness.

Rose felt responsible for her mother's illness and feared that growing up would reveal, to her, a similar fate. Rose's guilt and feeling of responsibility for her mother's illness were increased by her father's admonition to the family, just prior to her mother's return from the hospital, that any conflict within the family, any expression of anger or any discussion which might lead to tension within the family, would cause a repetition of Mrs. M's illness.

At this time, Rose felt abandoned, angry, guilty about the supposed effects of her anger, and unable to express this guilt or anger, except toward herself. It was at this time that Rose first began going to Mass each morning, hoping in some way to receive forgiveness for the sin which she felt she had committed against her mother.

After her illness, Mrs. M had to be extremely careful about her diet. Rose was especially sensitive to this issue of dieting and was afraid of becoming fat and ill like her mother. Becoming an adult meant becoming like her mother, a possibility which was particularly frightening to her since Rose was little able to differentiate between her mother and herself. She also felt that her mother was envious of the fact that she had reached womanhood at a time when her mother had just reached menopause. To grow up was to provoke her mother's jealousy, a theme which has been repeated throughout Rose's psychotherapy, but is nowhere as explicitly stated as in her story to a card in the Phillipson (1955) picture thematic series:

It seems like this mother, or whatever she is, looks very frustrated after having one of these fights with her daughter, who of course doesn't want her to go out, because she thinks that it's too early and she does not feel like doing anything. Because she was out really late the night before. And this mother was really jealous whenever her daughter does go out with some boyfriend or whatever. She just wants to beat her up in any way she can. And she wants to try to make her daughter very ugly by working her down to the bone. The daughter just lies there cursing her mother, not really giving a damn whatever she does or what she says. The daughter feels like if it takes killing her mother to go out, then she'll do it.

This somewhat confused story tells the story of a mother-daughter conflict of such intensity that one or the other must be destroyed. At the beginning of the story, it is not clear whether it is the daughter who does not want the mother to go out or the mother who does not want the daughter to go out. In view of Rose's difficulties in separating from her mother, it is consistent with her conflict regarding this issue of separation and closeness that she should resent her mother's own life and interests. Simultaneously, the mother in the story jealously resents her daughter's adolescence and her attractiveness to boys, in the manner described by Anthony (1970). The mother will retaliate like Cinderella's mother by working her daughter "to the bone" (surely, an important metaphor in an anorectic adolescent), and the alternative which the daughter sees to being killed by the mother is to kill her mother. The only means for avoiding a situation of either killing or being killed is not to grow up and become a woman, and one sure way of not growing up is not to eat.

Each of the issues of dieting and eating, fatness and slimness, and pregnancy and impulse control were involved in Rose's decision, shortly after her mother's return from the hospital, to go on a strict diet in which she ate one sparse meal each day. Since one is not supposed to eat before attending Mass, obviously Rose could not eat at breakfast. Lunch was hurried, between classes, so there was little time in which to eat. This left supper, which was always the same; thin slices of lean, rare roast beef, and red jello. Even the choice of these foods for a diet is interesting. Rose insisted upon lean beef in order to insure that she would not become "fat." Fatness meant both becoming like her mother and, ultimately, requiring hospitalization for hypertension and ulcers, together with the fatness of pregnancy which she had seen over and over throughout her childhood. Issues of eating, control, and pregnancy became confused in Rose's mind, as the following picture thematic story demonstrates:

> To me, this looks like someone's getting scared. This one looks like he or she is in despair or is going to eat this person or control it, or have a baby, or something. This picture here looks like someone who is just kind of helpless. I also think it's an ugly picture. (Examiner: What's going to happen, what's the outcome?) The person will eventually fall apart . . . the helpless person.

Rose's view of her mother's care was parallel with the Hansel and Gretel fairy tale: her mother provided her with food in order to fatten her up to eat her. For Rose, childhood is a process of slow torture in which the child is fattened up by the mother, and, as the victim, the child is slowly driven crazy by the mother's care. The way to prevent the catastrophe of being eaten is to turn passivity into activity and to diet, becoming nothing but unappetizing skin and bones. However, there is another component to this fear of being eaten, projection of Rose's wish to eat others (Klein 1932, 1952, Kernberng 1966). From this perspective, dieting serves as reassurance that the wish is not being translated into action. Rose was able to establish a compromise with this wish to eat others in the form of sacred and profane diet rituals. For Rose, communion was the most important part of the religious ceremony. She seldom missed an opportunity to receive communion and the wine and wafer which are said to represent the blood and the body of Jesus. Her diet of red jello and rare roast beef may be viewed as the profane parallel to the sacred communion diet.

This fear of loss of control and of cannibalism is enacted repeatedly in Rose's response to the Rorschach blots. Typical of these responses is her response to card II:

> II. 2. This part of it here (top red) reminds me of two parts staring into each other. Like one part, but it is split, being cut into half I guess. (Inquiry). The two faces you can tell, these are two faces, I'm sure of that, these are mouths and it looks like they are going at each other and they look more evil than happy. . . .

For Rose, control is necessary both as a protection against eating her mother, and as a protection against being eaten by her mother. Either outcome is equally possible since, in her mind, images of mother and daughter are fused. Interpreting her mother's continual pregnancies and miscarriages during her childhood as fatness, they provided confirming evidence for Rose's belief that her mother swallowed people. She had observed that first her mother became fat, then she went to the hospital, and finally came home with a new person who had been cut out of her. A strict diet protects against swallowing up another, although the content of the diet provides a compromise with the impulse to swallow and internalize the other. At the same time, if she is emaciated, she will not be a palatable object and can forestall the possibility of being eaten herself. *Dieting represents one means of defending against the symbiosis, for the concept of eating and being eaten is, in itself, a representation of a destructive symbiosis in which one no longer exists, except as a part of another.*

In Rose's life there was certainly evidence of a problem of separating from her mother. She began life prevented from being her own person and separate from her mother. Rose was born on the anniversary of her grandfather's death. From the outset, Rose already stood for another person of critical significance in her mother's own life. Then, to make matters even more difficult, grandmother first became involved with Mrs. M's children only at the time of Rose's birth, forcing Mrs. M to struggle for her own autonomy with her mother, which further deprived Rose of her mother's attention. It is especially important, in view of Rose's problems in establishing transference relationships in treatment, to note that she has never forgiven her mother for being so able to control her life, that, as she believed, her mother could even arrange for the date of her birth.

In view of these psychological issues, it is not difficult to understand why Rose's overt disturbance began at the time or in the manner that it did. Immediate precipitants included her mother's illness, her impending graduation from grammar school, which is a rite of passage marking entrance into the world of adolescence, her own physical development and beginning of menses, and her mother's almost simultaneous menopause. The fact of her mother's diet provided a means for Rose to emulate her mother's behavior and to use aspects of her identification with her mother as a means for fostering her own adaptation to both intrapsychic and intrafamilial conflict. Since dieting provided Rose with a means for dealing with her own conflict, it represented a truly significant achievement of the ego. Without the control provided by dieting and later by her anorexia, Rose believed she would have been flooded with anxiety, would have experienced complete psychic disorganization, and, ultimately, would have been devoured. Dieting represented an active solution where passivity would have led to inner chaos.

The alternative to chaos is the active struggle to prevent such disorganization which dieting, with its emphasis on active inner control, provides. Consistent with the observations of Waller, Kaufman, and Deutsch (1940), DuBois (1949), and Rowland (1970), Rose's fastidiousness and her ritualized activities, along with her diet, represented aspects of an obsessional defense against this anxiety about psychic disorganization.

EXACERBATION OF THE DISTURBANCES AND FIRST EXPERIENCES WITH PSYCHIATRIC TREATMENT

Mrs M returned home from the hospital late in the spring, with Rose attending the seventh grade. According to her mother's memory of events, Rose began her diet within a few weeks of her mother's return home, and rapidly lost weight. Rose's frantic activity, which also began at this time, represented a further attempt to lose weight, and during the summer months Rose spent nearly all her waking hours furiously peddling her bicycle, returning home only for supper. Mrs. M was aware of this weight loss and became increasingly concerned about it. However, her pediatrician assured her that there was no problem and told her not to worry.

By the following fall, Rose had begun to look seriously emaciated and, at this time, her pediatrician referred her for medical tests, believing that Rose was suffering from a serious physical illness. Only when all diagnostic tests returned negative was the physician willing to recognize the seriousness of Rose's emotional disturbance. Her weight now down to sixty pounds, Rose was hospitalized on the psychiatric ward of the same community hospital where, the previous winter, her mother had been a patient. Tube feeding was begun at once, and during the first days it took three strong orderlies to hold down the frail girl in order that the procedure could be instituted.

Rose was terrified of tube feeding. Since gaining weight meant losing control and being consumed, Rose viewed being forced to eat, rather than starvation, as threatening fatality. Confused about the meaning of body signals, she did not understand that she needed to eat in order to stay alive. As became increasingly obvious later during her residential treatment, Rose equated eating with death and starvation with life.

The hospital staff forced enough nourishment into her that Rose gained fifteen pounds. Since the staff did not realize how afraid she was of growing up and of becoming increasingly like her mother, which meant being part of mother, the staff believed that Rose would like to return home and graduate from eighth grade with the rest of her class. In their community, graduation from grammar school is celebrated with the same significance as is graduation from high school in many other communities. The grammar school graduates wore dignified robes, marched in solemn ceremony, and received engraved diplomas. Even though some parents thought this ceremony inappropriate, there was strong pressure for such an elegant graduation. Rose managed to march in the procession, but after the ceremony was completed became terrified, presumably of the transition to adolescence which this ceremony signified. In desperation, feeling overwhelmed and terrified, she fled into the girls' washroom where she broke a window and slashed her wrist. She was discovered almost immediately and rushed back to the hospital by ambulance.

This event was terribly painful for Rose's parents. In the first place, they were afraid that she would never recover since she had already been hospitalized for several months and had exhausted Mr. M's remaining hospitalization insurance; and yet there appeared to be little improvement in her condition. Not only did the M's feel depressed by their daughter's lack of progress, but, in addition, they felt completely humiliated.

Mrs. M recalls that, after her daughter's attempted suicide, she kept thinking that "if it's God's wish to take her, I only wish that he would take her soon." For Mrs. M, her daughter's death would have solved several problems. She believed that life was merely a preparation for an afterlife of reunion and comfort. Mrs. M felt that her daughter had already suffered enough. She wished that Rose could have the benefits of this better eternity as soon as possible. In this way, Rose could attain the status of the grieved, lost, ideal figure into which Mrs. M had already made her father. Rose sensed her mother's wish for her death and both wished for and feared death. To some extent, Rose's desire to die also represented a response to her mother's wish for her death, a wish determined both by her mother's desire to join her own deceased father, for whom she still mourned, and also by her frustration and anger at trying to deal with Rose. In response to this wish on her mother's part, Rose adopted an attitude of scorn and defiance which was expressed by the desire to be rid of her destructive and consuming mother by dying and finally achieving separation.

Given the mother's confused feelings, hospital visiting hours became a nightmare for the hospital staff, Rose, and the family. Rose would rush at her mother, accusing her mother of wanting her dead, and of trying to control her life and her body. She also accused her mother of being humiliated by her illness and of caring more for what the community thought than for her recovery. Rose was particularly sensitive to her mother's feelings, and these accusations were very painful for Mrs. M, who became visibly upset and developed additional gastrointestinal symptoms. As a result of such encounters, the administrative psychiatrist felt that it was essential for mother and daughter to be separated and recommended residential treatment where the family's visiting privileges could be controlled. In making this recommendation, the administrator echoed Charcot's (1889) admonition in treating anorexia nervosa in which he says:

> I have held firmly to this doctrine for nearly fifteen years, and all that I have seen during that time—everything that I have observed day-by-day—tends only to confirm me in that opinion. Yes, it is necessary to separate both children and adults from their father and mother, whose influence, as experience teaches, is particularly pernicious.
>
> Experience shows repeatedly, though it is not always easy to understand the reason, that it is the mothers whose influence is so deleterious, who will hear no argument, and will only yield in general to the last extremity. [p. 163]

Of course, in Charcot's time, there was little understanding of the concept of mother-daughter symbiosis and of the powerful role this symbiosis can play in intensifying the daughter's disturbance. Residential treatment is one powerful means for interrupting such an intense symbiosis, and it is for such reasons that the administrator of Rose's case had so strongly urged enrollment in residential treatment.

For a patient like Rose, feeling controlled by a world too complex for her to master, residential treatment is especially suitable, because, ideally, residential treatment provides an environment of only minimal pressure, in which the daily routine is sufficiently simplified that the patient can feel comfortable and safe (Bettelheim 1949, 1950, 1955, 1956, 1960, Bettelheim and Sylvester 1948, Noshpitz 1962). Separating the patient from his family and minimizing demands for socializing are often sufficient for symptoms to begin to disappear as the patient feels that his life is no longer in imminent danger, and control over the environment is, once again, asserted. Bettelheim comments, in discussing residential treatment:

> To begin life anew, the total extreme situation which destroyed autonomy must be replaced with a total living situation over which he can exercise control. As he was overwhelmed by his environment, he must now be able to control it. . . . This means that it must be simple; it

must not offer complex challenges nor make complicated demands. . . . When living under such conditions, even a very weak ego
can begin to function more adequately. [Kaufman and Heiman 1964,
pp. 516-517]

THE PSYCHOTHERAPEUTIC RELATIONSHIP IN AN INPATIENT SETTING: TRANSFERENCE AND EMPATHY

Rose strongly resisted the recommendation that she attend a residential
school for young people with serious emotional conflicts. Denying that she
had any problems, Rose refused the scheduled appointment to meet with
the staff, and only agreed to cooperate when her mother promised that
Rose's stay would be a short one and that she would be able to return home
by summer. Once she had been accepted into residential treatment, Rose
became upset at the possibility of separation from her mother. In part, she
worried about the possibility that her mother would once more become
pregnant and in her absence replace her with another child. This concern
was expressed primarily in terms of Rose's younger sister who, during
Rose's hospitalization, had also developed an ulcer and now shared a
symptom in common with her mother. Rose became convinced that her
mother would have a boy to replace her and said that if she had been born
as a boy, she would never have been rejected.

Given these fears, Rose's strongest reaction to enrollment in residential
treatment was that she would have to live in a dormitory with six other
adolescent girls, sharing, as well, a counselor-therapist with them. For
Rose, having to share with other young people was like having to share her
mother with her sister and brothers.

In observing the way in which she formed a relationship with her new
therapist, it was possible to gain new appreciation both of the manner in
which she had preserved her symbiosis with her mother and of her mother's
reaction to this symbiosis. From the outset, Rose was an important
presence in the dormitory. In the afternoon, when the girls returned from
school, they would gather around the group table, having snacks, and
discussing the day. The following observation is typical of Rose's reaction
to life in the group setting:

The group was sitting around the table discussing what they might
do during the afternoon. Rose, as usual, was pacing back and forth
around the dormitory. Occasionally, she would punctuate the
conversation with a remark like, "I really hate my body; it really

sucks." These remarks were made with considerable feeling, and were addressed directly to her counselor. Her counselor was unprepared to deal with such feelings at a time when the group was trying to decide upon its afternoon activity, and yet Rose's remark was offered with such emphasis that all other conversation stopped and the attention of both children and staff was focused on Rose. Her counselor attempted to console Rose and suggested that she come and sit by her and have some juice and cookies. Rose then said, spitefully, "Don't feed me any of that shit. I know you hate my body, you hate your body, and you are trying to make me fat like you are."

With this remark, tossed out in a tone of intimidation, Rose proceeded once more to pace back and forth across the dormitory. The silence continued as the attention of everyone in the group remained on Rose and her challenge to her therapist-counselor. "Look," she said, "you've got to realize you're trying to fuck up my body with that crap." Then, as a final challenge, she announced that her counselor-therapist couldn't help her get well. "You don't even know how to help me get well, do you?" Her counselor arose from the table, walked over to Rose, led her by the hand to the group table where she sat down beside her and continued the discussion with the group about feelings of helplessness, as expressed by Rose.

In this vignette, we can see how Rose succeeded in getting her therapist to leave the rest of the group, tend to her, and then managed to refocus the discussion from the afternoon's activity to a discussion of the problem of helplessness. This behavior in the group setting is similar to Rose's behavior at home. Her mother noted, for example, that the whole family might plan a Sunday outing, and just as they were almost ready to leave, Rose would announce that she was not going along. On the other hand, the family might decide on a trip to the forest preserve for a picnic, and just as they arrived at their destination and had settled down for the day, Rose would announce that she had to go home. Mrs. M complained that by such behavior Rose could throw the family into complete confusion.

In discussing Rose's behavior in the group, her counselor-therapist also noted how intense Rose was, and how she often felt that Rose was boring a hole into her with her gaze. The therapist's feelings paralleled those of Rose's mother, who felt that Rose was unlike the rest of the family in her serious, questioning approach to the world. Where other family members were concerned with prosaic, commonplace events, Rose asked serious life-and-death questions, which disturbed and annoyed the rest of the family.

Indeed, other family members expressed relief after Rose was first hospitalized and they no longer had to undergo her intent and questioning gaze as they went about their daily business.

For Rose, this intensity had an adaptive significance. In a large family, her intensity made it possible for her to be differentiated from other family members, not an easy task for a daughter involved in a symbiotic relationship with her mother. It made it possible for her to be noticed by her mother, a woman who was especially insensitive to subtle emotional nuances, and who had a difficult time distinguishing between her own needs and those of her daughter. Rose was sufficiently intense that even her own mother had to recognize her separate feelings and pay attention to her needs.

Rose's counselors spoke frequently of their reaction to this intense demand for recognition. One of her former therapists at the residential treatment center notes that although she would begin the session feeling that Rose's problems were different from her own, during the hour she would begin to question this. Rose would accuse her of being fat and of trying to make her fat. Having learned about the concept of projection, Rose would accuse her therapist of attributing her own troubles to Rose and would shout defiantly, "Why don't you get your own therapist? Why should I have to straighten out your head?"

Through the transference, Rose was repeating once more the conflict between her mother and herself in which her mother, unable to differentiate between her own needs and those of her daughter, had been unable to help Rose to see her own needs and her own personality as separate, thereby involving Rose in her own conflicts. Rose needed to try to make her problems into her therapist's problems and to bind her therapist to her by differentiating between their personalities. Most significant in this regard is her therapist's reactions to this effort to erase the differences between them. She reported feeling confused, completely smothered, and overwhelmed by Rose. Although she had always had a robust appetite, as she sat with Rose and tried to drink some of the milk which she brought to the session room she felt uncertain whether or not she was thirsty and, indeed, began to question whether she could interpret her own body sensations.

Terrified by feelings of merging with her patient, she had begun quite consciously to tell herself before starting the hour that she really was a different person from Rose and that it was she who was the therapist. Rose had succeeded so well in her attempt to merge with her therapist that her therapist, who had always had a regular menstrual cycle, now stopped menstruating, and reported the fantasy that she was pregnant with Rose who would live forever inside her body. As her therapist became increasingly afraid that she was losing her own self and merging with her patient, Rose became more disturbed, for she not only needed to be able to establish such a symbiosis as the only way she knew of being sure she would be cared for, but was also afraid of it. As long as she was a part of the therapist and a significant aspect of her therapist's personality, her therapist would have to take care of her. Simultaneously, she was afraid of being controlled, dominated, and "swallowed up." Despite this fear, there was an adaptive aspect to the way Rose made her therapist feel. As long as her therapist could accept these feelings, Rose could feel that it was her therapist who lacked a sense of self and who needed to get her head "straight." Simultaneously, Rose could feel strong and in control of a relationship rather than, as with her mother, being controlled by the relationship. If she could deposit her feelings with her therapist, Rose could begin to feel safe enough to examine these feelings, first about the therapist, then about her mother, and finally about herself.

It is only as a result of sharing in the patient's feelings and perceptions that the therapist is able to understand the significance of the patient's particular perceptions of self and others for the patient's adaptation and survival. Nowhere is this more important than in the treatment of anorexia nervosa where feelings of loss of a sense of separateness and loss of control are important in understanding symptom formation.

One of the advantages of residential treatment is that the issue of food and eating, and the transference and countertransference issues which it represents, may be studied directly, and conflict and symptom formation observed by both patient and therapist as it actually takes place. Observation of the patient's behavior at mealtime, over the course of many months, enables the patient's therapist to understand the complex meanings which the patient attaches to food and eating. This understanding, while not in itself sufficient to lead to major changes in the patient's behavior, is important in terms of the patient-therapist relationship, for it conveys to the patient her therapist's interest in knowing her as a person with individual feelings and beliefs. Our observations of these anorectic patients do not agree with Bruch's (1965, 1966) earlier observations that, in contrast to schizophrenic patients, anorectic patients develop few symbolic interpretations of food.

Our anorectic patients, of whom Rose is characteristic, all attributed a variety of complex meanings to food. One patient, the daughter of parents who were active in the antiwar movement, refused to eat all food manufactured or processed by companies having any association, no matter how remote, with the Vietnam conflict. She would only eat food processed by neutral countries, and would refuse lobster, steak, roast beef, or chocolate sundaes in favor of imported foods such as kidney pie. Rose, herself, refused to eat hot dogs or sausages, which reminded her of penises; all forms of casseroles, which reminded her of vomit; eggs, which reminded her of fetuses; and potatoes, which reminded her of brains. On the other hand, as we have already observed, she was willing to eat rare roast beef and jello, which she understood as profane parallels to the sacred host of the Mass. Her therapist's interest in Rose's unique understanding of these foods and in knowing why she accepted or refused particular foods was a first sign for this patient that her therapist cared about her, and wanted to understand her.

One central issue in the literature on treatment of anorexia nervosa concerns the advisability of forcing the patient to eat, particularly when her life is in danger. Bliss and Branch (1960), in their thorough review, note that two contrasting positions have been adopted by those who have treated anorexia nervosa on an inpatient basis. Some authors insist that the therapist should be authoritarian and should demand that the patient eat. Others believe that such aggressive treatment is disastrous. Bliss and Branch put this debate into a useful perspective when they note that:

> Unfortunately, these are dialectical exercises rather than scientific conclusions. They do point to the need to view the situations as an interaction between the physician and the patient, in which both parties, their needs, attitudes, and tolerances play a part. One can not simply study the patient who is receiving therapy since the treatment cannot be understood unless it is seen as related to the therapist and the setting in which the treatment is given.

Typically, the desire to see the patient eat arises as much from the therapist's concern about his professional reputation as from his concern for the patient herself. Since the patient knows that the desire for her to eat arises as much from institutional concerns as from the desire to help her gain greater autonomy, it is not surprising that she should have little desire to fit in with institutional requirements. After all, the symptom of not eating arises from the fear of loss of control and the need to maintain some autonomous control.

To the extent that the patient is not certain that she has such control, the symptom of not eating has adaptive significance. When the staff can acknowledge that their need for the patient to eat arises at least in part from their anxiety about their professional reputations, they may achieve greater success in their goal of helping the patient gain weight for, in such a circumstance, the patient may not so directly perceive the issue of eating as a power struggle (Sours 1969).

We have already seen that in Rose's life the refusal to eat had adaptive significance. It was the one area of her life where she could demonstrate both to herself and to others that she retained control and mastery. Attempts to force Rose to eat were met by the determined refusal of one in a situation of desperate fear for survival. In Rose's conception of the world, survival was equivalent to not eating; destruction was equivalent to eating.

Largely as a result of her own anxiety, acknowledged to Rose as such, Rose's counselor-therapist applied continual pressure to get her to eat. The following observation in the dormitory, just prior to supper, provides a good illustration of this pressure:

> Rose's counselor-therapist walked out into the hall, looked at the clock, and came back into the dormitory informing the group that it was five-forty, and that in five minutes it would be suppertime (all dormitory groups eat in a common dining room where supper is served at 5:45 each evening). Rose, who had been frantically wringing out her favorite sweater in the sink, came out of the bathroom at that moment to announce that she was not eating any of the School's "shitty supper." Her counselor replied that she wanted Rose to eat and that she (the counselor) knew that supper—fried chicken—was among Rose's favorite foods. Rose denied this and said that she had no favorite foods and, indeed, never intended to eat again.
>
> She began screaming that she hated her counselor-therapist, that her counselor didn't understand her and was trying to kill her by forcing her to eat, and that she refused to eat. Her counselor was frustrated by a difficult afternoon in which Rose had spent most of the time in the bathroom washing her sweater, pacing back and forth in the dormitory, cursing everyone in the group, and saying that she wanted to die. The cumulative effect of this on the counselor led her to scream back that she wanted Rose to live, and that Rose must eat. Rose flew at her counselor in a rage, and almost attacked her physically, before regaining self-control. By now, it was past supper time and the group started downstairs. Rose sat next to her counselor and ate two helpings of fried chicken, as well as dumplings and ice cream for dessert.

After the day was over and all the girls were in bed, the staff sat down to talk about the quarrel between Rose and her counselor. Several staff members observed that Rose ate better after she had had a quarrel about eating than at any other times. Some staff felt that this pattern of quarreling and eating showed that Rose should be forced to eat since, when she was forced, she was able to eat. However, such a position was clearly at odds with Rose's terror of losing control and of being required to eat. It was suggested that the fact that her therapist had become upset by Rose's refusal to eat proved to the patient that her therapist really cared about her and wanted her to live, a concern which was of obvious importance to a girl whose own mother had expressed the feeling that, if it were God's wish that she should die, then she should die as quickly as possible.

However, of at least equal importance was the fact that, in becoming involved with Rose in an argument just before each meal, as so often was the case, Rose was freed from being passive and controlled and now could be active and controlling. As long as her counselor-therapist could realize the importance of bearing these feelings (and she did indeed feel very much controlled and overwhelmed by her patient), Rose was able to let herself eat.

In time, as Rose began to experience being full, she could begin to feel the difference between this fullness and her previous feeling of emptiness. She could then begin to feel, for herself, the importance of eating for her survival. By providing an environment and persons whom she could control, rather than one in which she felt controlled, residential treatment made it possible for Rose to begin to give up her refusal to eat. At the same time, she could demonstrate her growing feelings of inner control in ways other than those related to eating. As the issue of eating and food refusal became somewhat less important, Rose's symbiosis with her mother emerged as the most critical therapeutic issue. Rose began to understand the basis of this symbiosis and, having been able to experience the symbiosis in the transference, was able to achieve a greater degree of individuation.

A significant breakthrough in the struggle to free herself from symbiosis occurred in the context of Rose's attempt to emulate her mother's preoccupation with weight as a means of mastering internal conflicts. Rose had been preoccupied with the fear of becoming like her mother. Not only was her mother controlled by grandmother but, additionally, she was domineering and burdened everyone in the family, especially Rose, with her problems. According to the patient, it was her mother's insistence upon telling Rose her problems that was the most difficult part of their relationship. Through her refusal to eat, Rose emulated one aspect of her mother's behavior; and while this in itself was frightening, she was particularly preoccupied with anxiety lest her fear (which was also her wish) would come true—that she would become fat like her mother. A part of this fear of becoming like her mother was that her father would then find her sexually attractive in the same way he found her mother sexually attractive and that, out of jealousy, her mother would destroy Rose. This was yet one more reason for not becoming like her mother and becoming fat, and one more reason for maintaining strict control. Any sign that she was becoming in any way like her mother terrified her. If her mother sent her a picture of the family, Rose anxiously asked her counselor-therapist whether she now looked more like her mother than before. This issue of becoming like her mother was finally put in perspective but, as the following incident shows, not before it had become a major crisis:

One morning, on arising, Rose inspected her body, as was her custom each morning, and asked her therapist if she thought that Rose looked any different that day. Her therapist assured her that she was still the same girl. She then went about the business of helping the girls to get dressed and prepared for the school day ahead. Rose's therapist gave no more thought to this apparently off-hand question as the group had breakfast and went off to school. Rose had not eaten much that morning.

Throughout the day, she was obviously downcast and upset. That afternoon, the group's other counselor was on duty, and Rose's counselor-therapist was out for the day. Rose was unwilling to form a relationship with anyone but her therapist-counselor (another manifestation of the development of a symbiosis in treatment), and therefore her other counselor tried to make her comfortable, but made little attempt to talk to her. That night, in her bath, she was seen crying. No one knew what to do, because when Rose's counselor-therapist was not on duty, the other counselor and the children in the group felt completely at a loss as to how to help her.

When the group was ready for bed and the counselor had turned out the lights, Rose refused to get into bed. At first, she was only stubborn, but soon became verbally abusive, and began accusing and threatening the counselor. By the time the director came through on his evening rounds, Rose and her counselor were screaming at each other; her counselor had tried to drag Rose over to her bed, and Rose had retaliated by hitting her quite hard in the stomach. The director took Rose outside in the hall. From the pallor on her face, it was apparent that she was in sheer terror. First she looked frozen in fear and then she began to scream in desperation and flung herself upon the director, already an important person in her life, screaming that she was going to die or be killed, and she would not survive the night.

After a long time consoling and quieting Rose, the following story emerged. That morning upon awakening, she noticed a slight corn on one of her toes. In fact, the corn was in exactly the same spot, and appeared to be identical in shape, with a corn on her mother's foot. Rose became convinced that, during the previous night, she had suffered a metamorphosis in which she had assumed a physical appearance which was identical with that of her mother. Her counselor's blithe reassurance had hardly sufficed to help her with this terror, nor had she been reassured by frequent visits to the bathroom where she studied herself in the mirror in order to be sure that she was still herself. She suffered a moment of panic during which she looked in the mirror and believed that the image was that of her mother. When she went to get into the tub for her bath, and inspected herself once more, she believed that she had become fat like her mother and, in fact, resembled her mother in each and every aspect of her appearance.

Terrified that the worst had happened, Rose was certain that her mother would murder her during the night out of revenge for her fantasies about her father. This concern, when expressed, provided considerable relief, and her awareness of the underlying wishes that contributed to her fear of becoming like her mother represented a first tentative step in her psychotherapy; Rose began to be able to decide for herself in what ways she did and did not want to be like her mother.

While Rose still had some difficulty being able to eat freely, her weight stabilized at about ninety-eight pounds, well within the normal limits for a girl of her height. With the anorectic crisis past, Rose and her therapist have started work on the many other conflicts which were inaccessible so long as this life and death crisis of the refusal to eat was uppermost in Rose's mind and in the minds of the staff members who worked with her.

While many factors contributed to Rose's first hesitant attempt at self-understanding after the most critical phase of her disturbance, perhaps the most important of these was her therapist's intuitive and empathic understanding of Rose's unique interpretation of her personal and interpersonal world. Her therapist needed to allow herself to feel controlled by Rose and to recognize this feeling of being controlled as the complement to the way in which her patient felt. This recognition made it possible to react not by attempting to put these feelings back on Rose, in order to avoid having to bear these feelings herself, but rather by allowing herself to be and to feel controlled by Rose, to serve as a depository for these feelings of being controlled. As a result, Rose felt free to yield some of her own insistence upon strict inner control and, no longer needing protection from a world beyond her control, she was able, gradually, to give up her symptoms.

Conclusions

Anorexia nervosa is a symbolic expression of a patient's desperate need to maintain control over an interpersonal and intrapsychic world which is felt to be beyond control. Because it provides a defense against feelings of being annihilated and destroyed, the refusal to eat of the anorexia nervosa patient represents an achievement of the ego which is not likely to be helped by manipulation aimed at making this symptom disappear while anxiety about loss of control remains. The anorectic patient becomes disturbed as a result of a life in which, almost from birth, body signals have been distorted and denied. The ordinary sensations of hunger and satisfaction are not correctly perceived and provide no means of signalling physiological distress. At the same time, like the proverbial Jonah in the Whale, the anorectic patient feels swallowed up by her controlling mother who incorporates her daughter into her psyche and uses her for her own ends. Seldom does the future patient exist as a person in her own right; she exists only as a means for satisfying her mother's needs (who in turn feels controlled by her own mother). Not having been able to achieve differentiation or individuation from her mother, the anorectic patient develops the feeling that she is only one aspect of her mother's personality and, like Rose's fantasy, that she will someday be transformed into her mother, a metamorphosis which she both fears and wishes.

The technical literature suggests that it is important to allow the patient to reexperience the original mother-daughter symbiosis in the transference. In the resolution of this symbiosis, the therapist must be prepared to be placed in the helpless position of being controlled by the patient. The therapist's acceptance of this development helps the patient achieve individuation, a sense of autonomy, and a consolidation of identity.

NOTES

1. Over the past several years, there has been considerable controversy regarding the effects of behavior modification in the treatment of anorexia nervosa. Stunkard (1972), reviewing previous research in this area, recommends procedures which require some deprivation, followed by rewards for weight increase. Favorable editorial comment in the *Journal of the American Medical Association* (May 8, 1972), followed by another favorable review (Agras et al. 1974) led to yet additional favorable editorial comment in that same journal by Hussey (1974), followed by critical comments by Feinstein (1974) and Bruch (1974), and letters of support by Spector (1975) and Wolpe (1975).

While some positive results have been reported using such behavioral techniques, including the even more recent reports by Halmi et al. (1975) and Garfinkel et al. (1973), it is the opinion of this author that such results are not as unambiguously positive as has been maintained, and that in order to create reinforcers, patients must first be subjected to such harsh deprivation that the regime becomes unmitigated punishment for the patient, as in the recent report by Werry and Bull (1975).

More recently, Minuchin and his colleagues (Liebman et al. 1974a, 1974b) have reported on a unique program using both operant techniques and family therapy. However, as Liebman (1974b) notes, success has also been reported by Minuchin (1970, 1974) as well as Palazzoli (1974) solely on the basis of family therapy. In the absence of a more complete empirical study of each modality together and apart, it would appear that treatment focused on issues of power and control within the family is at least as effective as that based on behavioral approaches.

2. Slade and Russell (1973) report that anorectic young women show a significantly greater overestimation of their body proportions than well women, and that the more rapid the weight gain while in the hospital, the less rapidly this body-image distortion is resolved. Less rapid weight gain is associated with a gradual diminution of body-image distortion. Crisp and Kaluch (1974) have, in general, replicated this study, although these authors find that even the well women in their study (on the average older than the women in Slade and Russell's research) tended to overestimate their body appearance. Crisp and Kaluch also note that overestimation is greater among women on a carbohydrate diet than those on a noncarbohydrate diet. These two studies suggest that helping the patient to maintain some feelings of control over their own weight gain is associated with lessened concern about weight and, presumably, enhances feelings of control over one's own life.

379

REFERENCES

Agras, W., Barlow, D., Chapin, H., Abel, G., and Leitenberg, H. (1974). Behavior modification of anorexia nervosa. *Archives of General Psychiatry* 30: 279-286.

Anthony, E. J. (1970). The reaction of parents to adolescents and to their behavior. E. Anthony and T. Benedek, eds., *Parenthood: Its Psychology and Psychopathology*. Boston: Little, Brown.

Bachrach, A., Erwin, W., and Mohr, J. (1965). The control of eating behavior in an anorectic by operant conditioning techniques. L. Ullman and L. Krasner, eds., *Case Studies in Behavior Modification*. New York: Holt, Rinehart, and Winston.

Berlin, I. N., Boatman, M. J., Sheimo, S., and Szurek, S. (1951). Adolescent alternation of anorexia and obesity: Workshop, 1950. *American Journal of Orthopsychiatry* 21: 387-419.

Bettelheim, B. (1949). A psychiatric school. *The Quarterly Journal of Child Behavior* 1: 86-95.

——— (1950). *Love Is Not Enough.* New York: The Free Press and MacMillan.

——— (1955). *Truants From Life.* New York: The Free Press and MacMillan.

——— (1956). Schizophrenia as a reaction to extreme situations. *American Journal of Orthopsychiatry* 26: 507-518.

——— (1960). *The Informed Heart.* New York: The Free Press and MacMillan.

———, and Sylvester, E. (1948). A therapeutic milieu. *American Journal of Orthopsychiatry* 18: 191-206.

Blinder, B., Freedman, D., and Stunkard, A. (1970). Behavior therapy of anorexia nervosa: effectiveness of activity as a reinforcer of weight gain. *American Journal of Psychiatry* 126: 1093-1098.

Bliss, E., and Branch, C. H. (1960). *Anorexia Nervosa: Its History, Psychology, and Biology*. New York: Hoeber-Harper.

Blos, P. (1967). The second individuation process of adolescence. *Psychoanalytic Study of the Child* 22: 162-186.

Bruch, H. (1965). The psychiatric differential diagnosis of anorexia nervosa. J. E. Meyer and H. Feldman, eds., *Anorexia Nervosa*. Stuttgart: George Thieme.

——— (1966). Eating disorders and schizophrenic development. G. Usedin, ed., *Psychoneurosis and Schizophrenia*. Philadelphia: Lippincott.

———— (1970a). Family Background in eating disorders. E. J. Anthony and C. Koupernik, eds., *The Child in His Family*. New York: Wiley.

———— (1970b). Psychotherapy in primary anorexia nervosa. *Journal of Nervous and Mental Disease* 150: 51-67.

———— (1970c). Changing approaches to anorexia nervosa. C. Rowland, ed., *Anorexia and Obesity*. Boston: Little, Brown.

———— (1970d). Instinct and interpersonal experience. *Comprehensive Psychiatry* 11: 495-506.

———— (1971a). Death in anorexia nervosa. *Psychosomatic Medicine* 33: 135-144.

———— (1971b). Family transactions in eating disorders. *Comprehensive Psychiatry* 12: 238-248.

———— (1973). *Eating Disorders: Obesity, Anorexia Nervosa, and the Person Within*. New York: Basic Books.

———— (1974). Perils of behavior modification in treatment of anorexia nervosa. *Journal of the American Medical Association* 230: 1419-1422.

———— (1975). Behavior therapy in anorexia nervosa. *Journal of the American Medical Association* 233: 317.

Charcot, J. M. (1889). *Diseases of the Nervous System, III*. London: The New Sydenham Society. Reprinted in M. R. Kaufman and M. Heiman, eds., *Evolution of Psychosomatic Concepts: Anorexia Nervosa: A Paradigm*. New York: International Universities Press, 1964.

Cohler, B. (1972). Individuation and the issue of control in the etiology of anorexia nervosa. Unpublished manuscript. Committee on Human Development, the University of Chicago.

———— (1975). Mothers and grandmothers: personality and childcare in three-generation families. Unpublished manuscript. Committee on Human Development, The University of Chicago.

Crisp, A., and Kalucy, R. (1974). Aspects of the perceptual disorder in anorexia nervosa. *British Journal of Medical Psychology* 47: 349-361.

DuBois, E. (1949). Compulsion neurosis with cachexia (anorexia nervosa). *American Journal of Psychiatry* 106: 107-115.

Eissler, K. (1943). Some psychiatric aspects of anorexia nervosa, demonstrated by a case report. *The Psychoanalytic Review* 30: 121-145.

Feinstein, S. (1974). Anorexia nervosa. *Journal of the American Medical Association* 228: 1230.

Flarsheim, A. (1975). The therapist's collusion with the patient's wish for suicide. P. Giovacchini, ed., *Tactics and Techniques in Psychoanalytic Therapy. Vol II: Countertransference*. New York: Jason Aronson.

Fliess, R. (1942). The metapsychology of the analyst. *Psychoanalytic Quarterly* 11: 211-227.

———— (1953). Countertransference and counteridentification. *Journal of the American Psychoanalytic Association* 1: 268-284.

Freud, S. (1909). Addendum to notes upon a case of obsessional neurosis. *Standard Edition* 10: 251-318. London: Hogarth, 1955.

———— (1912). Recommendations to physicians practising psychoanalysis. *Standard Edition* 12: 109-120. London: Hogarth, 1958.

———— (1915). Observations on transference love (further recommendations on the technique of psychoanalysis, III). *Standard Edition* 12: 157-171. London: Hogarth, 1958.

———— (1937). Analysis terminable and interminable. *Standard Edition* 23: 209-254. London: Hogarth, 1964.

———— (1938). Splitting of the ego in the process of defense. *Standard Edition* 13: 271-278. London: Hogarth, 1964.

Garfinkel, P., Kline, S., and Stancer, H. (1973). Treatment of anorexia nervosa using operant conditioning techniques. *Journal of Nervous and Mental Diseases* 157: 428-433.

Gifford, S. Murawski, B., and Pilot, M. (1970). Anorexia nervosa in one of identical twins. C. Rowland, ed., *Anorexia and Obesity*. Boston: Little, Brown.

Goodsitt, A. (1969). Anorexia nervosa. *British Journal of Medical Psychology* 42: 109-117.

Groen, J. J., and Feldman-Toledano, Z. (1966). Educative treatment of patients and parents in anorexia nervosa. *British Journal of Psychiatry* 112: 671-681.

Hallsten, A., Jr. (1965). Adolescent anorexia nervosa treated by desensitization. *Behavioral Research Therapy* 3: 87-91.

Halmi, K. (1974a). Anorexia nervosa: demographic and clinical features in 94 cases. *Psychosomatic Medicine* 36: 18-26.

———— (1974b). Comparison of demographic and clinical features in patient groups with different ages and weights at onset of anorexia nervosa. *The Journal of Nervous and Mental Disease* 158: 222-225.

————, Powers, P., and Cunningham, S. (1975). Treatment of anorexia nervosa with behavior modification. *Archives of General Psychiatry* 32: 93-96.

Hussey, H. (1974). Anorexia nervosa: treatment by behavior modification. *Journal of the American Medical Association* 228: 344.

Journal of the American Medical Association (1972). Behavior analysis and behavior theory. *JAMA* 220: 852-853.

Kaufman, M. R., and Heiman, M. (1964). *Evolution of Psychosomatic Concepts: Anorexia Nervosa—A Paradigm.* New York: International Universities Press.

Kernberg, O. (1966). Structural derivatives of object relations. *International Journal of Psycho-Analysis* 47: 236-253.

Klein, M. (1932). *The Psychoanalysis of Children.* New York: Grove Press, 1960.

——— (1952). Notes on some schizoid mechanisms. M. Klein, P. Heimann, S. Isaacs, and J. Riviere, eds, *Developments in Psychoanalysis.* London: Hogarth.

Kohut, H. (1959). Introspection, empathy and psychoanalysis. *Journal of the American Psychoanalytic Association* 7: 459-483.

Lang, P. (1965). Behavior therapy with a case of nervosa anorexia. L. Ullman and L. Krasner, eds., *Case Studies in Behavior Modification.* New York: Holt, Rinehart and Winston.

Leitenberg, H., Agras, W., and Thomoson, I. (1968). A sequential analysis of the effect of selective positive reinforcement in modifying anorexia nervosa. *Behavioral Research Therapy* 6: 211-218.

Liebman, R., Minuchin, S., and Baker, L. (1974a). An integrated treatment of program for anorexia nervosa. *American Journal of Psychiatry* 131: 432-436.

——— (1974b). The role of the family in the treatment of anorexia nervosa. *Journal of the American Academy of Child Psychiatry* 13: 264-274.

Mahler, M. S. (1968). *On Human Symbiosis and the Vicissitudes of Individuation, Vol. I.* New York: International Universities Press.

——— (1972). On the first three subphases of the separation-individuation process. *International Journal of Psycho-Analysis* 53: 333-338.

Minuchin, S. (1970). The use of an ecological framework in the treatment of a child. E. J. Anthony and C. Koupernik, eds., *The Child in His Family.* New York: Wiley.

——— (1974). *Families and Family Therapy.* Cambridge, Mass.: Harvard University Press.

Murray, H. (1938). *Explorations in Personality.* New York: Oxford University Press.

Nemiah, J. (1958). Anorexia nervosa: fact and theory. *American Journal of Digestive Diseases* 3: 249-274.

Noshpitz, J. (1962). Notes on the theory of residential treatment. *Journal of the American Academy of Child Psychiatry* 1: 284-296.

Palazzoli, M. S. (1970). The families of patients with anorexia nervosa. E. J. Anthony and C. Koupernik, eds., *The Child in His Family.* New York: Wiley.

———— (1971). Anorexia nervosa. S. Arieti, ed., *World Biennial of Psychiatry, I.* New York: Basic Books.

———— (1974). *Self Starvation.* London: Human Context Books.

Parsons, A. (1969). *Belief, Magic, and Anomic Essays in Psychosocial Anthropology.* New York: Free Press.

Phillipson, H. (1955). *The Object Relations Technique.* London: Tavistock Press.

Reik, T. (1937). *Surprise and the Psychoanalyst.* New York: Dutton.

Rowland, C. (1970). Anorexia nervosa—a survey of the literature and review of 30 cases. C. Rowland, ed., *Anorexia and Obesity.* Boston: Little, Brown.

Schafer, R. (1959). Generative empathy in the treatment situation. *Psychoanalytic Quarterly* 28: 342-373.

Slade, P., and Russell, G. (1973). Awareness of body dimensions in anorexia nervosa: cross-sectional and longitudinal studies. *Psychological Medicine* 3: 188-199.

Sours, J. A. (1969). Anorexia nervosa: nosology, diagnosis, developmental patterns and power-control dynamics. G. Caplan and S. Lebovici, eds., *Adolescence: Psychosocial Perspectives.* New York: Basic Books.

———— (1974). The anorexia nervosa syndrome. *International Journal of Psycho-Analysis* 55: 567-576.

Spector, S. (1975). Behavior therapy in anorexia nervosa. *Journal of the American Medical Association* 223: 317.

Stunkard, A. (1959). Obesity and the denial of hunger. *Psychosomatic Medicine* 21: 281.

———— (1972). New therapies for the eating disorders. *Archives of General Psychiatry* 26: 391-398.

Thander, S. (1970). Anorexia nervosa: a psychiatric investigation of 94 female patients. *Acta Psychiatrica Scandinavica* Supplementum 214: 194.

Thoma, H. (1967). *Anorexia Nervosa.* Trans. G. Brydone. New York: International Universities Press.

Waller, J., Kaufman, M. R., and Deutsch, F. (1940). Anorexia nervosa: a psychosomatic entity. *Psychosomatic Medicine* 2: 3-16.

Werry, J., and Bull, D. (1975). Anorexia nervosa: a case study using behavior therapy. *Journal of the American Academy of Child Psychiatry* 14: 646-651.

Winnicott, D. W. (1950-1955). Aggression in relation to emotional development. *Collected Papers.* New York: Basic Books, 1958.

Wolpe, J. (1975). Behavior therapy in anorexia nervosa. *Journal of the American Medical Association* 223: 318.

PART IV

PSYCHOTHERAPY OF ADOLESCENCE

EDITORS' INTRODUCTION

The following chapters deal with various treatment issues. Unlike the previous section, in which treatment was discussed principally in regard to specific psychopathology, we here focus on technical considerations in their own right and not necessarily on conditions undergoing treatment. Of course, this can only be a relative emphasis and adolescence has become associated with particular forms and manifestations of psychopathology.

Clinicians have considered acting out (which may or may not include delinquency) characteristically adolescent, and treatment techniques often are designed to cope with the special problems acting out universally presents. Some chapters are directed toward these issues.

Psychotherapists, in the past, have emphasized that adolescents, because of their tendency to act out and other characterological problems, are difficult to treat. As we learn more about psychopathology and technical factors, these issues do not seem to be as important as once believed. There are treatment problems, but, for the most part, these problems seemed to be involved in the treatment of most patients with whom we relate on a one-to-one basis. Furthermore, with our increasing awareness of countertransference responses, the adolescent patient may help clarify some of our own personality problems that would interfere with therapeutic capacities. Instead of hindering the treatment process, countertransference can be turned to therapeutic advantage. Thus, the treatment of the adolescent patient may be a useful experience reflected in our relationships with patients in all other age groups.

Jack Novick approaches the important issue of termination of treatment in adolescence. While the general impression is that adolescents interrupt rather than terminate treatment, they frequently resist by deciding to terminate prematurely. This must be dealt with by confronting the patient with the seriousness of his disturbance, the failure of attempts at self-cure, and the necessity to remain in treatment, giving up plans for unilateral termination. Dr. Novick writes that analysts of adolescents are in a unique position to observe and demonstrate that the oedipal conflict remains crucial as the phase from which termination can take place and further discusses important technical issues specific to adolescence.

Helm Stierlin focuses on the structure of the family of adolescent runaways. He describes centripetal (bound-up), centrifugal (expelling), and delegating families which produce various types of runaway patterns and notes that an adolescent's sudden absconding signals, almost always, a severe family crisis. In discussing the treatment of these situations he explores ideas on multigenerational fairness and empathy, the use of a third party mediator, and gaining control through acceptance of weakness.

Jarl E. Dyrud reflects on a case history of psychosis in the father and later in the son under similar stress. He discusses the metapsychology of Lacan and Faris around self-development and how symptoms may be passed from generation to generation with amazing fidelity.

Frank T. Rafferty and John C. Steffek recount a community mental health experiment where they approached a population of adolescent nonpatients. These teenagers, seriously deficient in social skills, academic achievements, and inner resources, were engaged in a group in an attempt to provide a corrective, ego developing experience. The authors provide a rich sense of ghetto culture, discuss technical aspects of group approaches, and outline their creative but not always successful strategies.

Luiz Osorio discusses technical limitations in the analysis of adolescents, particularly in the area of communication. He believes that adolescents have specific symbolic idiosyncracies expressed in language and behavior. These symbolisms are derived from the adolescent process which Dr. Osorio generally attributes to mourning the loss of infantile attachments. The treatment techniques used to approach behavior language are described in a series of analytic vignettes.

Therapists recognize that most psychoanalytic psychotherapy has less to do with resolving transference neurosis than in developing effective ego control, and that concomitant modifications of technique are in order. Myron F. Weiner and Joe W. King discuss the parameter of self-disclosure by the therapist to the adolescent patient. They believe that properly timed disclosures enhance interpersonal contact and help repress disruptive primary process material.

Reuven Kohen-Raz reviews the special education needs and approaches to handicapped adolescents. He disagrees with theories of cumulative developmental defect, and believes that early learning is far from irreversible. Dr. Kohen-Raz proposes approaches to the educable mentally retarded, the trainable mentally retarded, the physically handicapped, the organic brain damaged, the acoustically handicapped, the behavior disordered, and emotionally disturbed which can be used to stimulate motivation toward reeducation resulting in a life of independence and dignity.

23] TERMINATION OF TREATMENT IN ADOLESCENCE

JACK NOVICK

In the literature on the analytic treatment of adolescents there has been an understandable emphasis on the technique of getting adolescents into analysis (Aichhorn 1925, Eissler 1958, Harley 1970, Spiegel 1951) and of keeping them there once they are in (Geleerd 1957, Laufer 1974), but as yet there has been little written about termination of the terminal phase.[1] Except for a few articles on termination of child analytic cases (A. Freud 1970, Kohrman 1969, van Dam, Heinicke, and Shane 1975), the bulk of the literature is about termination of analysis of adults. Scattered, are a number of brief remarks pertaining to the fact that adolescents frequently interrupt rather than terminate their treatment (Adatto 1958, 1974, A. Freud 1970, Landauer 1970, Spiegel 1951). Reich (1950) notes that even those adolescents who do not break off treatment often do not show any of the features said to appear regularly in the terminal phase of adult analysis.

Discussions of termination include a wide range of clinical issues, from the question of analyzability (Rangell 1966) to the fate of the transference neurosis after analysis (Pfeffer 1961, Balkoura 1974). My aim is to initiate a discussion of a hitherto neglected aspect of the treatment of adolescents, and to examine some of the general issues involved in termination. I shall use material from the analysis of a boy who started five-times-weekly treatment at seventeen and terminated four years later.

George sought help because of a long-standing urination problem. He had never been able to urinate outside his home and recently had developed difficulties at home as well. He was enuretic until age eleven, and had a long history of multiple fears, anxiety attacks, somatic complaints, and school

Reprinted from *The Psychoanalytic Study of the Child*, Volume 31. New Haven: Yale University Press.

refusal. In early adolescence he had a brief period of transvestite behavior, feared being a homosexual, and there was a time when, as he said, he had "a crush" on his mother. He had always been bullied and teased as a child and now, as an adolescent, he was isolated and withdrawn.

George was the second child of working-class parents; his sister was five years older. He and his mother had a very close, almost incestuous relationship. They played a family game in which mother and father would be in the bedroom and she would shout for help. George would rush upstairs and pull his father away while shouting, "Unhand that maiden." In a variation of this game, mother and father were necking on the couch and mother would say to George, "Tell your father to cut it out."

At the beginning of treatment George had an idealized image of his mother. He saw her as a powerful, magical person who would protect him and grant all his wishes provided he was a good, passive little boy. She was, in fact, extremely sensitive to his infantile needs and totally accepted all his problems. She would take him into her bed whenever he was frightened, defend him against school bullies and sadistic teachers, nurse him through his panic attacks, and spend hours with play material to help him verbalize his fears. On the other hand, she reacted to the slightest sign of aggression or assertion by threatening to sell him and then refusing to speak to him until he begged forgiveness.

George's mother was the only girl in a family of seven boys, all of whom had been enuretic. She was a highly superstitious lapsed Catholic who believed that she was a reincarnation of Anne Boleyn. George's father was a passive, ineffectual man who worked nights and spent the days doing housework. He too had never been able to urinate in public toilets. George's sister was pathologically jealous of her brother, and from his infancy she took every opportunity to attack, hurt, and humiliate him. When George was fifteen, his sister had a psychotic breakdown and was hospitalized.

I will examine (1) the preconditions for the emergence of a terminal phase, (2) some criteria for deciding on beginning the terminal phase, (3) technical questions regarding the start of the terminal phase, (4) the terminal phase itself, and (5) the relation between the terminal phase and goals of treatment.

The Preconditions for the Emergence of a Terminal Phase

Since beginnings and endings are intertwined, one cannot talk about ending without looking at the beginning. Broadly, the terminal phase refers to the conclusion of the analytic process. The precondition for a terminal phase, then, is the existence of an analytic process, in particular the existence of a transference and transference neurosis and the capacity to experience and observe the transference rather than living it out as a current reality. Beyond this general consideration, however, there is a phenomenon directly related to termination which I have now observed in several adolescents and which I call *the unilateral termination plan.* Many adolescents plan a unilateral termination of treatment at the very beginning or soon after treatment has started. Sometimes the plan is explicit, as when they enter treatment in their last year of school with the stated intention of going to a university at the end of the year. This is not a "natural end" (Landauer 1970) to treatment, but the condition under which the adolescent enters and thus avoids the analysis. Often this plan is kept secret and then presented as an external event which unfortunately will bring treatment to an end. It is not a sudden, but a planned interruption, which is presented as a natural developmental step, as part of the adolescent's growth toward independence. Instead of separating from his parents, however, he often leaves analysis and ends up even more attached to them.

George's case was one in which the handling of this unilateral termination plan was crucial to the analytic process and a major precondition for the emergence of a terminal phase. His plan was overt, although the determinants were of course unconscious. He was in his final year at secondary school and had a provisional place at a college outside London. Although this was presented as an unfortunate external circumstance limiting the duration of treatment, it was, in fact, his condition for accepting treatment. The importance of this escape hatch, this unilateral termination plan, emerged only years later. By means of this plan he could control and limit the treatment, especially the quality and intensity of the transference. During the first year, I was for him an object onto whom he externalized the part of himself that wished to be free of his mother. In dreams I was a "spiv," a "wide-boy," a shady character who took him away from his mother and introduced him to women. He experienced independence as an aggressive attack on his mother. The battle was between his mother and me, while he stood by, a passive observer, ready to go along with the victor. In his relationship with me, other transference elements, notably rivalry, envy, and jealousy, led to homosexual submission in order to protect me from his rage and secretly steal my power. However, this could remain diluted and defended against by his awareness that our contact was limited. A most crucial limitation was the fact that he could avoid dealing with the separation experience by simply being the active one who left me. Nevertheless, despite or because of these limitations he made substantial progress during the year. From someone who had been completely isolated, inhibited, and constricted he became a young man who began to look and behave like an adolescent. He had friends, went to parties, had a girlfriend, played guitar, rode a motorcycle, smoked pot occasionally, and could experience critical, even angry feelings about his mother. Despite her active opposition, he passed his exams. Even though his mother cried for three days, he still managed to leave for college, where he shared a house with a number of friends. During the first year of college he continued to see me on weekends and during holidays. He liked this arrangement because he could now come and go when it suited him. Progress was maintained for most of the year and then, during the last term, I did not hear from him except for a letter telling me that he had decided to switch his course from science to psychology. He came to see me after the college year was over and without signs of distress described what was obviously a breakdown. He had become increasingly involved with drugs and at his final exams was so "zonked out" he could not read the exam papers and failed the year. He said that he had decided to take the year off, share a house with some friends, and practice his guitar playing. He readily accepted the idea of staying in London and coming back to analysis. However, once more it was with the understanding that he would return to college at the end of the year.

It took six months of work to make him aware of his depression, his rage, and the extent to which he lived in a delusional world in order to defend against these affects. It became clear that the immediate cause of his breakdown at college had been the realization that his parents were coping quite well without him and, in fact, seemed to be having a much happier time together. The pain and rage pushed him completely into drugs and he spent his last term of college "spaced out," as he called it, or, more precisely, out of touch with his feelings. Pot was one of his many attempts at "self-cure" (Khan 1970). After I had helped him wean himself from this antidepressant, we could focus more directly on how, in fantasy, he controlled and manipulated his family and me in order to feel that he was in the center of our world, that he was not excluded from anything, and that he had no reason for envy or jealousy since all his wishes were gratified. Coming back to analysis gave him the excuse to stay at home. In a series of dreams and associations we could also see that in collusion with his powerful mother he felt that he could steal whatever he envied in me.

Nevertheless, the work on his defenses took root and he began to experience the futility of his attempts at self-cure. As the underlying pain and depression became more accessible, he began to turn to me, not only as the omnipotent parent who would protect him and gratify his wishes, but as an analyst who could help him find different solutions. I could now take up the defense against the analysis itself—first, the denial of the extent and seriousness of disturbance, and from this the necessity to give analysis top priority above any other consideration, such as college, work, privacy, free time. In particular, if he wanted the treatment I was ready to offer, he would have to relinquish his attempt to control the process by unilaterally setting a termination date. At first he reacted with anger. He said I was putting him down, exaggerating things, but then he admitted that he was in a bad way, that I was right in pointing out that the future breakdown he feared had in fact already occurred. After a last-ditch effort to solve his problems on his own, with the aid of drugs and yoga, he announced that he had decided to put analysis first, and withdrew his applications to colleges outside London.

Discussing adolescence, Winnicott (1971) said that what the adolescent needs from the adult is not understanding but "confrontation." It is my view that, at some point during treatment, the adolescent must be confronted with the seriousness of his disturbance, the failure of his attempt at self-cure, and the necessity of accepting fully the analytic process by relinquishing his plans for unilateral termination. To echo Freud's classic paper on the subject (1937), analysis cannot be terminable until it is experienced by the patient as interminable.

After the confrontation and George's decision to undergo analysis, we could immediately see how the unilateral termination plan represented his way of rushing back to his mother, submitting to her, and thus feeling protected and gratified at all levels of development. It was only following the confrontation that his passivity and his intense attachment to his mother could be experienced and understood in the transference. Without the external mother to run to, I became both the powerful, envied father and the idealized protective mother. In his earlier work, George had withheld much, now he found that he was afraid that in analysis he would discover that he was really a girl and, more important, that he was really a killer. The interplay between these fears and their relation to his internalized parents could then begin to unfold.

George had a series of dreams involving rivalry with schoolmates. In one dream all the boys were comparing their penises and the little fellow had the biggest one, ten inches long. The girls then took their skirts off. He was consumed in the dream with envy and jealousy. I had become in the transference the powerful father with a ten-inch penis who took the mother away and left him lost, alone, jealous, and filled with rage. His earlier immediate response would have been to run to his mother, but now it was to my wife. He felt a flu coming on and he decided to stay home. He telephoned when he knew that I would be working, like his father who worked night shifts. The phone was answered by my wife and he told her that he was ill, as he used to tell his mother that he was frightened. Coming to the session the next day he saw my wife. In the preconfrontation period he had seen her a number of times (she is a child analyst and we share a waiting room) as an older woman and assumed she was my wife. Now he did not mention having seen her. I commented on this and he denied that he had seen my wife. He said he had seen a young girl who smiled at him and made him feel wonderful. He was now living out the fantasy that, in collusion with my wife, he could steal what was mine and reverse the situation. In another dream, he was sitting in my chair and I was lying on the couch. I told him that I was very anxious and would like to have a cigarette. He offered me a cigar.

With the fantasy that he had stolen my wife and my penis George felt active and powerful. He told me that he had played guitar all day, and could now do things with the guitar he had never been able to do before. He added that his sexual feelings had returned, he felt "potent," and when he masturbated he had a "super hard-on." The reaction set in very quickly. He became terrified of the destructiveness in his sexuality, guilty over what he had done to me, and frightened of my jealous rage. He then gave up all his activities, lost his sexual feelings, and in the sessions became extremely tense and blocked. We learned slowly that the tension reflected the struggle over his longing to submit to me sexually, but the homosexual position was untenable. To give in to his intense passive longings, with me as the powerful father, would mean being castrated and really becoming a girl. Instead he turned his passive anal wishes to me as his mother, who was a safer object. With his mother he could pretend that he was a girl and keep his penis, as he had done in his transvestite phase. Instead of being penetrated by the destructive ten-inch "super hard-on," he could be penetrated by suppositories. This anal masturbation fantasy related to the frequent experience of having had suppositories inserted by his mother. My interpretations were experienced as suppositories, providing relief by removing all the badness inside him.

As his tension was relieved and he relaxed in the session, a masochistic identification with the damaged female emerged. All the aggression was now in the external world. He told me of his fear of policemen on the motorway and of the nasty men at work, as he earlier had told his mother of the bullies at school. He made a mess of his activities in and out of the analysis; he felt my words wiped his bottom, my interpretations comforted him and fed him, and I became the magical mother he could keep and hold on to. He was also afraid that in analysis he would discover he really was a girl because he so wanted to be a girl. He told me that he had the fantasy that he was born a girl and doctored into a boy. As a girl he could avert the jealous destructive attacks of his mother and sister. As a girl he could evoke the sympathy, love, and devotion of his mother and keep her from leaving him, as she always did when he acted assertively. As a girl he could avoid dangerous rivalry with his father and steal the envied penis, as he felt his mother had done. At a point where the material centered on his envy of his mother and his wish to be a girl, he saw a television program about a man with an amputated leg. He afterwards dreamed that he was superman with an amputated leg, representing his fantasy that through castration he could become all powerful. Most crucial, however, was his use of the identification with the damaged woman as the defense against his murderous rage at his mother and his conviction that he was a killer.

There were many factors in George's history which could account for the intensity of his rage and his conviction of the omnipotence of his destructive wishes. The constant jealous attacks on his masculinity by his mother and sister in themselves account for much. As a child he was not only preoccupied with thoughts of death but felt responsible for any damage or death which occurred. A friend drowned, the brother of a boy who bullied him died, the Egyptian mummies in the museum were dead, and he felt responsible. His death wishes and his fantasy that he had damaged the women had, however, an additional determinant. Early in the treatment he told me of the death of a number of pets, events he presented as unrelated to him. Through his current material I could finally take up his fear of being discovered as a killer for he had, in fact, killed those pets.[2] This became an important focus of our work, as a result of which he could acknowledge the reality that now, as a tall and powerful young man, he was capable of murder.

What I have presented might be called the outline of the intrapsychic drama as it unfolded via the transference in the year of analysis between the point of confrontation and the setting of a date for termination. The confrontation allowed for the emergence and flowering of the transference neurosis, and it was by means of the transference and within the transference that elements of the drama could be experienced, observed, and understood.

Some Criteria for
Beginning the Terminal Phase

There are many ways to end treatment. In the previous section, I had discussed the unilateral decision made by the adolescent. The decision can also be made unilaterally by the analyst. It might be helpful to speak of these circumstances as decisions to stop or end treatment. *Termination* would then be reserved for a phase in the analytic process. The terminal phase can be defined operationally as the phase which follows the setting of a date for ending treatment. But what are the criteria for arriving at such a decision? Despite the fact that most of the articles on termination attempt to develop criteria, the relationship between these criteria and the terminal phase remains obscure. Although the criteria discussed in the literature have met with many criticisms, these are not criteria for initiating a terminal phase, but criteria of cure, determined in part by the work done in the terminal phase. I would suggest it necessary to consider criteria for deciding when to start a terminal phase, and that these criteria differ from those for assessing the outcome of treatment.

In George's case, the setting of the date was not based on a decision by one party or the other, but emerged in the space between analyst and patient. In fact, it was not a decision, but a mutual recognition and acceptance of an approaching end.

In his survey of British psychoanalysts Glover (1955) found that most of them relied on intuition as the basis for deciding upon termination. Although Glover was critical of this approach, I would counter that intuition can be seen as the preconscious operation of the analyst's skill and experience. The value of discussing a topic such as termination is to make explicit the preconscious judgments which enter into intuition and thus expand our skills. In looking over George's material leading up to the terminal phase, I can see three areas of change which contributed to "the clinical feel" (Rangell 1966) that time was ripe for initiating termination; changes in the transference, the working alliance, and the countertransference.

Most authors view the resolution of transference neurosis as the central task of analysis and the major criterion for termination (Firstein 1974). The work of Pfeffer (1961) and others (Balkoura 1974) in following up successfully analyzed patients raises the basic question whether the transference neurosis can be resolved in analysis, whether it is indeed ever resolved. However, if we accept the resolution of the transference neurosis as a major criterion for termination, we are left with the question of when this criterion applies. Do we wait for the transference neurosis to be resolved before the start of the terminal phase, or do we need a terminal phase in order to resolve the transference neurosis? On this topic, the literature is vague or ambiguous. The ambiguity can be seen in what Glover (1955) says about termination. In his discussion of criteria he cites resolution of the transference neurosis as a criterion of major importance, but then goes on to say that the transference neurosis can be resolved only when the touchstone of termination is applied to it. There is a further problem which relates to what is meant by resolving the transference neurosis. The word *resolve* signifies an ending or, more forcefully, an obliteration (Balkoura 1974). The Oxford English Dictionary defines *resolve* with yet another meaning: "To analyze (a force or velocity) into its components." We can thus speak of resolving the transference as analyzing the transference neurosis into its components. In this sense of the word, I could say that George's transference neurosis was resolved. However, psychoanalysis is not equivalent to physical analysis, for in psychoanalysis the process of investigation alters the object of investigation. Resolving the transference neurosis in the sense of analyzing and thus making conscious the underlying components results in a change in the intensity and quality of transference.

In the case of George, the transference neurosis had not concluded or been obliterated, but was in the process of changing toward ultimate resolution. As we worked on his pregenital conflicts, especially his early omnipotent rage at his mother and his masochistic submission to her as a defense, as an adaptation, and as a gratification, the transference became and increasingly remained oedipal in nature. This seems to me a crucial criterion for considering termination, especially in adolescence.

With the widening scope of psychoanalysis and our increased interest in the early phases of development,[3] we have tended, I believe, toward an artificial distinction between oedipal and preoedipal, and between narcissistic and libidinal (Rangell 1975). As analysts of adolescents we are in a unique position to observe and demonstrate that despite the degree or type of pregenital disturbance, the oedipal conflict remains crucial as the internal organizer of pathology, the immediate cause of adolescent breakdown, and the phase from which termination can take place.

Rather than further elaborating on these points, I shall limit my comments to say that in George's case, his ability to experience and increasingly maintain an oedipal level of psychic organization, as manifest in the transference, was a central criterion for initiating the terminal phase. The fact that a transference neurosis could evolve and be analyzed speaks for a multitude of significant changes such as an increased capacity to tolerate anxiety and frustration; a change in the quality, rigidity, and intensity of the defense system; increased availability of affects, wishes, fantasies, and childhood memories; an increased capacity to verbalize aggressive and sexual wishes and to change acting out into remembering; an increased capacity to integrate and synthesize hitherto incompatible parts of self and object representations; and, in general, an increasing capacity to take an analytic stance in relation to his inner world.

The experience of imminent termination was a necessary condition for resolving the oedipal transference in George's case, and I would suggest this holds true for most adolescents. In other words, I saw George's terminal phase as one in which considerable analytic work would have to be done, and be sustained by an existent working alliance. To illustrate the way in which George had begun to work analytically, I present material which shows how he dealt with a dream he had during a weekend. In the dream he was at a party and saw a lovely girl. He kissed her and put his tongue in her mouth. It felt good, though somewhat tight. He asked her to marry him and she agreed. He felt marvelous and was congratulated by a boy in a sailor suit. He woke up feeling "great" and felt that he was on the road to recovery. The dream, he thought, reflected an interest in normal sex with an appropriate person, revealing an ability to take the initiative, approach a girl, make a sexual advance, and feel sufficiently self-confident to ask her to marry him. He continued to think of the dream during the weekend, for he found that there were certain features he could not understand. He then realized, on his own, that despite the positive changes reflected in the dream, it was mainly a disguised version of his predominant fantasy. The tight sensation, he said, referred to his anal preoccupation and the persistent view of sex as an anal attack. The "boy in the sailor suit" referred to his father, who had been a sailor and was as short as I am. The woman was not an appropriate available girl but my wife, and being congratulated by me represented his masochistic fantasy that through his suffering and submission he would, without further effort, be granted the prize.

The working alliance is obviously crucial to the patient's capacity to do the further work necessary in a terminal phase. In addition, however, it indicates that a major obstacle to termination has been overcome. George could accept responsibility for the dream and make the links to his own infantile passive wishes. At an earlier period in the analysis when fantasies about my wife had first emerged, he had insisted that I put thoughts of my wife into his head.

Transference and the working alliance are interrelated phenomena (Novick 1970), and the analysis of adolescents provides further evidence that the two processes are intertwined. Oedipal envy, jealousy, and rivalry motivated George's intense resistance, but also motivated his wish to identify with my analytic stance and functions. Thus we return to the experience and maintenance of an oedipal transference as a central criterion for the start of a terminal phase.

I have so far emphasized criteria related to internal changes as reflected and observed in the course of analysis. These are what Hoffer (1950) referred to as psychological criteria. Starting with Freud's definition (1917) of mental health as the "capacity for enjoyment and . . . efficiency," there has been an equal emphasis on behavioral criteria for termination. Although we have become more sophisticated and justifiably suspicious of symptomatic and behavioral changes, we still rely heavily on these observable changes to justify the effort and cost of analysis. We have all had cases in which psychological and behavioral changes more or less coincide. These cases are most rewarding, and, I would emphasize, most reassuring to the analyst. I specifically chose to present George's termination because he was definitely not such a case. Despite considerable psychological changes after nearly four years of treatment and at the age of almost twenty-one, he was still living at home, had no girlfriends, worked as a laborer at a seasonal nighttime job, had given up all academic aspirations, and seldom discussed any plans for the future. His case forced me to distinguish between behavioral and psychological changes and to question the reliance we place on externals.

In George's analysis we had reached the point where the crucial oedipal and preoedipal conflicts had been interpreted and worked through, but external changes were minor and could not be maintained. The work increasingly focused on his inability to translate insight into action. I made many interpretations, but valid as they may have been, they were not to the point. I grant that he was envious and had to destroy my work; that my words represented the penis he longed for but had to reject; and, most central, that he was acting out a masochistic fantasy in which he was coming to me with his damage, and I would comfort, love, and stay with him. The point was that, despite all interpretations, he was in fact succeeding in his aim. Despite all the indications that termination was imminent, I could not consider letting him go. He wanted to stay with me but he also wanted to go. He could not go because I was having a countertransference reaction and I could not let him go. Like his mother who had fought the bullies for him, I had become narcissistically involved in and felt responsible for his external behavior. Parallel to the work done with George I, too, had to analyze and accept the extent and limits of my responsibility. I could then verbalize how I had become the anxious parent who was afraid to let him fight his own battles. Furthermore, I could share with him what I had worked out for myself: my responsibility extended to all aspects of his analysis, but his external activities were his responsibility. It was his responsibility to translate insight into action, his effort alone which would produce results in the external world; the pain of failure or the rewards of success would belong to him alone. There followed a brief period of testing me, of disbelief, and of depression. He then said that he realized that everything he did quickly turned into something he did for me.

The tempo of analytic activity increased, with a parallel, though limited change in his external behavior. One day he felt that he should start standing on his own feet, that he was using analysis as a crutch, and perhaps we should think of finishing in the near future. After further discussion of the work which remained to be done, George picked a date four months away with which I concurred.

Technical Questions Regarding the Start of the Terminal Phase

Termination should not be a unilateral decision, but a mutual recognition. However, someone has to make the first move; someone has to say that the analysis should end. In reviewing the adult literature on the question of broaching the issue and setting a date, Firstein (1974) says, "It hardly matters whether a termination date is broached by patient or analyst, for agreement between them is presumable." But for the adolescent it is an issue which matters greatly, for we are dealing not only with the termination of analysis, but with termination of his infantile relationships with his parents.

In George's case, he broached the subject of termination and I allowed him to choose the date for ending, but I felt that it was my responsibility to make explicit my thoughts about his termination. Before he chose a date I made it clear that I considered this to be a phase in which considerable work would have to be done. We discussed the work which had been done, and I spelled out some of the self-damaging ways in which he might respond to termination. We agreed that once he had chosen a date for ending the analysis, we would not, under any circumstances, alter it. The importance of this agreement in George's case will become evident when I present the material of his terminal phase.

There was another important consideration with regard to setting the date. I find it useful, especially with adolescents, to end the analysis at a time when I am still working rather than at a holiday. This seems to be a minority view in regard to the practice with adults (Firstein 1974), and indeed it is often more convenient for the analyst to have the end coincide with a holiday break. For the adolescent, however, it is important that the experience be one of active leave-taking rather than that of being left. Further, it is useful to have the reality balance of the continued existence and functioning of the analyst, a reality event which both relieves and pains the adolescent. Much of what I have said about my techniques of terminating may be seen as part of a personal style, but I view it as an aspect of the "confrontation and containment" (Winnicott 1971) required by adolescents. Earlier, I spoke of the confrontation necessary to get George into analysis, and now I refer to the confrontation necessary to help him terminate adaptively.

The Terminal Phase

During the sixteen weeks of the terminal phase the tempo of analytic work increased again. Resistances, defenses, regressions, and conflicts were intensified but short-lived. There were, as Gitelson (1967) notes, more "good hours," and the therapeutic alliance was at its maximum efficiency (Ticho 1972). During this period we recapitulated George's analytic and personal history, all centered now on the reality of the terminal date. Termination initially meant being active, independent, and masculine. He felt exhilarated, he said, by the experience of standing on his own feet and taking on more of the analytic functions. He then had a dream that he was "the great train robber." To take on my functions meant to take over, to steal everything. The activity was initially experienced in the context of a phallic rivalry—by being active he felt he was destroying me and stealing my penis. Later, in the terminal period he again had a dream of stealing after he bought some new and flattering clothes. He then experienced stealing in relation to his jealous sister and mother. He felt that he was stealing love and attention from his sister and depriving his mother of her need to be the active, intrusive, powerful one. To have initiated the process of termination was to George an act of aggression that would invite retaliation from all members of his family. His major fear was of being abandoned and left alone, and he again recalled the time at the age of four when he was lost on a crowded beach. That was the last time he had felt alone and never again until the analysis did he allow himself to experience this feeling.

During the terminal phase he again felt alone and spoke about a symptom which we had not completely understood. During the last year of treatment he had told me that he had a "weird, frightening, unsettling feeling" whenever he saw a statue. He now told me that what upset and frightened him about the statue was its density, its mass. He felt as if the weight of the statue was inside him. When I linked this with the bad, destructive fecal mass he held in with his tension he said that his current depression was due to the fear that all the things inside him would never be released. "Who will stick something up my anus? Who will give me the enema or suppository and get out all that dense material?" He regressed from the level of active independence, and the passive-masochistic regression which had been the central feature of his analysis became the major reaction to termination. First, he tried to regain the masochistic gratification of the analysis, coming to each session in a state of mental pain and constipation which was then relieved by my words. I interpreted his attempt to deny the finality of termination by reestablishing a sadomasochistic pattern where I insert my words into him. I said that this not only gave him pleasure, but he also felt it was giving me sadistic pleasure, a pleasure I would not want to relinquish. He then told me how much he enjoyed "having a crap," but it made him feel uneasy; it is a solitary pleasure, an independent activity. He wondered whether holding in his feces was the sadomasochistic pattern we were discussing. It gave him tummyaches, but got his mother to do something to relieve him of the pain.

The material then switched to another aspect of his anality, the sadistic messing which would force me to clean him, care for him, and break our agreement by keeping him in analysis. Each day he would tell me how terrible things were with him, all his activities were a mess, and perhaps we should extend the analysis. When I told him that I would not do so, he tried to have me alter my holiday or at the very least change the time of one of his sessions. As he felt his omnipotence challenged, his rage increased and one day he brought in, via enactment, the actual messing he had so far kept secret. Following one of his sessions I remembered that I had not replaced an ashtray in the waiting room. I found one of George's cigarettes stubbed out on the table. I confronted him with having made a mess and he became very angry. I was like a headmaster, he said, trying to put him down for a silly thing. He could not see anything wrong with what he had done. He left still feeling angry, but the next day he told me that he had been thinking about it all evening. He realized that he left a mess everywhere and expected people to clean up. When he uses the front sitting room at home, "there is shit everywhere." He often urinates on the carpet rather than in the toilet; and then, with much embarrassment, he told me that when he masturbates, he ejaculates onto a rug in front of his bed. When he returned on Monday he told me he had had "a great weekend, the best weekend I've ever had." He had also been thinking seriously of the mess he made; he had cleaned up the sitting room and had for the first time used a tissue when masturbating.

The working through and giving up of passive anal wishes became a turning point in the terminal process; simultaneously, his outside life became increasingly pleasurable and fulfilling. The attempt to control me and retain me by messing emerged once more, but this time in the form of a return of the original symptoms. He came in after a weekend filled with despair and misery. He was tense, angry, and depressed in the session. I said very little, and he described the return of all his old problems. He said that all his old fears, tensions, somatic anxieties, and urination problems had returned. He felt as he had when in the first year of treatment. I said that this had been the time he had left me and had gone to college. He had made a mess of things there and I had taken him back. He responded by saying, "I feel better now. It makes sense of the weekend."

He was almost ready to give up the fantasy of passive gratification in the transference, gratifications which were reflections of real past and current gratifications in the home, where his parents responded to his anal submissiveness and mess by feeding him. They also soothed him, penetrated him with suppositories, and offered him an easy oedipal triumph through the mother's endless variations on the game of "castrate Dad and I'm yours." He realized that these gratifications were infantile and ultimately frustrating. He wanted something more, he wanted the experience of real genital gratification, but could not yet relinquish these infantile gratifications. The fantasy of having all his passive wishes gratified allowed him to maintain the idealized image of his mother and an omnipotent image of himself. It was in relation to this issue, the idealization of mother and grandiosity of self, that the experience of termination was crucial. As I constantly exposed him to the reality of termination, his own infantile omnipotence began to crumble.

More important, however, was his gradual acceptance of the fact that whatever I did for him was not done for him alone. Whatever real and imagined gratifications he experienced were due to me and not to his omnipotent manipulations. I did what I did because it was part of me. I did it for others and I would continue to do it after he was gone. He said that it made sense logically, but it was hard to accept and believe. He then added that he knew I would probably fill his place the day after he left. But he did accept this and when, a few days later, he found that his mother had taken his infant nephew into her bed, his idealized image of her seemed to shatter completely. What she was doing to his nephew was destructive and done not out of love but our of her own "craziness." He talked now about a crucial historical event he had probably always known but had never been able to integrate. As we talked about his sister's abandonment of her child, George said that she was probably just like his mother, recalling that when he was three, his mother had left him with a neighbor and returned to work. We now had the historical basis for his lifelong fear that independence would lead to attack and abandonment.

In the last few weeks we focused on the extent to which the fantasy of magical omnipotence operated in his everyday life. He quickly picked up my comment and worked on it. He brought in numerous examples and said that it was amazing how much he acted as if everything was due to his magic. He worked in an ice-cream factory and the amount of work each night depended on the weather. Each day he would pray for rain and stand at his window in a tense state wishing for rain. The magical gesture, he said, was the tension of the anal retention of all his anger. Since it usually rains in London, his omnipotence was seldom challenged. Finally, he related a dream which contained elements of past, present, and future. The dream was set in George's garden. Mr. Hardwick was tuning a guitar and insects were flying in a V-formation over the sound-hole of the guitar. George got an apple seed from Mr. Hardwick and put it in a bird's nest. The seed then turned into an egg. In the dream George felt very good. His first comment about the dream was that it was a magical dream and a dream about magic. There was something magical in what Mr. Hardwick was doing, and turning the apple seed into an egg was typical, he said, of his magical beliefs. It was just like him to put a seed in a nest, leave out the fact that a bird had laid the egg, and he would then assume that he had made the egg appear himself. The obvious sexual content allowed us to work through his homosexual longings and the disappointments in not having transference wishes gratified. Other familiar analytic themes were contained in and worked through via the dream, but there were also new elements which surfaced in the last week. For the first time I was represented in the dream as an admired person and not a shady character or a little boy. The magic of the dream was also the magic of skill, mastery, and creativity. I was the admired adult male containing the seed women required. I could handle women and relate to them in a way neither destructive nor submissive. The insects referred to George's earlier nightmare of being attacked by them, a nightmare which had become a transient insect phobia. In the dream he was neither a child nor a superman. He was himself and he did not steal, but happily accepted what was freely given—the capacity to be a male who can produce babies. The egg represented the babies he will produce and also reparation for the babies he imagined he destroyed and the animals he actually killed.

What Menninger (1966) calls "the contract" was now over. At the end of our session George got off the couch, shook my hand, and thanked me for what I had given him. He said that he had gained a lot, that he had a lot. It was really a question now of whether he could use it.

Condensed as it is, this summary of George's terminal phase allows me to discuss a few issues regarding termination. There is of course no typical terminal phase, and each person creates something unique out of each aspect of the analytic process. Nevertheless, certain common features in the termination of adults have been noted (Glover 1955, Rangell 1966, Hurn 1971, Firstein 1969, 1974). Most of these features were present in George's terminal phase, which did not differ significantly from that described in the literature on adults. The phase was marked by the increase in tempo of the analytic work, a regressive intensification of the transference balanced by an increased efficiency in the working alliance. The frequently observed phenomenon of symptom revival occurred, as did increased planning for the future. It was a period of mourning, but also of hopeful anticipation. Although no new analytic themes appeared, new material previously defended against or withheld emerged and deepened our understanding. Like the terminal phase in the analysis of adults, it was crucial for the analytic resolution of the transference neurosis. I would suggest that the features of the terminal phase are independent of the age of the adolescent, but are rather a function of the interaction of a transference neurosis with the reality of ending.

I return now to the question of the relation between criteria for termination and the terminal phase. As stated, most relevant criteria cited are criteria of cure rather than indications of when to start a terminal phase. If, for example, the transference neurosis is resolved (obliterated), what then is there left to the terminal phase? Hurn (1971), after reviewing the literature on termination, says that the terminal phase is concerned primarily with the "disposition of the therapeutic alliance" and "deals extensively and primarily with the separation of the patient from the analyst as analyst." Using the material from George's terminal phase, I would argue that it is not the analyst as a real person, but as a transference object who is relinquished and mourned. It was only at the very end of the terminal phase that George could begin to experience and accept me as I really was; and in separating from me as analyst, he made me part of his ego ideal, thereby providing the possibility for future self-analysis.

Termination and the Goals of Treatment

If the criteria for termination are really criteria for cure or goals of treatment, what light does George's case throw on the issues involved? Most of the criteria suggested are irrelevant to clinical practice, since they are often ideals of mental health rather than goals set in the context of an individual pathology. The physician does not expect his arthritic patient to run a four-minute mile, but is satisfied if some movement can be restored and some pain alleviated. Freud's (1937) criticism of Ferenczi's criteria (1927) as too ambitious and unrealistic holds for many of the criteria put forth more recently. Often these criteria are, in Ticho's words (1972), "life goals" rather than treatment goals. The symposium on termination (Balint 1950, Bridger 1950, Buxbaum 1950, Hoffer 1950, Klein 1950, Milner 1950, Payne 1950, Rickman 1950) illustrates both the range of termination criteria and the extent to which goals of treatment can have a theoretical rather than a clinical base.

What suggestions, if any, can be derived from George's material regarding criteria for cure in the analysis of adolescents? One possibility is to consider his analysis a failure or, at the very least, a premature termination. We could say that he should have remained in analysis until certain behavioral criteria were met, such as leaving home, a shift of interest from home to the world of contemporaries, a commitment to work or school, the establishment of a heterosexual relationship. Partly I tend to go along with this view as I remain concerned about George and his future development. I did, however, receive a letter from him three months after the end of treatment. It was a long letter from which one point emerged clearly: the process of cure did not end at termination.[4] George left home, lived with contemporaries, and evidenced a realistic work commitment months after the formal end of analysis.

In his letter, George used the word *potential,* which raises in my mind the question: what is it we expect in the external behavior of our adolescent patients? Adolescence is a period of potentiality rather than actuality. During my adolescence, my friends and I had to contend with the anxieties of our parents and relatives, who found it difficult to tolerate the uncertainties of this phase. We were constantly asked if we had found a nice job, a nice career, a nice girl or boy, and "when," they would plaintively inquire, "are you going to settle down?" Is it then out of my own narcissistic needs and anxieties that I desire to see George settle down with a nice girl and a nice job? In the first section, where I dealt with the confrontation necessary to start the analytic process, I was implicitly saying that as analysts we should do more. Now in discussing criteria for cure, I am suggesting that we should expect less. In his letter, after mentioning some of his problems, George writes, "but after four years of treatment I know a great deal about myself and more than enough to sort myself out." He is saying, in effect, that he feels capable of self-analysis. I would suggest that self-analysis and all that this implies may be considered a major goal of psychoanalysis.

I would like to end this chapter with two quotes, one from Freud (1937): "The business of the analysis is to secure the best possible psychological conditions for the functions of the ego; with that it has discharged its task." The other is from George's letter:

> I saw Joe Pass at Ronnie Scott's the other week and that more or less set me on the road to be a jazz guitarist. Consummate virtuosity and taste don't come overnight but in hard work and in blossoming out one's personality. So that has me fixed up for the next ten years. I suppose that's why I have always admired you. All you have has been achieved through hard work, positive thinking, personality. The idea of success is an exciting one as is independence And to cut a long story short, I think I am making out O.K. Thanks and Happy Christmas.

Conclusions

This chapter is an attempt to initiate discussion on the hitherto neglected topic of termination of treatment in adolescence, using material from the four-year analysis of a seventeen-year-old boy. Termination issues were discussed under five headings:

1. *The Preconditions of a Terminal Phase.* Many adolescents plan a unilateral termination of treatment at the very beginning or soon after treatment has started. It is often the condition under which the adolescent enters and thus avoids the analysis. I suggested that at some point in the treatment, the adolescent must be confronted with the seriousness of his disturbance and the necessity of giving himself up to the analytic process by relinquishing the plan for unilateral termination. Analysis cannot become terminable until it is experienced by the patient as interminable.

2. *Some Criteria for Beginning the Terminal Phase.* Most criteria expressed in the literature are in fact criteria for cure and not criteria for starting a terminal phase. The start of the terminal phase is not a decision but a mutual recognition and acceptance of an approaching end. In the case presented, the mutual recognition related to significant changes in the transference, the working alliance, and the countertransference. A central criterion for starting the terminal phase was the adolescent's ability to experience and increasingly maintain in the transference an oedipal level of psychic organization.

3. *Technical Questions Regarding the Start of the Terminal Phase.* Implicit to this chapter is my view that termination is not only an important treatment issue, but is the central task of adolescence. Termination of treatment relates to the central task of terminating the infantile relationships with parents; thus the actual technique of starting the terminal phase is not a matter of indifference, but is crucial to the outcome of treatment of adolescents. It is important that the topic be broached and the date set by the adolescent. The date of ending should occur at a time when the analyst is still working rather than coinciding with a holiday. Once the date is set, it should not be altered.

4. *The Terminal Phase.* I presented material from the terminal phase and concluded that the features of this phase did not differ significantly from those found in the terminal phase of adults. The features of the terminal phase are a function of the interaction of a transference neurosis with the reality of ending. In this case, the terminal phase was crucial to the analytic resolution of the transference neurosis. Material of the case presented argued against the view that the terminal phase deals primarily with the separation of the patient from the analyst as a real object. Rather it is the analyst as a transference object who is mourned and transference wishes from all levels of development which have to be relinquished. The real aspects of the analyst, the function of the analyst, are internalized as part of the ego ideal and provide the basis for self-analysis.

5. *Termination and Goals of Treatment.* Most criteria for cure cited in the literature are irrelevant to clinical practice since they are often ideals of mental health rather than goals set in the context of an individual pathology. It is important, especially with adolescents, to distinguish between internal and external changes. In ideal cases, internal and external changes coincide. There are cases where external changes can occur without evident internal change (Eissler 1963). The case presented was one in which external changes were minimal despite significant internal changes. This is not unusual in the treatment of adolescents. The

translation of insight into action remains the responsibility of the adolescent. A major goal of treatment is self-analysis and all that self-analysis implies. With the capacity for self-analysis external changes can take place even after the end of treatment. In the case presented, important external changes occurred after termination of treatment.

NOTES

1. The idea for this paper arose at a postgraduate workshop on termination held at the Institute of Psycho-Analysis, London. My gratitude to Drs. Ilse Hellman, Moses Laufer, and Kerry Kelly Novick for their help.

2. I am indebted to Ilse Hellman, who alerted me to the finding that the killing of pets is a childhood feature in many adult killers.

3. See, for example, the work of Winnicott (1965) on the mother-infant unit, Mahler, Pine, and Bergman (1975) on the vicissitudes and stages of the separation-individuation process, and Kohut (1971) on the narcissistic disturbances.

4. See Milner (1950) and Menninger (1966) on the phenomenon of postanalytic cure.

REFERENCES

Adatto, C. P. (1958). Ego reintegration observed in analysis of late adolescents. *International Journal of Psycho-Analysis* 39: 172-177.

———(1974). Evolution of the transference in the psychoanalysis of an adolescent boy. In M. Harley, ed., *The Analyst and the Adolescent at Work*. New York: Quadrangle.

Aichorn, A. (1925). *Wayward Youth*. New York: Viking, 1935.

Balint, M. (1950). On the termination of analysis. *International Journal of Psycho-Analysis* 31: 196-199.

Balkoura, A. (1974). Panel report: the fate of the transference neurosis after analysis. *Journal of the American Psychoanalytic Association* 22: 895-903.

Bridger, H. (1950). Criteria for the termination of analysis. *International Journal of Psycho-Analysis* 31: 202-203.

Buxbaum, E. (1950). Technique of terminating analysis. *International Journal of Psycho-Analysis* 31: 184-190.

Eissler, K. R. (1958). Notes on problems of technique in the psychoanalytic treatment of adolescents. *Psychoanalytic Study of the Child* 13: 223.

————(1963). Notes on the psychoanalytic concept of cure. *Psychoanalytic Study of the Child* 18: 424-463.

Ferenczi, S. (1927). The problem of the termination of analysis. In *Final Contributions to Psycho-Analysis*. New York: Basic Books, 1955.

Firstein, S. K. (1969). Panel report: problems of termination in the analysis of adults. *Journal of the American Psychoanalytic Association* 17: 222-237.

————(1974). Termination of psychoanalysis of adults. *Journal of the American Psychoanalytic Association* 22: 873-894.

Freud, A. (1970). Problems of termination in child analysis. *Writings of Anna Freud* 7: 3-21. New York: International Universities Press.

Freud, S. (1917). Introductory lectures on psycho-analysis. *Standard Edition* 17: Part 3. London: Hogarth, 1963.

————(1937). Analysis terminable and interminable. *Standard Edition* 23: 209-253. London: Hogarth, 1964.

Geleerd, E. R. (1957). Some aspects of psychoanalytic technique in adolescence. *Psychoanalytic Study of the Child* 12: 263-283.

Gitelson, M. (1967). Analytic aphorisms. *Psychoanalytic Quarterly* 36: 260-270.

Glover, E. (1955). *The Technique of Psycho-Analysis*. New York: International Universities Press.

Harley, M. (1970). On some problems in technique in the analysis of early adolescents. *Psychoanalytic Study of the Child* 25: 99-121.

Hoffer, W. (1950). Three psychological criteria for the termination of treatment. *International Journal of Psycho-Analysis* 31: 194-195.

Hurn, A. T. (1971). Toward a paradigm of the terminal phase. *Journal of the American Psychoanalytic Association* 19: 332-348.

Khan, M. M. R. (1970). Towards an epistemology of the process of cure. In *The Privacy of the Self*. London: Hogarth, 1974.

Klein, M. (1950). On the criteria for the termination of an analysis. *International Journal of Psycho-Analysis* 31: 204.

Kohrman, R. (1969). Panel report: problems of termination in child analysis. *Journal of the American Psychoanalytic Association* 17: 191-205.

Kohut, H. (1971). *The Analysis of the Self*. New York: International Universities Press.

Landauer, E. (1970). Panel report: workshop on problems of technique in the analysis of adolescents. In Proceedings of the Fifth Annual Scientific Meeting of the Association for Child Psychoanalysis (mimeographed).

Laufer, M. (1974). The analysis of an adolescent at risk. M. Harley, ed., The Analyst and the Adolescent at Work. New York: Quadrangle.

Mahler, M. S., Pine, F., and Bergman, A. (1975). *The Psychological Birth of the Human Infant.* New York: Basic Books.

Menninger, K. A. (1966). Discussion. R. E. Litman, ed., *Psychoanalysis in the Americas.* New York: International Universities Press.

Milner, M. (1950). A note on the ending of an analysis. *International Journal of Psycho-Analysis* 31: 191-193.

Novick, J. (1970). The vicissitudes of the "working alliance" in the analysis of a latency girl. *Psychoanalytic Study of the Child* 25: 231-256.

Payne, S. (1950). Short communication on criteria for terminating analysis. *International Journal of Psycho-Analysis* 31: 205.

Pfeffer, A. Z. (1961). Follow-up study of a satisfactory analysis. *Journal of the American Psychoanalytic Association* 9: 698-718.

Rangell, L. (1966). An overview of the ending of an analysis. R. E. Litman, ed., *Psychoanalysis in the Americas.* New York: International Universities Press.

———(1975). Psychoanalysis and the process of change. *International Journal of Psycho-Analysis* 56: 87-98.

Reich, A. (1950). On the termination of analysis. *International Journal of Psycho-Analysis* 31: 179-183.

Rickman, J. (1950). On the criteria for the termination of the analysis. *International Journal of Psycho-Analysis* 31: 200-201.

Spiegel, L. A. (1951). A review of contributions to a psychoanalytic theory of adolescence. *Psychoanalytic Study of the Child* 6: 375-393.

Ticho, E. A. (1972). Termination of psychoanalysis. *Psychoanalytic Quarterly* 41: 315-333.

van Dam, A., Heinicke, C. M., and Shane, M. (1975). On termination in child analysis. *Psychoanalytic Study of the Child* 30: 443-474.

Winnicott, D. W. (1965). *The Maturational Process and the Facilitating Environment.* London: Hogarth.

———(1971). Contemporary concepts of adolescent development and their implications for higher education. In *Playing and Reality.* New York: Basic Books.

24] TREATMENT PERSPECTIVES ON ADOLESCENT RUNAWAYS

HELM STIERLIN

Adolescent runaways utilize a mode of separation which only an affluent, mobile, and noncohesive society offers. Effective treatment, therefore, would require substantial change in our society. But such societal changes are not at issue in this chapter. Rather, I want to focus on the runaway's family and what can be done with it.

As discussed elsewhere (Stierlin 1973a), runaways develop mainly in three major family scenarios, implying different patterns and types of runaways, different family dynamics, and different treatment approaches.

First are what I call "bound-up families." Here *centripetal* forces prevail: parents and adolescents cannot adequately separate and individuate according to the culture's timetable, unduly locking the adolescent into the "family ghetto." He may become bound either through excessive regressive gratification, or through mystification (i.e., is befuddled as to what he feels, needs, and wants), or through a deep and archaic loyalty which fosters massive breakaway guilt. Often these three modes of binding operate conjointly. And the more strongly they operate, the less likely will there be any running away. My studies showed that only two types of runaways emerge under similar circumstances: abortive and lonely schizoid runaways. Abortive runaways typically reclaim the parental orbit, usually within hours. They bounce away from, and back to, their families, as if held by a rubber leash. The very abortiveness of their runaway attempts attests their strong psychological ties to their families. Lonely schizoid runaways, on the other hand, often manage to get away from their families for longer periods. But, unlike most other runaways, they have no peers to run to as they are too scared or inept to sustain peer contacts. They roam on the fringes of the runaway culture, getting by on the spill-over from society's affluence, until they, too, return home or end up in penal or psychiatric institutions.

At the other pole, we find a family scenario dominated by *centrifugal* forces. Here parents, rather than delaying their adolescents' separations, push their precocious autonomy—often by insidiously rejecting and neglecting them. Instead of considering them to be assets they can exploit, these parents treat their children as nuisances and human surplus. Many of these adolescents—provided they are not damaged too badly—turn into "casual runaways." Unlike their lonely schizoid counterparts, these runaways have usually no difficulties in finding peers—and particularly sex partners—whom they can use (and also discard). These adolescents make up the rougher segments of the runaway culture, including its criminal fringe. Often they show little, if any, motivation to return to their parents. (It is estimated that 30 to 40 percent of long-term runaways never try to reunite with their parents, and are also not offered a reunion by the latter.)

Finally, there is a third family scenario in which centripetal and centrifugal binding and expelling dynamics blend. Here we find parents who entrust their adolescents (covertly) with missions to provide excitement, to act out the parents' disowned delinquent impulses, or to realize their grandiose ego-ideal. These adolescents are considered delegates of their parents (Stierlin 1972, 1973b, 1975, Stierlin and Ravenscroft 1972). In its original Latin meaning, the verb *delegare* means, first, to send out and, second, to entrust with a mission. Many a delegate's missions are incompatible with each other. For example, a boy might have to vicariously provide thrills—smoke pot and take part in sex orgies—and also realize the parents' virtuous ego-ideal—study for the ministry. Many a delegate is subject to intense loyalty conflicts as when, loyalty bound to one parent, he might have to destroy the other parent, a situation for which Hamlet provides the paradigm. This family scenario mostly produces crisis runaways—adolescents who typically run in response to complex and conflicting family pressures. To the extent that they remain delegated—are sent out yet held on the long leash of loyalty—they are likely to return home sooner or later, yet will run away again unless the family scenario changes or the crisis resolves.

Clearly, these differing family and runaway patterns demand different treatment strategies. However, before taking up these differences, let me briefly dwell on those aspects which they all have in common. These aspects interweave and relate to the central fact that by the time an adolescent can or does run away, his family system requires major alteration.

Such alteration implies that members have new options for careers and relationships outside the family. Particularly, an adolescent who reaches an age of twelve or thirteen can now opt to live without his parents, without school, and without the difficulties that go with both. For, provided there is spillover from society's affluence and a reasonably warm climate, it is unlikely he will physically perish. Middle-aged parents may also decide to break away from entrenched family relations or professional dead-ends, and to make new starts elsewhere. Side by side, and interweaving with the runaway culture of adolescence, there exists nowadays a similar culture of middle-aged parents. The therapist of adolescent runaways must therefore consider the centrifugal or runaway tendencies not only of these youngsters, but also of their parents.

Along with facilitating or requiring new starts outside the family orbit, change in the family system implies a rebalancing of emotional and geographic closeness and distance between the generations. We must keep in mind that achieving geographical distance—by running away—does not necessarily diminish emotional distance, as the contrary is often true.

Further, by the time adolescents can or do run away, the generations need to renegotiate their mutual rights and obligations. This process is not automatic, but requires active and clear communication, an accounting of merits, as described by I. Boszormenyi-Nagy and G. Spark (1973), and involves mourning and reconciliation by all members.

Finally, and interweaving with the above, the balance of power within the family system will shift. This change, too, has far reaching implications for treatment approaches. To understand what is involved, we must examine the differences in these three family and runaway scenarios.

Unbinding of Bound-up Families

In turning first to bound-up families, we find they present only marginal runaway problems, limited to those of abortive or of—relatively uncommon—lonely schizoid runaways. While such abortive or schizoid runaways may galvanize the whole family into seeking treatment, their individual vicissitudes are less important than the underlying familial pathology. I have elsewhere (Stierlin 1974) outlined the therapeutic principles involved in the unbinding of such bound-up families. Suffice it to say that here a prolonged and successful running away might indicate progress rather than reaction, as it attests a loosening of family ties.

On the Treatment of Delegated Runaways

Runaways who serve as their parents' delegates (Stierlin 1975) suffer from conflicts of missions and loyalties. To intervene constructively, we must take account of the whole family drama. For example, I was called by a mother whose thirteen-year-old daughter—I shall call her Mary—seemed ready to run away on a large scale. According to the mother, the girl was ever harder to control, had strayed away from home frequently, and had taken to marijuana and sex. Rather ominously, Mary also talked about running away for good. When I saw the parents with Mary, I found a precociously blossomed girl whose radiant vitality contrasted with the boredom and gloom which her mother—a pale, dried out, and bitter woman—presented. The mother's worried face lighted up, however, when she reported on Mary's alleged sexual exploits. It was then obvious how much Mary served as her mother's thrill-provider, yet it became equally evident that Mary had to live up to her mother's conventional, virtuous ego-ideal—that is, had to go to school and do well. Hence Mary's conflict of missions. As her thrill providing mission was more central to her mother than her student mission, it was no wonder that Mary's academic work lapsed. But besides such (and other) conflicts of missions, there were also conflicts of loyalties. Mary's father was an alcoholic, seemingly bent on destroying himself, and Mary, as her mother's ally, abetted his self-destruction. Yet as Mary also felt loyal to and protective of her father, she was intensely conflicted. It was thus only too understandable that she attempted to run away for good, and that she lashed out against her parents and the stress of family life. While she detailed her runaway plans during the joint meeting, she sounded cocky, defiant, and castigated her parents for having messed up her life. She finally announced that she would not attend further sessions.

This vignette brings into view major dynamics which must influence our treatment of such runaways and families. I consider central the dynamic importance of the parents' shame and guilt. Typically, Mary's delinquency and her—so far, mild—runaway ventures dramatically advertised her parents' failure as parents, as she delivered herself now as the living proof of their badness. Besides making them feel helpless and furious, she caused them excruciating humiliation. Yet, by so doing, she (almost) nipped in the bud any chances for successful treatment. For the parents, reeling under their shame and guilt, were now loathe to seek professional help as this, to them, further confirmed their failure as parents. Also, they were now almost bound to view me as an accusatory prosecutor rather than a potentially helpful agent. To be sure, to appease their guilt, they were ready to do penance. But this, of course, would not help Mary, as it further confirmed her power over her parents while also increasing her guilt over wielding such power.

Typically, runaway adolescents will, under such circumstances, do any of three things (or a combination of them) to appease their guilt. They can (1) ferociously blame and attack their parents and any psychiatrist they might choose, (2) try to do repair work by working harder at their missions, or, (3) punish themselves by making a mess of their lives. And the modern runaway scene, we well know, provides plenty of opportunities for the third option—as when girls, in passing their bodies around, can covet pregnancies or venereal diseases, or when runaways of both sexes manage to ruin themselves through drugs, malnutrition, or mere drifting. Fortunately, through all this, they may not only succeed in punishing themselves, but also make sure they are eventually retrieved home.

Faced with the above scenario, a family therapist confronts several immediate tasks. He must counteract the parents' expectations that he is out to blame them or put them to trial. He must convey to them that he wants to understand them, assist them, and be a fair mediator. He must then focus on how the runaway has strategic leverage to subject his parents to excruciating shame and guilt. In so doing, the therapist pursues a double purpose. He effectively reduces these parents' shame and guilt (Boszormenyi-Nagy and Spark 1973). This, in turn, enables them to look less defensively and more objectively at their real contributions to their adolescent's runaway problem, revealing how they exploit him as their delegate. This, then, can foster a process of assessing and redistributing disowned problems and obligations within the whole family. In Mary's family, for example, the mother, rather than recruiting Mary as her thrill-providing delegate and ally, would eventually have had to cope with her own depression, emptiness, and deadlocked marriage.

Treatment Problems Posed by Wayward Expellees

A major group of runaways—causal runaways—are found to spring primarily from parental rejection and neglect. They can be considered wayward expellees, suggesting expulsion as well as escape. Such wayward expellees divide into two groups. One group comprises drifting "street youngsters" (Miller 1974). They have few marketable skills and have experienced so much failure they are benumbed, even afraid to aspire. Like the typical skid row person, the issue is just getting through the day. Often children of blue collar parents, they are frequently from broken homes. The other group, by contrast, appears more activist. The brutish, callous youngsters of the film *A Clockwork Orange* seem typical. Like the passive drifters, they feel rejected by their families and society; but, unlike them, they lash out against their real or seeming rejectors with retaliatory sadistic fury. (The louts in the film subjected a villa named "home" to a sadistic rampage, clearly treating its owners as standins for their own expelling parents.)

Whether such runaways turn into skid row drifters or destructive tough guys, they pose formidable treatment problems. Ordinarily, it makes little sense to try to reunite them with their families. Their family experience has been simply too traumatic and chaotic, and neither parent nor runaways seem able or willing to seek and maintain that minimal investment in and good will toward each other that successful family therapy demands.

Essentially, three treatment issues appear. First, an instant rescue operation is often needed. We must find for these expellees some sort of haven that provides shelter, protection, and a base for new starts. Runaway houses, foster homes, residential treatment centers, and—if they are run humanely—detention homes can fulfill this purpose.

Second, on a long-term basis, we must offer opportunities for reparative growth and for the experience of those caring, nonexploitative relationships they failed to obtain at home. This, then, allows the development of capacities for concern, genuine guilt, and object love. But this task will most likely overtax even the most dedicated professionals. For they now come into the firing line of all the distrust, rage, and retaliatory fury engendered by what these youngsters have experienced at the hands of their own parents. Rather than receiving from them (the parents) what should have been their birthright—a sense of being important, and an attentive concern for their needs, rights, and well-being—they were found to be negligible surplus, often not even worth exploiting. Here the mental health professional can empathize with many school teachers, correction officials, and probation officers, who are also called upon to absorb the sequelae of earlier rejection and neglect.

There is—and this brings me to my third point—no easy answer to this dilemma. The focus, though, must be on prevention—the improvement of the fabric and quality of family life in our society. However, I for one see ominous trends. In a recent feature article, "The Child's World," we read, for example, that "many fathers and mothers today see themselves more as individuals and less as just parents." The same article alerts us to the fact that "the growing number of divorces is now accompanied by a new phenomenon: the unwillingness of either parent to take custody of the child. All this suggests that the United States is beginning to be less child centered than it used to be" *(Time* 1973). To me this suggests primarily that children are more easily neglected and abandoned, that hordes of wayward expellees are therefore likely to grow, and that, sooner or later, society will have to pay a terrible price.

Some General Perspectives on the Treatment of Runaways

The following treatment perspectives do not apply to runaways and their families only, since they bear on a wide range of separation problems—be they runaways or not. However, when adolescents run away, they sharpen the issues under discussion.

THE NEED FOR MULTI-GENERATIONAL FAIRNESS AND EMPATHY

Running away, more than other adolescent problems, can split a therapist's empathy along generational lines. If he is himself middle-aged, he can easily identify with the abandoned and slighted parents (the more so when he struggles with runaway adolescents of his own). In this case, he will underestimate, and underempathize with, the runaway's real difficulties and grievances. The opposite holds true for those younger therapists whose age and experience move them closer to their adolescent patients. Many of these therapists serve with runaway houses, community mental health centers, listening posts, and the like: places where they confront many a runaway's acute plight and distress, and also might give undue credence to stories of cruelly impervious, traumatizing, and expelling parents. Rather than working toward a reconciliation with these runaways' parents, they then tend to shelter them from the latter's supposedly destructive reach.

THE IMPORTANCE OF THE THIRD PARTY MEDIATOR

Spiegel (1971), among others, has stressed the role of the third-party mediator in situations where communication bogs down and the parties stalemate in frustration and mutual blame. Runaways and their parents often desperately need such mediators. The available mediators are frequently not psychiatrists but social workers, teachers, clergymen, various types of counselors, and police officers. Yet I believe that psychiatrists can help here by strengthening the mediating roles and skills of these groups of professionals. Two things seem crucial: first, that the mediator empathize fairly with both opposing parties and, second, that he actively structure the interpersonal field so as to allow the parties to communicate from positions of articulate separateness.

BRIDGING THE EXPERIENCE GAP

To have multigenerational empathy, the mediator must grasp the different levels of experience and, hence, different perceptions of reality which the opposing generations present. He must constantly remind himself that contemporary parent and offspring generations often live in different experiential worlds. The new affluence and permissiveness combined with the threatening prospects of nuclear holocaust, overpopulation, global scarcities, and environmental devastation create experience gaps often so deep they tax to the utmost the mediator's empathy and capacity to be fair and just.

GAIN OF CONTROL
THROUGH ACCEPTANCE OF WEAKNESS

By running away, we found, an adolescent often delivers the decisive proof that his parents, contrary to what they might think, are really powerless to control him. Hence, their frequent experience of excruciating shame and rage. Such sense of powerlessness in parents then has its (mild) counterpart in that of the psychiatrist who wants the runaway to show up for family sessions, while the latter, true to his status as runaway, does not oblige. Yet such a blow to the parents' and the therapist's sense of power can also, paradoxically, usher in a more realistic and effective use of parental power. It is a common observation that parents become more effective as parents the very moment they can face up to—and admit to their children—their weakness, helplessness, or mistakes. For such admission of weakness, far from definitively alienating the adolescent, ordinarily makes the parent more realistically appraise and utilize his remaining (and increasing) leverage over the child. As a result, he may, for example, plan and execute a step-by-step strategy for dealing with the child's breaking of curfew. In so doing, he will very likely realize that his main enforcement problem lies not with the child but with his spouse who was, or still is, using the child as delegate and ally. This shift from an intergenerational to an intermarital problem focus will eventually further decrease the adolescent's reasons for, and rewards from, running away.

Conclusions

Runaways generally operate under the assumption that one can solve problems by avoiding difficult situations. But the effects of guilt and shame prove this assumption is largely wrong, at least as far as crisis runaways are concerned. For them, geographical distance does not increase emotional distance. Rather, a more workable balance of closeness and distance hinges on how the parties achieve positions of articulate separateness and, hence, create psychological boundaries through an ongoing dialogue. The therapist must foster this dialogue.

An adolescent's sudden running away signals, almost always, a severe family crisis. This crisis can either resolve itself in a tragic yet familiar alienation, or it can trigger positive reconciliation within the family. For mental health professionals this often means they have the opportunity to help avert life-long estrangements between family members. Here even a brief intervention can be decisive.

REFERENCES

Boszormenyi-Nagy, I., and Spark, G. (1973). *Invisible Loyalties.* New York: Hoeber and Harper.

Miller, H. (1974). *The Street People of Berkeley.* Forthcoming monograph.

Spiegel, J. (1971). *Transactions. The Interplay Between Individual, Family, and Society.* New York: Jason Aronson.

Stierlin, H. (1972). Family dynamics and separation patterns of potential schizophrenics. D. Rubinstein and Y. O. Alanen, eds., *Psychotherapy of Schizophrenia. Proceedings of the IVth International Symposium on Psychotherapy of Schizophrenia.* Amsterdam: Excerpta Medica.

———(1973a). A family perspective on adolescent runaways. *Archives of General Psychiatry* 29: 56-62.

———(1973b). Interpersonal aspects of internalizations. *International Journal of Psycho-Analysis* 54: 203-213.

———(1974). An introduction to family therapy. Unpublished manuscript.

———(1975). The adolescent as delegate of his parents. *This Annual* 4: 72-83.

———, and Ravenscroft, Jr., K. (1972). Varieties of adolescent 'separation conflicts.' *British Journal of Medical Psychology* 45: 299-313.

Time Magazine (1973). "The Child's World/Christmas 1973." December 24, 1973: 60-67.

JARL E. DYRUD

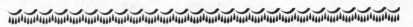

An observation we all have made is that case material dictates to a considerable extent the aspect of theory we find congenial to it. There is always therapist bias in what we select to pay attention to, but in psychoanalytically oriented psychotherapy we hope there is always, predominantly, the bias of the material itself (Maskin 1960).

In this instance to be recounted, I found myself fascinated with the specificity of words lost to consciousness, words that needed to be given to the boy by his parents, or more accurately, by the analyst as intermediary, so that he could emerge from the crippling restrictions of his father's fantasy. As many will no doubt recognize, this is the rhetoric of Jacques Lacan. I must admit, to read Lacan (1966) is an exercise in futility if one seeks the content of his thought, either in the original or in translation (Wilden 1968). It eludes us until we recognize that the form is there, namely his concept of the unconscious (Mannoni 1970, 1972, Bär 1974).

Some years ago I saw a young man freshly discharged from the army after serving only six weeks, the last month of which had been spent in the hospital. He had completed law school, married, and was drafted within a month or two prior to his illness. Separated from his wife, he quickly developed an acute paranoid reaction focused around pain in his testicles. He was confused, assaultive, and convinced that separation from his wife would destroy him. Following discharge from the hospital he appeared still pretty shaken and somewhat suspicious, but the pain was gone following reunion with his wife. Review of his hospital record confirmed my impression that his madness, confused or not, had been powerful enough to spring him out of the grasp of the United States Army.

As our work progressed it became apparent that he had reason enough to be determined to control his own destiny. His father was a crippled—he had only one leg—immigrant shoemaker who never owned his own shop, never learned English very well, and went through long periods of unemployment. His mother was a strong, beautiful woman who worked and was unfaithful to her husband as opportunity permitted. He grew up with the conviction that a man must never be as helpless as he knew his father to be. His parents both supported him in his ambition to be an adequate male, but there was no adult role model available. His mother made it very clear that what she liked about him did not resemble his father. He grew up on the streets of Chicago; intelligent, cynical, and able to dominate his group with his fists. He had friends, but they were admirers rather than confidants. He went to college and law school full-time, and worked to support himself. The girls he slept with were objects of contempt, except for an occasional one whom he saw as a threat to lure him into marriage and interrupt his education. Leaving home for the first time after graduation from law school, he went to another city to work. After a whirlwind courtship he married a very pretty, serenely quiet girl who had just completed nurses' training. They rented an apartment and had begun to decorate it when he was drafted.

In four years of psychotherapy, I developed from a once-a-week reality oriented counselor to a three-times-a-week dynamically oriented psychotherapist. I saw my patient relax into being much more human both at home and on the job. As I look back over my notes I am impressed, however, that friendships did not seem to emerge either at work on in the neighborhood. His wife was his friend, and except for the relationship with me he seemed to need no one else. Near the end of our first year of work their only child was born, a boy. He insisted that his wife stop work when she became pregnant and staunchly opposed her going back to work for the next fifteen years. He explained this to me by saying that he knew what it was like to have a working mother. At one point, several years later, I noted that he still referred to his son as the "baby," as if the boy had not yet acceded to the role of a member of that household. When his son was three, he commented that they had taken the boy to the hospital to be operated on for a painful, constricted foreskin. Otherwise, in the three years of his life I spent listening to his father, there were no notes to suggest that the boy had emerged as a person.

Ten years after we had terminated, the father called me in great distress to say that his son had gone into a panic over beginning school in the fall of his freshman year of high school. He would not go to school without carrying a hunting knife to protect himself from the other boys, whom he feared. Through the eighth grade his school had been close to home, high school was a bus trip away. In our brief review of the history, he had been a model boy, courteous, helpful around the house, had a number of neighborhood acquaintances, but no really close friends. Although he spent a good bit of time around the house, he did not have any hobbies. No incident that they knew of could have precipitated this fright.

When I saw David, his panic and confusion were such that I decided to hospitalize him at once. During the acute phase he was confused and physically assaultive to ward personnel. Treated with chlorpromazine and a supportive environment, he slowly reconstituted in a matter of several months, then stayed on as a night patient throughout the school year. Curiously enough, during his psychotic phase he was reported as saying that his father was a cripple, his mother an unfaithful woman, and he was in danger of physical harm. While he was hospitalized, his therapist was the resident on the service, but he was particularly insistent on getting back to see me.

When David came to see me it seemed as if the chlorpromazine had removed all the positive signs of schizophrenia, but had left the negative signs. In a flat and apathetic fashion he explained that he needed to see me because I knew his father and thus could help him. This theme was worked and reworked as we picked up clues that his mother did not want him to be like his father, but did not offer any alternatives other than the notion of being warm and responsive. Both parents had emphasized to him that going to high school was a big step. He would now have to be more on his own, and take care of himself in an external world that they perceived as hostile.

In the nine months we spent together, particularly after we had phased out the medication, we had an increasingly lively time reviewing his past life. We dealt with his memories of "the trouble with his penis," separating the real from the imaginary, his mother and father's words from his own, including separating mother's anxiety over his going to high school from his own. What had been a worried, morbid, fantasy ridden childhood became something much clearer and at times even amusing to him. It was very clear that I was a representative, a spokesman for his father, as well as a mediator with the family. He knew I had seen his parents the year he was away and that I had encouraged his mother to go back to work. The work question had realistically come up in regard to their medical bills, but it had led into discussion of their life style, which they shared with David on visits. His parents had learned to talk to each other and to David the year he was away. Our work was terminated by David's decision to go to a boarding school for his last two years of high school. Since then I have seen or heard from him occasionally as he went to college, graduated, got a job, married, and now has a young son.

This rambling case account is bound to be somewhat unsatisfactory, since it includes too much as well as too little. The arrows of significance seem to point in a variety of directions. My reason for trying to make such a presentation is that I think this is what most of our cases are really like, and the vignette streamlined to support only one hypothesis so often fails to come alive for the reader unless he has an identical bias.

From the biological-genetic point of view we have the father-son incidence of acute psychosis; convincing in the son's case, less so in the father's. As far as could be determined, there is no other record of psychosis in the family. Both father and son are mesomorphic, well-coordinated, with no reported problems around birth or the neonatal period. Thus, I would consider the genetic contribution minor.

From the family dynamics point of view, there is considerable evidence of a boundary problem between mother and son, as well as between father and mother. The father's dependency on his wife as a substitute for his mother was not challenged in treatment. In that sense we might say only his induction into the army challenged that symptom with rather spectacular results.

It is well within the realm of possibility that the father's projective identification of his son with his own unacceptable traits could have played a part in symptom development in David. The point I hope to make is that we need not and do not as a rule treat etiology. The way you get into a situation may have very little to do with how best to get out of it.

My treatment of the father was in large part ego-supportive, including using the therapist as a model of a less punitive superego. I do not mean to denigrate this sharing of benevolent affects, but I do think there was a lack of work in the imaginary realm that could have enlivened the dream content of ruling fantasies of earlier life that still restricted his autonomy.

Outstanding in the work with David was his need to talk out past experiences. Words not said, centering around the operation on his penis, often became the subject of our interaction. Mother didn't speak much; she simply took excellent care of him, anticipating his every wish. Father simply laid down requirements: no negotiation, no dialogue. As I reread my fragmentary notes on the two cases I was struck by the differences in technique, dictated, I think, more by demand characteristics of the two situations than by any a priori reasoning.

The traumatizing factor in a neurosis is not the real event itself, but what was said or left unsaid about it by the people concerned. In this case, it was mostly words unsaid between mother and son, and father and son, that needed reviving in fantasy, completing the frustrated act. This notion of the frustrated act was described by Faris (1940), who defined the action as follows:

1. Immediate acts—drop a pin and pick it up.
2. The delayed act—one which calls for an intermediate step that requires some adjustment, foresight, or reasoning.
3. The frustrated act—one which begins, but fails to achieve closure. A beginning, a middle, but no end. This leads to the retrospective act which means running the frustrated act over and over again in fantasy, in all likelihood experiencing the bafflement and pain a thousand times instead of once.

I quote further:

The "mechanism" of the retrospect lies importantly in the fact that we take the role of the other and it is by taking the role of the other and only by this method that a conception of the self is formed and the attitudes of personality and character are organized.

For the self, as experienced, is defined by the actions of responses of others, although the actions and reactions, the responses and gestures of the others are not sufficient in and of themselves to produce the result. In order that the actions and responses of others shall affect the personality it is necessary for the self to assume them on his part. The function of the retrospective act lies just here. It is in the rehearsal of the past event that one takes the attitude of another, because he is repeating what the other has said. This is seemingly the reason the infant in the prelinguistic stage does not feel resentment or hold a grudge. Because there is no language, the past cannot be recalled in symbolic ways. When, however, one can talk to one's self and answer his own talk, he necessarily takes the role of the other for no one can talk without being talked to beforehand. The mother tongue is acquired from the mother and all language is a social product. It is only after some one has spoken to me that I can speak to myself. And when I have learned to speak to myself, I have a self and not till then. A self is best defined as a subject which is its own object. One takes an attitude toward one's self. The "me" appears in experience. The very formation of the self is dependent on the retrospective act.

The child who suffers a feeling of isolation may be hard to reach, but he will usually respond with eagerness to the well-considered approach. If the isolation is overcome, the retrospective act is not prevented, for retrospection is universal and normal. But when wrongs or hurts or failures or frustrations are talked over instead of brooded over, a great gain is had.

Faris also shows some remarkable similarities in his thinking to that of Lacan (1966) in his *Discours de Rome*. Lacan's mirror stage corresponds well to the concept of the developing self, and the healing dialogue Faris describes is not far removed from Lacan's examples of the dialectic of analysis where the phenomenon to be investigated is the envelope of collective utterances in which the child is caught up. Faris sees fantasy in treatment not as the image or trace of an experience lived through, but as words lost that must be regained.

Conclusions

Several recent studies have shown the amazing fidelity with which symptoms are passed on from generation to generation with some subtle changes occurring in each generation, until the symptoms finally disappear (Fisher and Mendell 1956). This clinical material is suggestive of such a possibility. From Lacan's point of view the oedipus complex is the expression of an unsolved problem of the parents in regard to their own parents, of which the child, by his symptom, has become the representative signifier. He sees the analyst as standing at the center of the words brought to him by the child and his family attempting to recover words lost that needed to be said not in order to relive experiences lived through, but to settle them so as to achieve a symbolic order in which each person's truth is distilled out of the family drama. In this role Lacan brings us back to Freud (1905) and Klein (1932), for whom the most introspective work is at the same time outside in the structure of the language.

REFERENCES

Bär, E. S. (1974). Understanding Lacan. L. Goldberger and V. H. Rosen, eds., *Psychoanalysis and Contemporary Science*. New York: International Universities Press.

Faris, E. (1940). The retrospective act. *Journal of Educational Sociology* 14: 79-91.

Fisher, S., and Mendell, F. (1956). The communication of neurotic patterns over two and three generations. *Psychiatry* 19: 41-46.

Freud, S. (1905). Jokes and their relation to the unconscious. *Standard Edition* 8: 9-236. London: Hogarth, 1960.

Klein, M. (1932). *The Psycho-Analysis of Children*. London: Hogarth.

Lacan, J. (1966). *Ecrits*. Paris: Editions du Seuil.

Mannoni, M. (1970). *The Child, His "Illness," and the Others*. New York: Pantheon.

——— (1972). *The Backward Child and His Mother*. New York: Pantheon.

Maskin, M. (1960). Adaptations of psychoanalytic technique to specific disorders. J. Masserman, ed., *Psychoanalysis and Human Values*. New York: Grune and Stratton.

Mendell, D., and Fisher, S. (1956). An approach to neurotic behavior in terms of a three generation family model. *Journal of Nervous and Mental Diseases* 123: 171-180.

Wilden, A. (1968). *The Language of the Self*. Baltimore: Johns Hopkins Press.

FRANK T. RAFFERTY AND JOHN C. STEFFEK

It is our intention to share some ideas evolved out of clinical experience in a
lower socioeconomic ghetto of Chicago, where we functioned in a
catchment-area community mental health team. The ideas are twofold.
First, we suggest there is a population of adolescent nonpatients who
neither ask for treatment nor are referred by parents, schools, or other
agencies, but who are so seriously deficient in ego skills as to be potential
school failures or criminals, mentally ill or socially inept at a later time
when social demands become more exacting. Second, there must be a
technique to engage these youngsters in a group process that will provide a
corrective, ego-developing experience, since one-to-one intervention seems
impractical.

The Population

Our subjects live in the Near West Side of Chicago, an area that was
ravaged, in 1968, by fire and racial turmoil. The housing is now almost all
public and about half of that is of the hated, high-rise variety characterized
by long corridors, stairwells, and sometimes working elevators where street
gangs and less well-organized groups of two and three molest weaker
individuals. The dominant themes of the area are economic survival, fear of
personal injury, religious moralism, and take your pleasure when, where,
and how it might appear, since it won't last or return.

Many of the children are raised in an atmosphere of fear for individual
safety. Spatial, social, and intellectual explorations are restricted. As small
children, their play area is limited to the immediate vicinity of the mother
since to go further exposes them to danger. Even by adolescence, many of

the youth have not been out of the tightly circumscribed neighborhood. Most of these youngsters attend a vocational high school across the street from the mental health facility. The average reading score is in the 7.5 percentile of national averages, the lowest score in a school district with notoriously low marks. A considerable portion of the neighborhood is channeled into the police, juvenile justice, and correctional system. Few of these children are referred to the mental health center. In other settings, children and adolescents are brought by parents or referred by schools, but both parents and schools in this area are overwhelmed, burdened, and fatigued with the magnitude of problems. Symptoms of distress are so prevalent that only major disorganization and threat elicit response. Whether it can be considered tolerance of pathology, absence of social demand, or sheer depressive defensiveness and loss of hope in the face of overwhelming threat, the fact remains that the children and adolescents are not referred, and are not identified by themselves or others as patients. The important facet of this absence of patient status is the concomittant absence of motivation to seek therapeutic alliance, to be prepared to observe and reveal self, and to tolerate threats of group process for the hope of relieving suffering.

Our experience with this population extends over six years. In 1968, we offered afternoon use of our gym to four or five local youths known to be on probation, and suggested they invite their friends. Within a few months there were regularly fifty to seventy boys on the rolls and the number had to be restricted to fifty. Subsequently, without any additional advertisement or recruitment, a similar number has shown up each September.

Basketball has always been the major attraction with snacks a distant second. It is difficult to convey the idealized, magnetic, romantic, starstruck attraction of basketball. It is the fantasied and real route to superstar success, wealth, college scholarships, positive self-image, personal success, social entry to any group, and protection from local gangs. It is also the one role which can compete with the idealized view of the pimp, his girls, and the Eldorado. If the community divides along these lines into two cultural ideals, then we obviously appeal to the basketball faction, though frequently a youngster will proclaim that he is ready to stop trying and plans to go out and get himself some girls.

Since only minimum social data have been collected, it is not known how this faction compares with boys who do not come in. The thirty-one boys who remained in the program throughout this year range in age from fourteen to seventeen. Sixteen of them live with both parents, nine with mothers only, and six have other family patterns. Twelve have been arrested at least once. While at our facilities, the youths exhibit little obvious classical psychotic or neurotic symptomatic behavior. Nor do we observe the more florid, dramatic, aggressive, explosive, uncontrolled ego deficits so vividly described by Redl (1957). Rather, they present a picture of low self-esteem and lack of self-awareness. They mistrust themselves, their peers, and adults; information is distorted by this mistrust. They identify no problems within themselves, and view their peers as experiencing the same life space and events. They appear to trust only immediate gratification and manifest little frustration tolerance. Their reaction to frustration is more likely to be withdrawal than explosive violence, while they do not anticipate any gratification in new equipment or activities. The pressure for immediate gratification is served by an opportunistic, manipulative style of relating, and a continual sensitivity to issues of dominance and control, but with a more passive tone.

The Program

Although basketball and snacks have remained most important at various times, efforts have been made to offer counseling and tutoring. These attempts, however, are met with indifference. Racial sensitivities, the Black Power movement, reciprocal black-white fear and mistrust, and a dearth of black professionals have been influential in the program goals and management. The recent major goal has been to move a population of black males, age twelve to seventeen, from an outreach recreation program using basketball and snacks as immediate, familiar gratifications into an ego-development program using group process—while being acutely aware that these young men have not applied or been referred for treatment.

Theoretical considerations demand that we locate our efforts with respect to the two major traditions of group theory and practice. Yalom (1970) compared the T-group and therapy group on a variety of parameters. Since our effort is focused on a population not classically defined as patients nor motivated toward personal psychological growth, it would be helpful to review group methodologies within our context.

Group therapy arose as a form of treatment of individuals afflicted with some disease, disorder, or disability. Administered by a person in an authoritarian role with an aura of healing power, it is aimed, minimally, at relieving the suffering; maximally, at modifying the causes. Attendance is nominally voluntary, although frequently individuals attend under the coercive influence of their parents, the institution in which they live, or their own suffering. By contrast, the T-group (as also, sensitivity training, encounter groups, etc.) was clearly derived from an educational tradition. The group participants are voluntary, generally well-functioning members who expect to gain knowledge and skills that increase personal and occupational effectiveness. The group leader presents himself as a teacher of theory and skills which the members are capable of acquiring with facility equal to the leader.

The basic task of the T-group, the acquisition of interpersonal competence, requires a degree of interpersonal skill most psychiatric patients do not possess. Ordinarily, T-group trainers expect their members to be able to send and receive information about themselves and others with a minimum of distortion. This requires a relatively high degree of self-awareness, self-acceptance, and adequate personal security to seek change. Members must be able to trust enough in others to believe the group will fundamentally constructive and to be willing to consider new ideas, attitudes, and behavior.

By contrast, these attributes are sorely lacking in the patient who has a relatively low level of self-esteem and self-awareness. Their initial attitude can be an expected mistrust of others and defensiveness of their belief system for the sake of survival. The survival oriented patient does not give or accept accurate feedback and usually seeks experiences to confirm his belief system. Since he experiences feelings of suspicion, fear, distrust, anger, and self-hate, he fears any directions that are open, honest, and trusting.

To repeat, our target population does not have the voluntary or even coerced motivation of either of the discussed groups, but prominent ego characteristics are similar to that of the patient. Perhaps, based on their lack of motivation and the probability of therapeutic failure, one might argue that these adolescents should not be treated. For years we have struggled with a type of reverse racism which proclaims these youth are not sick, but are well adapted to their culture and community and that we have no right to force an alien culture on them. We agree that these young men are not sick, and are adapted to their culture, but we not feel experienced enough to deny their circumstance as an authentic Black culture. Rather, it is a situation characterized by fear of failure and personal injury. The strengths of the Black family—their warmth and interpersonal relatedness, religious faith, verbal and artistic skills, and humor—modify but do not eradicate this fear and mistrust. Alternative modes of coping with the pervasive characteristics should be developed in order that these adolescents become able to cope effectively with a broader culture and society.

After several years of offering simple recreational activities, we decided to give our youth an alternative opportunity to expand their coping methods knowing full well that their fear of failure and insecurity might prohibit effective utilization of such opportunities.

From previous experience, we were confident of attracting the usual collection of fifty young men enticed into the gym and cottages of what used to be a residential treatment facility by the opportunity to play basketball and have an aftergame snack. This provides access to them from two-thirty to four-thirty P.M. each week day through the school year. The pool table and ping-pong table have always provided overflow activities for those of lesser status, usually the younger. Spontaneous, unguided interaction of previous years never led to anything that could be considered goal directed groups, and nothing ever happened that could remotely be called group therapy. We knew that they came faithfully, returned the next year, seemed to develop personal attractions to the group leaders, and on occasion would individually ask for some tangible help. From this basic level of gratification we decided to move into an imposed structure of guided group interaction around activities and goals with leaders to provide not only the structured pressure to achieve a goal, but to explore the decision making process along the way, and to serve as transparent role models.

The use of white professionals as group leaders was negated by the time involved, the unwillingness of most to accept a position in this setting, and by the anticipated rejection by the adolescents because of the implication of mental illness. The use of black professionals was rejected for the same reasons, especially that of time; there is a need to conserve the time of these unique resources.

Three black, nonprofessional men in their early twenties were chosen to be group leaders with the expectation of on-job training to function as models and educators in the T-group sense. One of these was on the staff and had had program responsibility for several years, another was a four year participant in the program, the third was a college student from a nearby community college employed on a part-time basis. A fourth informal, but important, contributor to the program has been the black security officer stationed in the building who has long term experience with this program and with church organizations. The immediate supervisor was an experienced black social worker. Two child and adolescent psychiatrists, both white, were consultants.

The essential premise of the program was that optimal growth and development is facilitated by participation in multiple group experiences.

The characteristics of these groups included engagement in activities covering a moderate range of interests and tasks, the provision of opportunities for participants to be both a leader and a subordinate in an appropriate dominance structure, and the opportunity to develop and experience an array of social participation skills such as the ability to interact, share, trust, and depend on others in the service of goal achievement. Our evaluation of these adolescents was that they had missed enough similar opportunities to produce a relative lack of ego skills. The program was designed to remedy the deficiency of experiences which are ordinarily available during preschool and latency years.

Our procedure was to offer enough structure to support peer interaction, to generate some anxiety, but not to force individuals to flee. The gratification of basketball and snacks was augmented with the suggestion that if they organized, determined their interests, and developed subgroups to plan activities, a rich array of opportunities would unfold. It was expected that a satisfying selection of other activities in addition to basketball could be generated at our facility, but also that an organized group could well approach the local business and academic communities for as yet unimagined benefits. The focal message was that individual gratification and self-fulfillment were available through participation in and development of a cohesive group effort. Since efforts to achieve group cohesion would be attended by fear, resistance, and repetition of habitual patterns of interaction, the opportunity to deal with these in a safe setting, at one's own pace, with adult support, would constitute the core therapeutic experience.

In the choice of leadership style we chose low authority, absence of the healer mystique, personal transparency, peer modeling, and the participatory educational approach. We focused on real tasks, accomplishments, working in the group, trusting others, and honesty about self. There was to be one weekly session of at least an hour, initially called a "rap" group. The population was divided into three loosely bound, age-related groups, providing the structure sharper definition and offering the opportunity to introduce more definitive group therapy as young men entered into some degree of alliance with the staff.

The Process

It was expected that difficult problems would occur in the transition from a nonchallenging recreational program focused on the beloved basketball game to a task oriented self-development group. Clearly over the years, the gate keepers of the institution had made entree extraordinarily easy. Beyond the time frame, and some minimal behavioral controls, the community youth had obviously established a tradition of territorial control over the basketball court. Now the institutional gate keepers were changing their roles from that of playmates and low profile symbols of institutional values to clearly designated group leaders with the power to demand, if ever so gently, different behaviors and goals with the intention of converting the aggregate of fifty adolescents into cohesive groups with clearly structured tasks to accomplish. Based on our prediction that these adolescents would resist increased performance demands of identifiable authority and program structure, the decision was made to introduce new expectations gradually, after the youth were involved in basketball, rather than to erect a new institutional gate. The purpose was to achieve a delicate balance of gratification and frustration. The tenuous nature of such a balance cannot be underscored enough. We believe that our concern was justified by the fact that over the first few weeks the attendance gradually dropped from fifty to thirty.

Initially, there were several groups. The older, larger group contained returnees from previous years who had some tradition about ownership of the basketball court, and who strongly exerted their dominance over the younger by excluding them from the game and from court time. Although attendance held up for the first few weeks, their major attitude was one of passive compliance to imposed structure and resistance to involvement in the suggested task that "Project Opportunity" could be something greater and better if the adolescents would start to talk about it, to reveal and express their interests, and to develop initiative toward a new goal of self-development and individual fulfillment. The group leaders tried to balance our power maneuver of gently but firmly imposing the new task, with the counter position of being nonauthoritative group leaders who try to generate self-expression and self-direction. Not only was there passive resistance to change, to structured meetings, to discussion of possible activities and plans, but there was an inability to anticipate any gratification in future activities. The immediate gratification of basketball overwhelmed any possible lure of other activities. In addition, what appeared to be sociability, friendliness, and warmth of individual interactions turned out to be a superficial mechanism of social distancing, defending against an inability to trust others in any kind of real interdependency. This was explicitly revealed in the passive resistance and refusal to participate especially prevalent in the older group who came alive only on the basketball court.

An alumnus of a number of years in the program, who had worked as a leader before and who was expected to be a valued transition leader in the new program, finally said, "I think that they are just waiting it out, hoping it will go away." As it became apparent that "it" was not going away, the older ones drifted away silently one by one with no major effort to rebel, fight, defend, or discuss their position. Subsequently, this same leader acknowledged his lack of commitment to the new program and asked to be relieved of his responsibility. This young adult continued, however, to come daily as a member, although his participation remained unfortunately restricted to playing basketball.

The backbone of the program, the discussion sessions were initially characterized by silence, chaos, and erratic attendance. Interactions between group members took the form of either nonverbal cueing or flurries and rounds of signifying. Signifying is a rather special form of interaction among black adolescents that demonstrates a number of potential ego skills and strengths, but also major weaknesses. A definition is beyond standard English usage. The following example is typical even though slightly laundered:

> In a group meeting when one of the members was apparently breaking ranks and starting to participate in a discussion of the significance of playing basketball, one of the other members proclaimed loudly, "Hey, bird, what are you doing talking? The only thing you know how to do is suck my dick!"
>
> The quick reply was was, "Well, I knew enough to screw your sister ten times last night." This was followed by a flurry of similar exchanges by a number of persons around the room.

The effectiveness of signifying as a prohibitor of group discussion is evident. It has no group task orientation, but simply maintains personal contact and status. The adaptive value of signifying is as a sociable interchange, expressing hostility that is not responded to except by a similar kind of dampened symbolic retort. Signifying serves to recognize and validate the presence and importance of others, but still provides distancing against intimacy or interdependency. Use of signifying is not limited to the program and groups. It is the primary form of peer interaction wherever the boys are, and serves as an exchange of aggressive competitiveness that, fortunately for these youngsters, seems to replace fighting.

Nonattendance, silence, disruptive behavior, and signifying were clearly challenges to the dominance of the leader, and, therefore, to the structure and purposes of the program. This then represents the familiar dilemma in leadership style. If the leader forcefully set limits, quashed the challenges, and insisted on moving toward the designated task, he risked playing out the anticipated transferred role of authoritarian teacher or parent and further risked generating fantasies of omnipotent leadership. On the other hand, failure to structure and to exert dominance would maintain the chaos or allow the process to settle back into the nondemand, nondeveloping, recreational status quo. The leaders would walk this tightrope of leadership style only if they could couple their limit setting with the promise and hope of real need gratification.

This in turn presented another problem choice for the leaders. Presumably, ego developing activity was to confront the boys with a potential gratification if they would tolerate the anxiety of defining their own interests and needs, planning group action, and initiating their own role and leadership activities. We were surprised by their apparent inability to conjure or anticipate activities, or to hold the fantasied gratification in mind long enough to develop and carry out plans. Leaders were tempted to infantilize, patronize, and suggest activities and procedures and, therefore, reinforce the group's dependency, stifle any budding autonomy, and inhibit any leadership initiatives. Again and again the leader had to resist this temptation and support and trust the group process to define tasks, roles, leaders, and develop trust, interdependency, and eventual cohesion. The following vignette highlights various aspects of the group process:

At one point a group was able to focus on the deficiencies of the program and of the group leader. The leader was able, with support from his consultant, to withstand the assaults of various members and to encourage open communication. One youth finally said, "You don't do shit. You just sit around and wait for us to do all the work." Several of the more assertive members of that group then went to the project director and asked to be transferred to another group. They were listened to but encouraged to return to the group and deal directly with the leader. Their expression of anger through thinly veiled jokes continued for several more weeks. "It's O.K., he's just a stupid mama's boy and don't know what to do in here."

Ultimately, after several months, the group showed some consistency, and certain individuals began making bids for leadership while accepting some of the values of the group leader. However, the members continued to resist trusting their peers. The mere act of volunteering to make out a basketball schedule would cause four or five others to signify the volunteer down. Then they would appeal to the leader that only he was capable of making out a schedule

One group moved more rapidly toward cohesiveness than others. The middle age-group progressed furthest. The younger group had difficulty in finding a territory of its own, while the oldest group controlled the gym. The middle group established ownership of a recreation room with television, pool table, and ping-pong.

The younger boys' rap group consistently concentrated upon the themes of impotence, alienation, and abandonment. They tried to disperse and join other groups, but were rebuffed. Possibly this group needed more direction, structure, or direct gratification to deal with special developmental needs. A counter suggestion, however, might be that more self-determination and peer interaction were maintained in the middle group. Thus, it is possible that rather than the younger group needing more direction and gratification, they in fact needed more consistent facilitation of their own differentiation and determination.

A variety of subtle personality differences between group leaders may also have contributed to the different group reactions. The leader of the middle group was more of a peer in age, dress, and demeanor. By virtue of his part time employment, he was less a part of the institution, felt less anxious for the success of the program, and without the burden of role responsibility apparently felt freer in avoiding taking a directive and authoritative position. He also had had no previous experience with the program, and because of this lack of experience, he was receiving more consultative support. Surely the reasons for the accelerated process in the middle group were a combination of these and others, including the characteristics of the individuals forming that group. Though advanced beyond the others, even this group displayed only occasional cohesion. The discussion groups could not be considered group therapy or T-groups, but they did evolve a considerable distance from the silent, chaotic, passive resistance of the first months, the signifying rounds of the middle months, and the leadership baiting efforts of more recent time. The following vignette portrays one of the higher points in the group interaction:

Fifteen-year-old Bart became known to the group as a sneaky thief, as one not to be trusted. The boys were talking openly about Bart's lack of conformity to the implicit ethic that one does not "rip off" friends.

On one occasion, a relatively valuable object disappeared. There was open recognition that Bart had struck again, quietly disappeared from the scene, and not returned. Later in a rap group, after a brief round of signifying, one youngster gave the new group *coup the grace*, "I don't trust you any more than Bart Jones." In an attempt to continue the themes of trust and values, the leader raised the hypothetical moral issue of what might happen if any of the group members found a wallet. Displaying a transparent model, the leader revealed what he would do. As so frequently happened when he revealed some moral standard, he was ridiculed for being a fool. On this occasion, however, the group did not stop with ridicule, but went on to an extended discussion of the ethics of the situation. Each member of the group participated, revealed his own moral code, and confessed his own stealing. In fact, it would appear that cohesion and conformity were so important that some individuals might have confessed to stealing when in fact they did not. The level of moral development specified was that one does not steal from friends, but otherwise it's good luck to find money. It is always acceptable to be opportunistic and acquire things of value as long as friends aren't hurt.

In nine months, Project Opportunity showed some development. Loss of membership had dwindled by the end of the first three months. Several of the activity or interest groups then solidified. Basketball and chess tournaments were scheduled. With staff support a group of boys interested in art instruction mobilized and found equipment and a volunteer teacher. But much as in the past, summer has terminated the program's activities. Basketball is played on every street corner and housing project plaza. Our gym is hot and the staff not cool enough to compete with the familiarity and seductiveness of basketball and the summer sun.

Conclusions

Several characteristics of a population of adolescents, which we feel has been lost between systems, are presented. Major emphasis is placed on the deficiency of effective socialization skills within the group and the lack of motivation to rectify this deficiency. A program focused on remediation through the formation of cohesive task oriented group, subgroup, and varied group role experiences is proposed. In conjunction, the type of staff leadership necessary for such group experiences is defined through a discussion of the various features of therapy and T-group leadership utilized. The process of the group intervention program is described through the use of vignettes and problems of management are reflected. Only modest gains toward increasing social skills were noted in the short term. Frequent reasons for such moderate results include issues of utilization of the limited staff resources, meager financing, and abbreviated process time to accomplish the remediation of experiences that have occurred over a lifetime for the adolescents. These features can be at least partially adjusted in future intervention attempts. The most important of these seems an expansion of group process time and continuity for the resolution of the tremendous mistrust of self, others, and future fulfillment which became so evident in the population.

The other major focus in such projects must remain the described lack of participant motivation for change, which in most instances was pervasive enough to effect the attraction to most any program enticement. The fine lines between enticement and coercion, or gratification and frustration which were traversed on numerous occasions by the rap group leaders are the similar, but possibly more subtle, lines upon which all therapists must tread when undertaking the treatment of adolescents. Questions surrounding the evaluation of motivational forces which largely determine the outcome of any intervention with adolescents are crystallized in the staff and adolescent relationships within this program. How much motivation, toward what goals, disparate or congruent, and emanating from which of the interacting sources are important issues in determining the critical quantum necessary for change in the direction of personal growth and concomitant social adjustment. Further dissection of these forces and the strategies utilized to deal with the less than optimally motivated patient are necessary for a more complete understanding of the dilemmas with which we are confronted in the morass of motivations and agendas common to therapeutic work with hapless adolescents in the community mental health setting.

REFERENCES

Brown, J. S. (1961). *The Motivation of Behavior*. New York: McGraw-Hill.

Cofer, C. N., and Appley, M. (1964). *Motivation: Theory and Research*. New York: Wiley.

Hill, R. B. (1971). *The Strength of Black Families*. New York: Emerson Hall.

Lewis, O. (1966). The culture of poverty. *Scientific American* 215:19.

Marana, A., and Lourie, R. (1967). Hypothesis regarding the effects of child rearing patterns on the disadvantaged child. J. Hellmuth, ed., *Disadvantaged Child*, Vol. 1. New York: Brunner/Mazel.

Redl, F., and Wineman, D. (1957). *The Aggressive Child.* New York: The Free Press.

Rafferty, F. T. (1961). Day treatment of adolescents. *Current Psychiatric Therapies.* New York: Grune and Stratton.

Rafferty, F. T., and Bortcher, H. (1963). Gang formation in vitro. *Journal of Nervous and Mental Disease* 137: 1: 76-81.

Yalom, I. (1970). *The Theory and Practice of Group Psychotherapy.* New York: Basic Books.

Yamamoto, J., and Coleman, W. (1973). Adolescence and poverty from little Tokyo to black housing projects to the heartland of America. J. C. Schoolar, ed., *Current Issues in Adolescent Psychiatry.* New York: Brunner/Mazel.

LUIZ CARLOS OSORIO

While many analysts question whether or not adolescents can be successfully analyzed, growing experience has begun to indicate that many doubts about this method of treatment relate to a lack of technical understanding of the adolescent patient's mode of communication (Alves, Osorio, and Piccoli 1972).

Analytical work with children became possible because of the development of technical procedures facilitating infantile communication. Play, an important means of communication of the child's unconscious fantasies, became the central element of Klein's technique. Therapy with adolescents may also require new technical procedures to make it easier to reveal the adolescent's intimate feelings. In my opinion, the treatment of adolescents cannot employ a technique that is simply an extrapolation of techniques applied to children and adults, and definitely not a ludicrous combination of both. The procedures used in the playroom, as well as in the consultation room, are inadequate for the analysis of adolescents.

The difficulties in the technical handling of adolescent patients are, to a large extent, derived from the concept that adolescence is merely a phase of transition between infancy and adulthood. This belief leads to the uncertainty as to whether we should treat adolescents as children or adults.

Adolescents present problems in communication that are related to peculiarities, from the adult viewpoint, in symbolization. Idiosyncrasies in symbolizing during adolescence cause may clinicians to equate adolescence with psychosis and to consider them, like psychotic patients, as unanalyzable.

The study of symbols and their pragmatic functions by theorists on communication has opened new perspectives for the understanding of the interactive phenomena which take place during the psychoanalytic process. The words "communication" and "conduct" are regarded as virtual synonyms since the word communication includes not only verbal symbols but their concomitant nonverbal symbols as well, part of which comprise "body language" (Kusnetzoff 1973).

It is commonly known that adolescence is fundamentally characterized by an identity crisis and that the transition from childhood to adulthood results in a number of complementary losses and gains: loss of infantile bisexuality, gain of adult heterosexuality; loss of infantile dependency, gain of adult autonomy; loss of infantile language or method of expression, and gain of symbolic verbal communication at an adult level. These losses are accompanied by mourning, which shapes the depressive situation essential to the adolescent process.

I believe that defensive concretizing of adolescent thought as well as the frequent blocking of verbal communication constitute, so to speak, the semantic expression of grief for the loss of the infantile condition. The significant commitment of verbal expression toward the mourning process stresses the importance of understanding nonverbal expression in the adolescent patient.

Adolescents express themselves through a language of action which, in my opinion, embraces much more than simple body expression. It is a behavioral language composed of action, affects, and thought elements which demands of the therapist recognition and comprehension of the symbolization process that this language expresses. To each behavioral manifestation of the adolescent's communication there should correspond a behavioral explanation. Such understanding also depends on the therapist's capability of establishing good communication with his own unconscious, adolescent aspects.

It seems that the greatest initial difficulty met by those who decide to carry on analytic treatment with adolescents is understanding all the paraverbal nuances and modulations used to convey their feelings to us. When we complain about the difficulties in working with adolescents because they don't make themselves understood it is because we are not able to cross the barrier of conventional verbal expression and understand their "behavioral language."

I undertook the treatment of a fifteen-year-old adolescent following hospitalization for drug abuse. His clinical picture indicated hysterical-psychopathic features. He kept expressing an interest in treatment but complained that the didn't know what to talk about. After the first few sessions, in which a long silence followed every laconic bit of information

443

about daily events, he told me about some songs that he and some friends had composed. (I later learned he was talented and had won a prize in a popular music festival.) From that moment the sessions became a colorful musical panel. He sang songs he had composed and brought a tape-recorder to play the latest musical arrangements he composed with his group.

At the beginning I interpreted such behavior as resistance to treatment. He was dissatisfied and perplexed. His reaction made me realize that he was seriously attempting to communicate with me. In other words, he was offering me a method which enabled him to express himself in a creative fashion and simultaneously maintain his self-esteem. I was finally able to establish a relationship between the melodic line of the songs he sang in session and his attitudes about his life situation. Initially, I felt that the lyrics of his songs, even though they represented modes of communication, were sealed off and part of a private autistic reverie. Gradually, I saw them in a new light which allowed me to gain comprehension of unconscious conflicts to which I had no access through conventional verbal communication.

I thought of the hermetic quality of the lyrics, which sometimes gave me the impression of a disintegrated schizophrenic monologue hidden under the tonal clothing of pop music—the impressions some of us form when listening to much modern musical composition is not different.

When an adolescent says, "It's useless to talk with adults because they don't understand me," he is referring to much more than just a difference in opinion between himself and his parents. Implicit in such a statement is a process of linguistic and semantic divergences which parallels the widening ideological gap between generations.

Slang, as an adolescent mode of communication related to an identity crisis, requires scrutiny. With all of its kaleidoscopic proteanism, it confounds us and demands a permanent and never satisfactory updating with regard to neologisms and to the new symbolic connotations of words which already have an established meaning. It is necessary for a therapist to be acquainted with adolescent dialect in order to establish the rapport absolutely essential to analytic work.

Slang is a perversion of language. I use the word *perversion* deliberately in order to analogically refer to what occurs during infantile development. The perverted polymorphic disposition defines infantile sexuality in the same way slang defines adolescent language. Normal adults use slang only occasionally; its systematic use is a deviation in linguistic behavior. Discounting the influence of social and cultural factors, one could say that the use of slang by adults corresponds to a partial and occasional replacement for a complete and satisfactory verbal communication. In an adolescent, however, it is a form of expression peculiar to his linguistic identity.

Similarly, the adolescent, in his anxious search for an emergent identity, establishes pseudoidentifications which he embodies partially or abandons later on and acquires linguistic idioms which barely and transitorily suit his purpose of conveying ideas and feelings which otherwise could not be verbalized. Slang is the verbal expression of the adolescent's process of differentiation and his eagerness to recognize himself and his equals as holders of an identity which is their own and distinct from that of parents and adults in general.

Adolescent slang acquires an hermetic, mysterious character for adults as a defense against the younger generation's attempts to destroy their comfortable genre. It is not surprising to note an increase in the use of slang when the adolescent patients' resistances are increased in the context of the transference regression.

The progressions and regressions that characterize the pubertal process are reflected in the adolescent's lexicon. Beside the large number of words which are oral, anal, or phallic residues of infantile language, one finds certain neologisms and speech mannerisms that are identified with adult sexuality and are manifestations of youth's creative potential.

The clinical observation of slang phenomenon and its psychopathological significance among adolescents allows us to verify that the degree of saturation of slang words in this language is related to the predisposition to acting out conflicts instead of expressing them in words. Slang would be, so to speak, the verbal modality of acting out. On the other hand, I have found that a decrease in usage of slang occurs when progress is made and conflicts are verbalized rather than acted out.

I have referred to the adolescents' behavioral language and to the correspondent behavioral interpretation made by the therapist. I would like to clarify these concepts by presenting some brief clinical material.

An adolescent male whose clinical picture showed a dominance of manic and psychopathic features and who, from time to time, used drugs to seek relief from depressive feelings began a session by lighting up a marijuana cigarette. It was evident that he was more interested in my reaction to his behavior than in the effects of the drug. He began to describe the stages of his "trips" with an abundant use of slang. He showed great interest in knowing whether I had previously seen the effects of marijuana in a patient in spite of the fact that we had discussed marijuana in an earlier session.

445

I realized that he was reexperiencing his original introduction to the use of drugs and was using language to repeat this event. At first I remained silent, observing but not indicating much curiosity. The scene struck me as quite grotesque because of the avid, almost simian, manner in which he was sucking the cigarette and inhaling its smoke.

In order that the patient not feel that I was aloof and withdrawn, I interpreted that in the same way he had shown great curiosity in knowing the effects of the drug before trying it, he must have imagined I would be curious, since he knew that I had never witnessed a patient smoking marijuana. I suggested he was offering a demonstration in order to satisfy my supposed curiosity. He replied, "Yes, but it is no fun to do it in front of you . . . you remain so locked up in yourself, so uninterested. . . . I even realize now that this marijuana thing is not as exciting as I was promised."

I believe that the effect of the interpretation occurred more as a result of my attitude than the verbal content. My conduct, which I conceptualize as a behavioral interpretation, enabled the patient to acquire insight into his disappointment with the effects of marijuana. My own feeling that the patient would be disappointed if I had remained uninterested in what he was doing corresponded to his own growing disinterest in the drug and to his own disappointment with its effects.

Regarding the verbal aspects of interpretation—until now I have made reference mainly to its non-verbals or para-verbal aspects—it should be emphasized that, besides not getting involved in intellectual discussions with patients, interpretations should be of a level of abstraction that corresponds to what the adolescent has achieved developmentally. It is well described that many adolescents have not progressed beyond the level of concrete operations (Piaget 1967), and the use of abstract conceptualizations in interpretations may increase resistance to the analytic process. The following fragment of a session will illustrate these ideas.

A female adolescent patient felt both submissive to and envious of me. She mentioned that my armchair was more comfortable than hers. I interpreted that she regarded my position of analyst as more comfortable that hers of patient, making reference to previous data. I added that the discomfort she was feeling was caused by her envy of what she called my "capacity for being calm" as well as her defensive, submissive attitude toward me, an attitude that characterized the transference. Apparently, my interpretation as well as subsequent interpretation had no effect. The patient remained tense and insisted that her chair was less comfortable than mine. I reminded her that she could make herself more comfortable by lying down on the couch, something she had so far refused to do. With a sudden expression of relief she exclaimed, "It's true, if I wanted to I could be much more at ease. This means I keep pushing myself. My feeling comfortable depends only on me, doesn't it?" She then chose the more comfortable position of lying on the couch.

Here again, as is so common with adolescents, one is confronted with a particular mode of communication. The patient expressed rather complex feelings by dealing with symbols, in this case, a sequence of symbols such as chair-discomfort, couch-comfort, in a concrete fashion.

Conclusions

For many years, the psychoanalytic treatment of adolescents has been neglected. This has, in part, been due to the therapist not being alert to the specific methods of communication such patients employ. Here, I have emphasized two characteristics of their communication patterns. One deals with peculiarities of verbal content, the abundant use of slang expressions which the therapist has to learn to understand in terms of subtle emphasis and idiosyncratic context. The other deals with the adolescent's propensity to orient his thinking in concrete terms and to use symbols in a somewhat literal sense. Subtle emotions are concretized and material objects represent very complex feeling states. Unless the therapist understands these elements of communicative mode and responds appropriately, interpretations will be ineffective and therapy will remain at a standstill.

REFERENCES

Alves, F., Osorio, L. C., and Piccoli, B. (1972). Adolescent psychoanalysis. Presented to the Porto Alegre (Brazil) Psychoanalytic Society.

Blos, P. (1962). *On Adolescence.* New York: The Free Press.

Buxbaum, E. (1970). Psychology of the adolescent. *Revista Argentina de Psicoanalisis* 27: 3.

Kalina, E., and Roscovsky, A. (1972). A review of adolescent psychoanalysis: technical and theoretical aspects. *Revista Argentina de Psiquiatria y Psicologia de la Infancia y de la Adolescencia* 3: 2.

Knobel, M. (1971). Adolescence and the psychoanalytical treatment of adolescents. A. Aberastury, ed., *Adolescencia.* Buenos Aires: Ediciones Kargieman.

Kusnetzoff, J. C. (1973). Approach to the theory of communication to the brief psychotherapy of children and adolescents. *Revista Argentina de Psiquiatria y Psicologia de la Infancia y de la Adolescencia* 4: 1.

Osorio, L. C. (1971). Psychotherapy in adolescence. Presented to the South Brazilian Meeting on Child Psychiatry, Porto Alegre, Brazil.

——— (1972). A review of adolescent psychoanalysis: technical and theoretical aspects. *Revista Argentina de Psiquiatria y Psicologia de la Infancia y de la Adolescencia* 3: 1.

——— (1972). Slang as a verbal expression of the identity crisis during the pubertal process. Panel on identity in adolescence. Latin-American Congress of Psychiatry, Punta del Este, Uruguay.

Piaget, J. (1967). *Six Psychological Studies*. New York: Random House.

Watzlawick, P., Beavin, J., and Jackson, D. (1967). *Pragmatics of Human Communication*. New York: W. W. Norton.

28] SELF-DISCLOSURE BY THE THERAPIST TO THE ADOLESCENT PATIENT

MYRON F. WEINER AND JOE W. KING

The traditional neutrality of the psychotherapist has been strongly challenged in the last twenty years. Existential psychiatry, introduced into this country in the 1950s, and the humanistic psychology movement which arose in the 1960s have advocated that the therapist reveal his own thoughts and feelings during the treatment hour to reduce the impersonality of the treatment situation and to make it more of a person-to-person encounter. The existential method encourages the therapist's open reaction to the patient in order to diminish the distance between them rather than perpetuate the patient's already troublesome condition of alienation (Havens 1974). Rogers (1961) argues that open expression of feelings by the therapist facilitates communication. Jourard (1964) believes that the therapist's openness helps patients become more trusting and provides a healthy role-model of interpersonal behavior. Freud (1912) and others in the field of psychoanalysis have questioned the value of revealing oneself as a person to patients on the grounds that it distracts from the exploration of the patient's unconscious and focuses attention on the therapist and the therapist-patient interaction. Weiner (1972) has described some of the advantages and disadvantages of self-disclosure with patients and advocates that decisions about self-disclosure be based on the therapist's knowledge of himself and his patient's treatment methods.

There are many objective studies of the effects of self disclosure between persons in laboratory and social settings (Jourard 1971). In general, they indicate that openness begets openness. There are, however, few objective studies of openness with patients in psychotherapy. Whitehorn and Betz (1954) report more positive outcome of treatment of schizophrenics by therapists who display a lively, personal interest in their patients. Truax and Carkhuff (1965) postulated that patients who disclose more of themselves to their therapists tend to improve most, and that disclosure of therapists to their patients, by facilitating patient disclosure, would also result in greater improvement. This was true with a population of hospitalized schizophrenics, but not with a group of institutionalized juvenile delinquents.

Barrett-Lennard (1962), in a study of clients in a college counseling service, was unable to demonstrate a correlation between therapist openness and positive outcome. Weiner, Rosen, and Cody (1974) were also unable to demonstrate that leader disclosure enhanced patient disclosure in four short-term therapy groups. Otstott and Scrutchins (1974) demonstrated that self-disclosure by the therapist is less effective in stimulating patient disclosure than open invitation to talk and confrontation. Leiberman's (1973) study of encounter groups demonstrated that psychological casualties could be attributed in part to leaders' displays of feelings expressed without regard to the individual needs of group members.

There are only two studies of the effects of therapist disclosure to adolescents. Both are studies of group therapy. Truax and Carkhuff found an inverse relationship between leader disclosure and positive therapeutic outcome with a group of forty institutionalized delinquents. In Kangas' study (1971), leader disclosure did not stimulate disclosure by members of an adolescent group, but did enhance disclosure in two short-term experimental student groups.

It is evident from the above data that patients in therapy (and especially adolescents) respond differently to self-disclosure by a therapist than do nonpatients in laboratory or social situations. Self-disclosure per se is of little value in promoting openness by patients or in ameliorating treatment results. Leiberman's (1973) study shows that what is disclosed and under what circumstances are of greater importance. He found, for example, that self-disclosure was useful when it conveyed personal interest and positive feelings and was part of a larger cognitive frame of reference. It was destructive when it conveyed negative feelings at a time when there was little support and little cognitive frame of reference.

The literature on the psychotherapy of adolescents includes suggestions that the therapist serve as a model of adult behavior (Meeks 1971) and that he correct patients' misconceptions about daily living by giving information based on personal experiences (Holmes 1964). Other therapists share information about their own past adolescent concerns about peer acceptance and dating (Forgotson 1974). Some tell of experiences with other patients who have faced similar situations (Brien 1974).

This chapter attempts to set forth parameters to help the psychotherapist make rational judgments concerning the use of himself as a person in the psychotherapeutic process. These parameters are dependent upon: (1) the goal of treatment, (2) the real relationship between therapist and patient, (3) the ego strength of the patient, (4) the nature of the patient-therapist alliance, (5) the patient's feelings about the therapist, and (6) the therapist's feelings about the patient.

Goal of Treatment

The treatment goal for most adolescent patients is to increase the adaptability of the ego. This does not come about primarily (as in the adult neurotic) by working through primary process material in a regressive transference neurosis, by analyzing resistances to transference, or by analyzing transference resistances other than those which interfere with a positive alliance between the healthy ego of the patient and the therapist.

It is our impression that certain properly timed disclosures and communications to adolescents enhance their contact with interpersonal reality and lead away from primary process material, which most teenagers find disruptive. The therapist of the adolescent frequently takes a direct approach to strengthening the ego of his patient. He advises. He shows that a person can live with his feelings rather than deny or be overwhelmed by them, and he shows the capacity to regulate and control his own behavior. He shows that he is able to conform to social norms when necessary and to deviate when they violate individual integrity. He is able to understand the adolescent's feelings, but is unwilling to be seduced into allowing more freedom than the patient's ego can tolerate. With ego growth reality-testing improves, the capacity for delay of gratification increases, the need for immediate discharge of instinctual drives diminishes, and pathological ego defenses are less readily mobilized.

The Real Relationship
Between Therapist and Patient

Evaluation situations. When a person is referred for evaluation and recommendations and a report is required by the referring individual or agency, the therapist needs to disclose to the patient that he is responsible to the referral source and will have to share his evaluations with them. Withholding such information invites retaliation and may destroy the interviewee's potential for constructive use of psychotherapy in the future.

451

On the other hand, the therapist is obliged not to reveal his findings unless he has the specific consent of the individual or agency requesting the evaluation.

Adolescents are frequently referred by parents or by school authorities. The most common adolescent defense is to claim that nothing is wrong— it's the school, his parents, or a mistake. In this situation the therapist accepts the child's lack of motivation, states that he is nevertheless a problem for others, and asks the child's cooperation in obtaining information for the people who are concerned.

A sixteen-year-old girl, seen as an outpatient, declared herself not interested in therapy. After her cooperation was sought so that information could be gained for use in working with her parents, she returned for six sessions on the premise that she, too, might gain some useful information.

Treatment situations. Other considerations arise when both therapist and patient agree that treatment is indicated and that they will work together. In this situation, the therapist establishes that he is the agent of the patient. Confidentiality is an issue with many patients. With the adult neurotic, it is usually possible to promise strict confidence. Adolescents who experience difficulty with impulse control or with countering strong regressive urges must be told that the therapist reserves the right to breach the confidentiality of the relationship and to interfere actively in the patient's life should he deem the patient unable to cope adequately with a dangerous life situation. Self-disclosures, other than the above, have little place in the first few interviews. When made, they usually relate more to the personal needs of the therapist than the therapeutic needs of the patient. At most, they suggest vulnerability, self-centeredness, and a wish to display one's self. At the very least, early self-disclosure suggests unwillingness to listen to the patient. The following illustration suggests the appropriate time for a disclosure of the therapist's reaction to a patient's parent and of the therapist's feeling about the patient herself.

Miss F, an eighteen-year-old girl, was brought to treatment by her father, a quarrelsome, suspicious, emotionally volatile man. As soon as the therapist (M.W.) felt that she had a strong commitment to work with him, he said he feared her father might act impulsively and destructively toward her. She, too, expressed concern that her father might hurt her during an outburst of rage. At this point, the therapist also told Miss F that he had been angered by her tendency to argue with him. He suggested that if her attitude angered him she could imagine the inflammatory effect on her father, whom she knew to be in constant danger of exploding. M.W. hoped that the disclosure of his reaction to her father would help support her reality testing. He hoped that disclosure of his anger would be more helpful than a simple statement that he found her to be argumentative, because it demonstrated her provocativeness with such immediacy that it left no room to argue whether or not she was argumentative. She understood.

Later, when Miss F's father decided (over her objections) to terminate her therapy because he "didn't want her working with a Freudian psychiatrist," the therapist shared his sense of loss with her, made some speculations about the father's motivation, and expressed hope that she would continue in therapy at some time in the future. Within six months, recognizing that she was alienating her friends, she was able to persuade her parents to allow her to continue in treatment with another therapist.

The Ego Strength of the Patient

There is little doubt that the greater the impairment of ego function the greater the need for persons in the patient's environment to be seen as real people, interested in the patient and actively involved in attempts to help him. This can be demonstrated in many ways, including personal openness on the part of the therapist.

Every patient, whether suffering a mild or severe emotional disorder, has some area of distorted or compromised reality testing. In dealing with both neurotic and borderline adolescents, revealing the therapist's awareness of their defective reality testing is a sensitive undertaking. With the exceptionally provocative patient it is best to suppress one's spontaneity. One can tell the patient, who is usually impatient for a reaction, that a few moments are needed to consider an answer. When accused of calculating an answer, the therapist can reply that the patient is owed a thoughtful response so that therapy will be helpful rather than destructive.

The following illustrates a negative reaction to a therapist's self-disclosure. Miss D, a negativistic, rebellious, seventeen-year-old high school senior, had been caught lying about an all-night rendezvous with her boyfriend, a young man who had recently been released from prison. She was angry with her parents for discovering her, but not with her boyfriend for "pushing" the drugs which helped precipitate a state of near-psychosis. Her therapist suggested, angrily, that she might more appropriately be upset with her boyfriend than with her parents. She then said she had previously decided that this session would be her last. In spite of opposition, she was adamant and did terminate at the end of the session. Neither the therapist's anger nor his opinion were of therapeutic value at that point. He was obviously identified with her parents and this, coupled with her concern over dependency, added to her determination to flee.

It is useful to support the perceptions of hospitalized adolescents, especially in relation to important people in their lives. Once, when one of the authors (J.K.) was undergoing a personal difficulty, one of his patients told him she was concerned because he appeared depressed. He admitted he was disturbed by events in his own emotional life, but that they were unrelated to his dealings with the patient or his work at the hospital. The patient appreciated his honesty, and no subsequent difficulty was encountered in her treatment because of this disclosure.

One problem of adolescents with impaired ego function is the belief that fantasy and action are inseparable. The therapist may deal with this maturational hurdle by disclosing examples of his own fantasies.

A hospitalized sixteen-year-old related that she dared not have sexual or aggressive fantasies lest she act on them. Rather than only reassure her that act and fantasy are not always directly connected, the therapist told of his own use of fantasy; for example, the fantasy of a pleasant social evening or of an upcoming vacation to keep his spirits up during a particularly trying day. In this way, he helped his patient to see that fantasy can be used as a substitute gratification rather than as an impetus to action.

The Nature of the Patient-Therapist Alliance

The ideal therapeutic alliance is between the rational, observing ego of the therapist and the rational, observing ego of the patient. With adolescents, the therapist must address himself to helping the patient build sufficient ego strength to deal with pathological ego defenses, superego, instinctual drives, and to maintain an alliance with this tenuous new structure. Pathological alliance is, unfortunately, too common.

There are patients who seek out incompetent therapists in the hope that they will continue successfully in the gratification of id impulses. A smile in response to an adolescent's defiance of his parents may suggest an unwitting alliance between the therapist's unexpressed instinctual drives and the instinctual drives of the adolescent.

Those who are attempting to reinforce their own primitive superego introjects may seek a harsh, judgmental quality in the therapist. Those who seek to enhance intellectual defenses may look for the tendency of a therapist to explain. The therapist, by explaining the etiology of his patient's behavior, may unwittingly help the patient rationalize or continue the same behavior.

A therapist who is strongly self-disclosing early in therapy may well reveal his liabilities, for example, his tendencies to condone impulsive action, to have a punitive attitude, or to promote rationalization. Having tipped his hand in this manner, he makes himself an easy mark for manipulation as therapy progresses.

In the development of a therapeutic alliance trust is a crucial issue. The patient decides upon the trustworthiness of his therapist. No amount of disclosure of past successes or of deliberate expression of goodwill is necessarily convincing. The patient decides for himself whether the therapist has what he wants. There is no substitute in this situation for the therapist's own sense of competence, self-awareness, and capacity for understanding and establishing limits, all of which is communicated nonverbally and involuntarily.

Finally, one must ask to what end the alliance is formed. In theory, the alliance is to the end of helping the patient to understand and change himself. Self-disclosure can subvert this end by changing the focus of the relationship from the patient to the therapist, and to pull patient and therapist toward gratifying each other's object needs and instinctual needs rather than working out the patient's problems.

The Patient's Feelings About the Therapist

The patient's feelings about the therapist are an important determinant of what and how to disclose. Early in therapy, another eighteen-year-old girl pressed her therapist (M.W.) to tell her that he liked her. He felt that in the transference she identified him with her parents, whom she derided by assuming that anyone who liked her was no good himself. She also manipulated, using the formula; if you like me, you will do me a favor. He refused to tell his feelings about her, choosing instead to say that there were times, when they talked, that he felt good—leaving the interpretation up to her. In other situations, aware that we were engaged in transference gratification, both authors have told adolescents that they like them. In these situations, the patient-therapist relationship was positive, and the therapist's acknowledgment of liking the patient supported their reality testing.

The Therapist's Feelings About the Patient

The therapist must take care that his self-disclosures are not a vehicle for acting out idiosyncratic countertransference feelings. This requires that the therapist have considerable self-understanding. The therapist needs to be aware of his usual style of relating to patients and to examine changes in his style (like the urge to be more self-disclosing) in the light of his conscious and unconscious feelings about the patient. The latter may come to light through investigation of the therapist's dreams, fantasies, and slips of the tongue. Self-disclosures by the therapist may provide a vehicle by which the countertransference can be brought into the open and discussed by patient and therapist together. Holmes (1964) describes a therapist who disclosed his wish to do a patient's bidding as a means of understanding and working out his countertransference.

It is tempting to self-disclose to an adolescent whom one respects as a means of conveying a sense of human equality. One must be careful, however, not to abandon a position of expertise and unconsciously denigrate or discard one's professional awareness. Becoming a pal can undermine the therapist's necessary status as a professional.

Expressions of liking or of anger have little place early in treatment, but may be appropriate and meaningful as treatment progresses. Disclosures of information about the world or about how people in general feel in given situations or at a particular point in life may be manifestations of the therapist's need to be seen as knowledgeable, but are appropriate at many points in treatment, especially when the patient's ego is becoming overwhelmed. Stories of similar feelings from the therapist's own past may also have a place in the treatment of severe ego decompensations as a means of reassuring a patient that he is not totally deviant (Long 1972).

Miss G was an eighteen-year-old high school senior. After treatment for a year, her initial attitude, that her parents were her problem and that only faith in God could help, softened to the point that she could admit her provocation of her parents, and use her faith to help her toward constructive action rather than passive expectation. She had little experience with dating. She was highly moralistic and would only date boys of similar religious convictions with whom she felt there was a possibility of developing a boy-girl relationship. The notion of dating to get around socially or for companionship was out of the question. She liked a boy at school. After much hesitation, she initiated a conversation with him one day at the water fountain. He responded well. She asked her therapist if she had been overly bold, fearful of rejection and desiring to know what made the boy unwilling to approach her first. The therapist felt she was asking for information and reassurance rather than baiting him, and he was glad that she had turned to him for information he could provide. He told her that he did not feel she had been too bold, and said that from what he knew of boys, and from what he could recall of his high school days, the boy was probably as afraid of rejection as she. She assimilated this information without difficulty, and excitedly reported the following week that he had telephoned her and asked her out.

Indications and Contra-Indications

Self-disclosure by the therapist is indicated if it helps the adolescent to become more aware and deal more effectively with various aspects of his interpersonal and intrapsychic reality (Weiner 1974). For example, the therapist may wish to demonstrate that he is a real, feeling person who recognizes the patient also as a real, feeling person. Indications for such a disclosure are: (1) a severe crisis in the patient's life which calls for an expression of human concern, such as a loss which the therapist knows to be of great significance to the patient, (2) to help a patient with markedly impaired ego function and reality testing perceive the therapist as a separate person rather than as a projection of his own fears and wishes, and (3) as a means of entering the emotional life of a patient who defends against emotional growth by detachment from others.

The therapist may use himself as a model to demonstrate that one can experience feelings without being overwhelmed or acting on them, to distinguish between act and fantasy, and to demonstrate that one can be potent without being omnipotent. For example, admitting to a patient that he is not physically able to restrain him can be a form of limit setting based on the therapist's actual physical limitations.

When in doubt, it is better to wait until a clear picture of the transference-countertransference situation and the therapeutic alliance becomes discernable. There must also be adequate time available to work through the sequelae of a disclosure. The patient's ego strength must be adequate to assimilate the disclosure. It is not useful to disclose for the sake of honesty alone. Honesty can demean the patient and suggest that he is less potent or in some way inferior to the therapist. On the other hand, one must not be dishonest, especially with expressions of positive feelings toward the patient.

Conclusions

In recent years, personal openness by therapists has been advocated to increase patient disclosure and enhance therapeutic outcome. Mutual openness does heighten interpersonal disclosure and intimacy in the laboratory and social settings. With few exceptions, studies of psychotherapy do not show increased disclosure by patients or enhancement of therapeutic outcome as a result of the therapist's personal disclosures. What is disclosed, and in what context it is disclosed appears more important than self-disclosure per se. Self-disclosure by the therapist distracts from acting out unconscious impulses, promotes positive or negative identification with the therapist, and focuses attention on interpersonal reality. These characteristics make self-disclosure less useful in working through a regressive transference neurosis and more useful in the type of therapy most appropriate for adolescents—increasing the adaptive capacity of the ego by education, identification with the therapist, strengthening the ego's defenses against the unconscious, and developing suitable displacements and sublimations.

Self-disclosures by the therapist are most useful to show the therapist as a real person, apart from the patient and his parents, who can recognize the adolescent and respect him as an individual. In allowing himself to be seen as a real person, he also offers his patient an opportunity for identification with constructive attitudes and approaches to life's problems. Disclosures are not helpful when they change the focus of therapy from the patient to the therapist, when they serve the therapist's personal needs rather than the patient's treatment needs, and when they move the patient away from constructive change by gratifying neurotic needs.

REFERENCES

Barrett-Lennard, G. T. (1962). Dimensions of therapist response as causal factors in therapy change. *Psychological Monographs* 76: 562.

Brien, R. L. (1974). Personal communication.

Forgotson, J. H. (1974). Personal communication.

Freud, S. (1912). Recommendations to physicians practicing psychoanalysis. *Standard Edition* 12: 111-120. London: Hogarth Press, 1958.

Havens, L. L. (1974). The existential use of self. *American Journal of Psychiatry* 131: 1-10.

Holmes, D. H. (1964). *The Adolescent in Psychotherapy*. Boston: Little, Brown.

Jourard, S. M. (1964). *The Transparent Self*. New York: Van Nostrand.

———(1971). *Self-Disclosure: An Experimental Analysis of the Transparent Self*. New York: Wiley-Interscience.

Kangas, J. A. (1971). Group members' self-disclosure: a function of preceding disclosure by leader or other group members. *Comparative Group Studies* 2: 65-70.

Lieberman, M. A., Yalom, I. D., and Miles, M. D. (1973). *Encounter Groups: First Facts.* New York: Basic Books.

Long, R. L. (1972). Personal communication.

Meeks, J. E. (1971). *The Fragile Alliance.* Baltimore: Williams and Wilkins.

Otstott, R. L., and Scrutchins, M. P. (1974). Therapist behaviors preceding high degrees of client self-disclosure. Unpublished Master's Thesis, University of Texas at Arlington.

Rogers, C. R. (1961). *On Becoming a Person.* Boston: Houghton-Mifflin.

Truax, C. B., and Carkhuff, R. R. (1965). Client and therapist transparency in the psychotherapeutic encounter. *Journal of Counseling Psychology* 12: 3-9.

Weiner, M. F. (1972). Self-exposure by the therapist as a therapeutic technique. *American Journal of Psychotherapy* 25: 42-51.

————(1974). Self-disclosure by the therapist. *American Journal of Psychiatry* 131: 930.

————, Rosen, B., and Cody, V. F. (1974). Studies of therapist and patient affective self-disclosure. *Group Process* 6: 27-42.

Whitehorn, J. C., and Betz, B. J. (1954). A study of psychotherapeutic relationship between physicians and schizophrenic patients. *American Journal of Psychiatry* 13: 383-400.

REUVEN KOHEN-RAZ

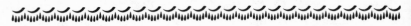

In spite of the conspicuous advances in the area of special education as science and profession, the peculiar psychological and educational needs of exceptional and handicapped adolescents comprise a relatively neglected field in research and service. Since even so-called normal adolescence has been a difficult and controversial subject in clinical theory and practice and if, in addition, handicaps and developmental aberrations must be taken into consideration, the issue seems to be of an overwhelming complexity.

There are, however, other reasons for the still prevailing scarcity of information on this subject. One is the fixation of educational and psychotherapeutic models to the paradigm of cumulative, developmental defect. Impacts of early disturbance or traumatization are supposed to increase in depth as age progresses. Consequently, efforts to diagnose and to treat must be concentrated at early childhood or even infancy. On the other hand, reeducation at adolescence may be too late and eventually futile, hence the relatively low priority given to the exploration of educational problems of the handicapped at or after puberty.

Another obstacle to the appreciation of special education needs at adolescence is the evaluation of educational and scholastic failures on the basis of requirements laid down by the traditional regulations and curricula of the normal elementary school. These are, as is well known, literacy, basic arithmetic, and elementary knowledge in history, geography, science, and the arts. It is also assumed that the child is able to adjust reasonably to a classroom routine. Children who do not meet these requirements will be put, sooner or later, into special classes. Here they will be tutored to catch up with the program, even if they have reached adolescence or passed it—whatever the relevance of such a curriculum to their future life and career. Consequently, the exploration of their specific educational needs as adolescents remains a matter of little concern to educational administration and counseling.

Additional difficulties are managing exceptional adolescents in school. While retarded, disturbed, and handicapped elementary school children will be ready to accept classroom discipline within reasonable limits of control as well as respond to instructions and teaching methods, most deviant adolescents (of various clinical types) have outbursts of rage, episodes of bizarre behavior, low or complete absence of motivation, a strong desire to abscond from school, together with a host of symptoms which disrupt class and teacher-pupil interaction.

Another problematic aspect of exploring educational needs of deviant adolescents is the relative ignorance concerning effects of physiological puberty on the abnormal human organism. There may be direct neurophysiological correlates of deviant pubertal maturation as well as secondary psychological problems indirectly caused by the impact of the pubertal process on the self-image and social maturation of the handicapped adolescent. The elucidation of these problems seems to be of basic importance to the understanding of many educational and psychological aspects of abnormal adolescence.

A Systematic Approach to Special Education Needs at Adolescence

A systematic, scientifically based approach to the educational problems of exceptional and handicapped adolescents should stress the following: (1) a thorough clarification of the etiology of the handicap in order to evaluate its impact on the adolescent's physical, mental, and emotional development. Whenever possible, information should be gathered on effects of the physiological pubertal process on the handicapped organism. (2) A careful design of an adequate and comprehensive curriculum which meets the peculiar emotional and intellectual needs of the handicap or disturbance. This should be supplemented by an intensive program of social learning and sex education. (3) An appraisal of the adolescent's urge for existential expansion, involving the planning and structuralization of his future.

An exemplary design for such purposes is the Illinois Program (1958) based on a two-dimensional model of educational aims: (a) involvement in "life situations" providing opportunity for pragmatic confrontation and theoretical information (examples of these life situations are citizenship, home and family, leisure time, materials and money, physical and mental health, safety, and social adjustment), and (b) development of knowledge and skills in arithmetic, language, fine arts, crafts, science, and social relationships. These two types of aims can be combined and focused around central themes such as "Post-Office," "Airport," "Supermarket," and "Traffic Police." By creating in this way intellectual and practical contact with life situations, the adolescent will be motivated to apply his knowledge in arithmetic as well as language and communication skills, and thus implicitly be trained in what the traditional curriculum considers basic school subjects without the feeling of being treated as a low elementary grader. It should be stressed that in the special education curriculum, art and physical training, as well as most extracurricular activities should be considered as a carefully planned and integrated component of the general educational program.

Handicapped and exceptional adolescents have to face special problems. They suffer from a basic dilemma created by aspirations to be equal, and possibly superior, to normal adolescents on the one hand, and the awareness of their impairments and handicaps on the other. Obviously, the self-image and inner security of the exceptional adolescents is deeply shattered by failures to find friends and by rejection by peers, especially by those of the other sex. Often the anticipation of such rejection is so strong that no real contact is sought and the imagined rejection becomes a determinant of social behavior patterns. The handicapped and deviant adolescent will also find himself in painful situations of being pitied, avoided, or treated with artificial concern, especially by adults.

Another matter of serious concern to the educator is the handicapped, retarded, and disturbed adolescent's difficulty and frequent unwillingness to realistically envisage his future as an adult. Obviously, vocational and professional careers, which the normal adolescent is able to imagine and anticipate, are often beyond his abilities. Still there are many avenues to satisfactory and remunerative work open to the handicapped. Without systematic vocational education, however, they remain unknown to the youngster and thus cannot provide any basis for a realistic perspective of his future.

As any other adolescent, the handicapped suffers from sexual tensions. However, these tensions are more difficult to tolerate as the handicapped as has less outlets.

Some aspects of these problems may be dealt with by individual talks or group discussions. However, some will require a realistic encounter with life situations. Eventually, artificial situations may have to be arranged in order to provide corrective emotional experiences. Psychodrama and sociodrama are important techniques which will stimulate social learning.

In certain cases, psychotherapy and education will have to be coordinated in order to treat individual problems. However, it should be kept in mind that psychotherapy at adolescence cannot proceed and succeed in an educational vacuum, that is, without keeping the adolescent in an educational setting and without involving the educator, directly or indirectly, in the therapeutic process.

The third aspect of special education problems at adolescence, the concern for existential expansion, seems at first sight to be a metaphysical question without practical pedagogical implications (Fromm 1950, Parsons 1955, Muchov 1962). However, it would be fallacious to assume that the problems of exceptional adolescents are limited to psychosomatic complications and social conflict. In order to appreciate the task of existential expansion as an educational problem, the full worth of the handicapped adolescent's life as equal to that of any other human being must be fully recognized by the educator. Such worth is totally independent of external educational objectives, such as vocational and social adjustment. Existential expansion means that at the crossroads between childhood and adulthood the adolescent views his future as an independent and free individual striving to be active and creative; interrelating with culture and society in an innovative, original manner; transcending the status ascribed him as a member of his family of origin; and searching for value systems different from those taught him at home. At first sight it may seem farfetched to assume that physically handicapped and mentally retarded adolescents can strive for autonomy, freedom, innovations of their life style, and creation of values. Obviously, the scope of the handicapped's existential expansion is limited in comparison to that of normals. However, within such limits, it must be recognized, respected, and taken into consideration as an integral component of the educational program. It should by no means by overshadowed by educational approaches.

I shall now discuss the peculiar educational needs of the most frequent types of exceptional disorders suffered by adolescents: mental retardation, behavior disorder, emotional disturbance, physical handicap, organic brain dysfunction, and auditory impairment. The problems of the blind and visually handicapped are very specific and are not within the scope of this chapter.

The Educable Mentally Retarded

The educable mentally retarded do not suffer from gross central nervous system damage, although "minimal brain dysfunction" may be an accessory but not central component. Genetic factors may be involved, manifested in the significantly higher incidence of educable retarded children in families where parents and siblings are mentally deficient (Chiva and Rutschman 1971). Still, educable mental retardation is closely linked with sociocultural deprivation. Actually, there is no clear line of demarcation between the culturally disadvantaged and the educable retarded, and this has caused considerable confusion in educational research and administration.[1]

In spite of the predominantly nonneurological basis of educable mental retardation and cultural deprivation, these populations show a high incidence of visual handicap, defective speech, weak lateral dominance, deficient bimanual coordination, motor instability, and poor control of synkinetic movements. These neurogenic dysfunctions may become serious obstacles to adjustment and work and therefore must be taken into account when planning educational programs for retarded and disadvantaged adolescents.

Puberty occurs at the appropriate age (Rundle and Sylvester 1973). However, one often encounters evidence of delayed pubertal maturation in the more severely retarded among the culturally disadvantaged (Kohen-Raz 1973). Language development is conspicuously retarded and the acquisition of reading, writing, and basic arithmetic is slow. The educable retarded child typically shows lack of school readiness at the age of six or seven. He may, however, reach the psychomotor and cognitive levels of the normal first grader at preadolescence, i.e., a delay of two to four years. Often this scholastic immaturity is concealed and somehow tolerated for two or three years in a regular class. Then, at the fourth grade, somewhat paradoxically, the educable retarded child is expelled from normal school, just when he appears to have attained school readiness. Thus, in a strict sense, he starts school at preadolescence and adolescence—a circumstance which should be seriously taken into account as an important point of reference to special education programs for retarded adolescents.

Keeping the basic educational and psychosocial needs of the educable retarded adolescent in mind, the following principles of curriculum construction may be proposed, principles that will require some modification of the traditional elementary school curriculum. Essentially this means that the learning of reading, writing, and arithmetic is not the core of the learning program, notwithstanding the fact that Western society values literacy and makes it a prerequisite for most occupations above unskilled labor. It is a fact that the effort spent to teach educable mentally retarded subjects the "three Rs" at the lower and medium grades is ineffective and many reach junior school age at a level of practical illiteracy. It seems futile to go on tutoring educable mentally retarded adolescents in reading, spelling, and arithmetic after they have responded so poorly and they may have developed negative attitudes toward these subjects.

Instead, it seems advisable to introduce a core curriculum of communication skills, which obviously would include reading, writing, and manipulation of numbers, but only as one method of communicating, placing similar, or even greater emphasis on training in other types of communication. Among these alternatives, language should first be mentioned. This means, in practical terms, acquisition of manners in everyday social contact: what, how, and when to say whatever is to be said, habits of listening to other people, and the like. The use of the telephone is an important part of this type of teaching program.

Another aspect of the oral language curriculum is the ability to express inner needs and mental states verbally. The retarded adolescent has difficulty in verbalizing affective tensions, which he therefore tends to act out by clownish poses or physical aggression.

The use of expressive movements and gestures has been recently explored scientifically under the title of "sign language" (Long 1963). The wealth of material accumulated in this area, and hitherto exploited chiefly in the context of teaching programs for the deaf, should be adapted and applied also to the communication curriculum for the retarded. This would include the use of audiovisual techniques as a communication medium supplementary and eventually alternative to written and printed language. Whatever the degree and type of the adolescent's reading problems, he should be taught to decode such vital outdoor signs and inscriptions as traffic signals, designations of shops and offices, destinations of public transport, announcements, warnings, and important posters. This may be achieved without exact recognition of individual letters.

Besides communication skills and their variations, essential parts of the curriculum should be dedicated to the acquisition of cultural and moral values, including the appreciation of fine arts, music, and literature. This seems, at first sight, to be a somewhat far fetched recommendation as it is assumed that the mentally retarded adolescent, because of his intellectual limitations and somewhat shallow emotions, is unable to understand art and enjoy artistic activities. However, experience has shown that this is an unsubstantiated prejudice. Besides giving lessons in music, art, dance, drawing, and sculpture, it seems also important to stimulate interest in literature by translating classics into shortened versions with simple

465

language, enlarged print, and rich illustrations. Obviously, the use of audiovisual aids could again be of great assistance.

Basic arithmetic and geometry should be included in the learning program. This, however, could be integrated in a more comprehensive curriculum of handling money and quantities, orientation in two and three dimensional space, evaluating and measuring distances, and discrimination of forms and spheric bodies. Special attention must be paid to the training of those cognitive skills which are the prerequisites to the conceptualization of the euclidian space and number system, such as seriation, reversal of sequences, multidimensional classification, conversation of substance and quantity, field independency, discrimination of right and left, the perception of diagonals, angles, and slanted lines. These processes have been described in detail by Piaget (1952a, 1952b, 1956), Werner and Kaplan (1963), Werner and Wapner (1949), Olson (1970), and Cratty (1969).

Perception of time is another important component of a learning program involving cognitive skills. The retarded adolescent learns about evaluation of past events in correct sequence, realistic anticipation of imminent events as well as structuralization of the more remote future, planning and maintaining a daily schedule, fixing and keeping appointments, being on time, and understanding and estimating short temporary spans, such as quarters of hours and minutes. These activities lead to the attainment of "concrete operations" (Piaget 1956) and, therefore, all exercises and teaching units which directly or indirectly foster the development of these mental structures are desirable components of the curriculum for retarded adolescents.

I turn now to the training of psychomotor abilities. The relationships between cognitive and psychomotor skills are rather complex and cannot be discussed in detail within the context of this chapter (see Kohen-Raz 1965, Cratty 1969, 1972). However, some general findings seem to be of peculiar relevance to the educational needs of retarded adolescents. For example, mentally retarded subjects show a conspicuous lag in the development of synergetic motor skills, that is, the capacity to execute two or more simultaneous movements of different pattern and direction, such as performing a circular movement with outstretched arms while tapping with both feet, manipulating two knobs simultaneously or handles of a tool (Kohen-Raz 1965, Rey 1952). Furthermore, the ability to suppress unnecessary motor reactions to the sudden or startle type of stimuli is conspicuously weaker in retarded than in normal subjects,[2] and there is a definitive relationship between static balance ability and cognitive school readiness (Kohen-Raz 1965).

These manifest or latent interactions between intellectual and motor functions seem to justify an intensive motor training program for retarded adolescents which should be designed according to principles of integrative visual spatial and motor stimulation (Kephart 1971, Cratty 1974, Keogh 1969).

Within the context of motor training, some efforts should be directed to strengthen and to develop the retarded adolescent's attention span, resistance to fatigue, and reaction speed. It is also obvious that the training of bimanual versatility (intimately linked with the ability to perform synergetic and to supress synkinetic movements) is of fundamental importance to prepare the retarded adolescent for semiskilled or skilled work with standard machinery.

Turning now to problems of social learning, several independent studies conclude that the vocational adjustment of retarded adolescents and young adults is much less related to their level of intelligence than to their ability to adapt to the social stress involved in work and cooperation with peers and superiors (Kraus 1972, Sali and Amir 1971, Gold 1973). Thus, the adolescent should learn to perceive and to interpret adequately the social responses of superiors, peers, and clients, as well as how to shape and control his own reactions, especially how to inhibit his typical free-floating affectivity and proneness to outbursts. The retarded adolescent tends to blur social relations by infantile projections of parent and sibling figures. Being often unable to reduce or to withdraw these projections, he will induce conflicts into his job relations (especially with foremen) which may jeopardize his employment.

It appears that certain forms of group work, especially activity group therapy, might be a suitable approach to these problems. Efforts should also be made to teach employers and foremen how to treat the retarded adolescent at work and how to assist him to establish satisfactory job relationships. Experience has shown that a sufficient number of employers are able and willing to cooperate in this respect.

Another central theme of social learning is behavior in public places. Modern technology has created conditions which oblige retarded persons, characterized by weak attention, reduced alertness and vigility, and low reaction speed, to be confronted with machinery and communication systems constructed for normal functioning brains. This discrepancy between a slowly responding mind and a high rate of environmental stimulation creates many problems for the safety of retarded persons.

Another aspect of the social education of adolescent retardees is the appropriate use of leisure time. Unlike the normal youngster, the retarded adolescent frequently lacks initiative and is inhibited. His inner world is prone to impoverishment, and given free time, he is seldom able to enjoy it. Therefore, the proper structuring and guidance of his leisure activities must be viewed as an indispensable part of the social learning curriculum.

In line with the general objectives of contemporary special education, the educable retarded adolescent is considered able to lead a more or less normal social life. There is therefore no reason he should not be eligible for marital partnership—morally as well as legally. Consequently, family and sex education has become an essential part of the social learning program. It should be noted that the educable retarded adolescent seems much more aware of the facts of sexual life and its problems than is anticipated (Hall 1973; Alcorn 1974). Actually, his preoccupations, conflicts, and queries are much the same as those of the nonretarded youngsters (Arnan 1973). Obviously he has additional problems. The boy resents his intellectual and vocational inferiority and feels the limitations of his prospective psychosexual status as a male in a technological culture in which weak intellect is depreciated. For the more passive type, seduction and eventual fixation to homosexuality is a potential danger. The retarded girl has less reason to suffer from feelings of inferiority. As a woman in our society her psychosexual role of motherhood is not threatened by her intellectual weakness. Eventually, supported by appropriate counseling, she may become a reasonably functioning mother and housewife. She also is able to perform in such jobs as domestic aide and baby sitter, as well as in a considerable number of unskilled and semi-skilled occupations. However, in spite of her less impaired self-image as a retarded adolescent girl, she needs to be protected from seduction and exploitation, and her essentially insufficient controls from within should be supplemented by external support and supervision in the form of specially organized social-work services, which should be available beyond the period of compulsory education.

Finally, in the context of social learning, the problem of coeducation of mentally retarded girls and boys must be considered. Although in most special schools and classes for the retarded coeducation is widely practiced without particular problems, its deeper implications are not fully recognized.

The process of coeducation should help the educator explain sex-role differences, and their impact on social relations as well as on marital partnership. He should try to sensitize the adolescent to perceive such differences and to teach respect for the other sex in its otherness, as well as to understand the behavior of the retarded boy and girl. This is important, as retarded adolescents, if eligible and ready to establish a family life of their own, will in the vast majority of cases marry partners of similar intelligence. In some rare exceptions, retarded girls may be chosen as spouses by men of normal mental level.

As to the third aspect of adolescent educational needs, the urge for existential expansion, one must consider the adverse effects of being labelled retarded; these menace the adolescent's striving for independence, undermine his self-confidence, and obscure his perspective on the future. Superficially, it might seem the retarded adolescent possesses insufficient insight and foresight to worry about either his future and independence or his diagnostic label. Any such appearances, however, are misleading. He should have the opportunity to express his feelings, anxieties, and apprehensions. On the other hand, he has to be told the truth about his abilities, limitations, and prospects. In spite of the generally accepted opinion, retarded subjects will respond to counseling and therapy based on verbalization of conflicts.

Another obstacle to existential expansion is the tendency of many retarded adolescents to remain fixated to infantile behavior and to be unable to overcome their overdependency on parents or parent substitutes—which, to a large extent, is the result of the general overprotective style of educating retarded children at home and at school. Thus, steps must be undertaken to assist the adolescent to become independent; emotionally, socially, and intellectually. Such independence will be fostered by offering opportunities to leave home for excursions, by participation in extracurricular activities with normal adolescents, by letting the adolescent make decisions, take responsibilities, and perform chores and duties of some importance. The tradition of evaluating the educable retarded on the basis of his intellectual and scholastic performance has led to a gross underestimation of his social competence and to considerable reluctance to grant him freedom for independent judgment and action, thus curtailing the possibility of existential expansion.

The Trainable Mentally Retarded

In contrast to the educable mentally retarded, the trainable type suffer from general damage or dysfunction of the central nervous system, caused by inherited disease, chromosomal aberrations, or early pathogenic processes. Ability to use symbol systems in human communication, is limited as is concept formation. The development of receptive as well as of expressive language is conspicuously delayed, and there is great difficulty in mastering reading and writing, even in a rudimentary form. Motor functions are underdeveloped, especially bimanual coordination. Physiological puberty is retarded, the maturational delay being roughly correlated with the degree of mental retardation. Intellectually, the level of concrete operations is not reached. Other results of basic neurophysiological handicap are: low resistance to stress and fatigue, weak affective control, problems of continency and if more seriously retarded, assistance is needed in daily routines of dressing, eating, going to bed, etc. Emotionally, fixation is on the response level of a three- to four-year-old child and relationship to adults (including the educator) is as a toddler clinging to his mother. In a strict sense, the trainable mentally regarded is neither emotionally nor intellectually ready for school, even during adolescence and adulthood.

For all these reasons, the trainable retarded has been considered noneducable. In the light of such a perspective, education during adolescence was viewed as a simple aspect of custody. However, this pessimistic viewpoint has changed and learning programs have been established. It may be stated that the modern approach is based on the belief that the trainable mentally retarded is able to achieve partial social and economic independence, and even if he cannot become literate he is capable of acquiring a considerable inventory of perceptual, motor, and cognitive skills.

Social learning should concentrate on the acquisition of elementary manners and habits of social interaction, besides the obvious objective to educate towards independence in all matters of daily routine. Sex education will generally have to be limited to simple, straightforward explanations, as well as to the extinction of habits endangering the adolescent's social acceptance, such as masturbation in public, acts of exhibitionism, and physical clinging to persons of the other sex. Appropriate means must also be sought to protect the retarded adolescent, especially the girl, from seduction. On the other hand, outlets for physical activity and movement must be offered, as the sexual tensions of the trainable retarded are chiefly manifest in diffuse aggression, tendency to clownlike behavior, and bizarre acting out.

In the cognitive sphere, the adolescent curriculum should concentrate on the development of language as an indispensable means of elementary communication and orientation in daily life. The teaching of reading and writing skills may be limited to the recognition of important inscriptions, warning signals, as well as to copying names and simple forms.

Attention should be paid to the improvement of manual skills and reaction speed. The understanding of primary spatial relationships should be developed, involving perception and discrimination of forms and distances in two and three dimensions. The aim of cognitive (and necessarily motor) reeducation should be a thorough preparation to perform productive and remunerative work, predominantly on the level of unskilled occupations.

In the case of trainable mental retardation, the issue of existential expansion seems to be hardly meaningful at first sight. However, it will appear quite realistic if formulated as a question of how to provide a realistic future perspective to the adolescent, and how to ensure—in pure pragmatic fashion—his appropriate living conditions during adulthood without lifelong custody or institutionalization as the last and only alternative. Obviously, even from the most optimistic view, the trainable retarded will not be able to lead an entirely independent existence, although he may be capable of partially supporting himself. The laudable establishment of sheltered workshops does not solve problems of emotional and social life during all those hours he is not at work. He might stay with his family of origin, but besides the psychological problems created by such an arrangement, he will probably outlive his parents since the life span of the severely retarded has been considerably extended.

Trainable mentally retarded adolescents are now being placed in flats and houses located in residential neighborhoods, preferably at the outskirts of the city. Here they form carefully selected groups destined to grow up and live together throughout their youth and adulthood. In these homes they remain under permanent supervision of responsible educators who guide them, live with them, and secure all their material, social, and cultural needs.

The Physically Handicapped

The category of physically handicapped includes first of all those types of impairment of the nervous system which cause a manifest dysfunction of gross and fine motor responses, especially impediments in postural control, walking, coordination of arms, hands, and fingers. Another subcategory are gross or minor malformations, not necessarily linked with CNS defects. Minimal and medium brain damage not leading to gross disturbances in static balance and in limb movements would be included in the category of brain injury treated in the next section.

The educational problems of the physically handicapped adolescent are multi-dimensional and complex. They may be divided into three types: (1) problems linked with the direct impact of puberty on the physical handicap, (2) problems of pubertal changes in the self image and their implications on social and psychosexual relations, and (3) problems of vocational habilitation. It should further be noted that there are at least three subpopulations of the physically handicapped, whose respective educational problems differ essentially, and thus need to be treated separately: (1) the normally intelligent, but multiply handicapped, characterized chiefly by sensory deficits and language disturbances, (2) the physically handicapped and also mentally retarded, and (3) the predominantly physically impaired but intellectually gifted, sometimes with a tendency to overcompensate their physical handicap by striving for mental superiority.

The impact of puberty on physical handicaps (or vice versa) is still insufficiently explored. In certain cases, surgical procedures must be carried out necessitated by pubertal growth and by alterations of the already existing defects and malformations. Prosthetic devices must be re-adapted and refined, especially those constructed for the purpose of manipulation and fine coordination needed to handle tools, doors, locks, typewriters, and communication media. These instruments require special training during adolescence, as in many cases it is only at this age that the physically handicapped may attain the physical strength, mental level, and social maturity necessary for mastery. However, there is still a great need to explore the more intricate relationships between pubertal, hormonal changes and the specific physiological responses of the physically and neurologically impaired organism.

From a psychological viewpoint, the impact of puberty on the self-image of handicapped youth causes an overall sensitization of the body resulting in an increased awareness of the physical defect. Also, the handicap, already experienced throughout the middle and late childhood as a general stigma, is now perceived with an additional negative valence, as sexually repugnant. The delicate social situation of the handicapped adolescent is, in addition, ill affected by the embarrassment he creates in his social environment. The healthy adolescent's peers, themselves under the impact of sexual conflicts, unconsciously associate the cripple with castration fears, and this impedes their spontaneous, natural contact with the handicapped person. Activating defense mechanisms, they try either to avoid contact or to demonstrate artificial concern and pity. Both responses evoke resentment and bitterness in the handicapped adolescent, who wishes nothing more ardently than to be treated as if his handicap did not exist.

The most efficient way to rehabilitate his impaired self-image is to establish mixed youth clubs where normal and handicapped adolescents meet and enjoy common recreational activities. The social readjustment of a crippled youth can be achieved by working through his problems of physical handicap with the normal adolescent. In this way, the prejudices and fears of the healthy peer group may be overcome and new avenues opened to create an adequate educational atmosphere for an integration of the handicapped in a normal social environment.

As to sex education, with the aim of achieving adequate sexual and marital relations, pioneer work has been recently undertaken, with promising although not yet fully evaluated results (Nordquist 1972, Cook 1974).

In the case of the intelligent, but multiple handicapped type, the combination of visual, auditory, and linguistic problems often requires individual tutoring, usually in special classes. Still, great care should be given to improve, as far as possible, the communication skills of these handicapped youngsters, and in spite of the high degree of specialization (and subsequent segregation needed to ensure their proper education), contact with normal adolescents should be established and maintained as much as possible. The use of modern mass media is of great help in overcoming the isolation of these difficult cases, and the use of sociodrama and acting is by no means beyond the scope of their abilities.

For the physically handicapped with retardation, no adequate solution has yet been found. They are generally placed in institutions or classes for the severely retarded or severely handicapped, and sometimes in psychiatric hospitals, as their poor reality control tends to break down under the pressure of adolescent drives. They need specialized care, either in residential treatment centers or in open homes. The combination of physical and mental handicap seriously limits the prospects of vocational rehabilitation, and the danger of extreme isolation resulting in psychotic breakdown is considerable.

The third type, characterized by normal and above normal intelligence, should be placed in normal classes, with eventual support of auxiliary lessons. The main problem with these adolescents is their social adaptation to normal adolescents.

Regarding the problem of existential expansion, the situation of the

473

mentally retarded and physically impaired is difficult since he may be doomed to lifelong custody and institutionalization. The best solution, in my opinion, is the planning of group homes like those recently established for the severely retarded. The normally intelligent types, in order to gain a realistic future perspective and to motivate them to establish a free and independent existence, may require individual or group psychotherapy.

Minimal and Medium Organic Brain Damage

This category includes a broad spectrum of clinical types supposed to have a common etiology of minimal or medium organic brain damage, which, in many cases, cannot be clinically substantiated. The symptomatology of these cases is extremely variable. As a general basis for our discussion, I cite Cruickshank's (1966) formulation based on the definition of Task Force One of the joint study of the National Institute of Neurological Diseases and Blindness and the National Society for Crippled Children and Adults. He states:

> Brain injured children have intelligence levels from below to above average and are characterized by learning and/or certain behavioral abnormalities, ranging from mild to severe, which are associated with subtle deviant function of the central nervous system. These may be characterized by various combinations of deficits in perception, conceptualization, language, memory and control of attention, impulse, or motor function.

The clumsiness, stubbornness, scholastic failure, and affective outbursts of the brain injured child put him in a marginal position in his family as well as at school. Sometimes he is openly rejected, at other times simply ignored. Relatively devoted and conscientious parents often fail in their educational efforts because they tend to relieve the organically damaged child from chores and duties since they have no confidence in his skills and versatility. On the other hand, they overburden him with all kinds of extra activities and treatments, remedial lessons, art, gymnastics, and psychotherapy. The child is overprotected and develops feelings of dependency, inadequacy, and insecurity. Frequently he becomes the scapegoat of family conflict and develops a neurotic superstructure. Under extreme social and emotional stress, the brain injured adolescent partly or temporarily looses reality control and shows symptoms of psychotic breakdown.

The middle-class adolescent with minimal organic brain damage and normal intelligence is generally reasonably adjusted to educational settings. Psychomotor clumsiness, if present, need not become an obstacle to a normal scholastic and vocational career. By contrast, the student with medium organic damage who is also of lower intelligence poses serious problems. Being a black mark on his family's pride and reputation, he is overstimulated and irritated on the one hand, and overprotected on the other. He has great difficulty in becoming emotionally and socially independent, and typically behaves in a demanding and sometimes aggressive manner. Although behavior therapy and behavior modification is often recommended, family therapy is a more adequate solution. Even though the focal problem seems to be neurological, the breakdown of communication between the unpredictable personality of the brain injured youngster and his parents is often at the core of his difficulties.[3]

It is possible to reeducate and rehabilitate the minimally brain damaged and culturally disadvantaged youth, and to activate their essentially normal intellectual potential (Kohen-Raz 1974). Their reading and arithmetic skills must be developed by applying remedial techniques aimed at their typical organic deficits; perceptual and motor difficulties (Cratty 1969, Frostig 1964, Fernald 1943). Special efforts must be dedicated toward developing the ability of concrete operational thought. Some pupils may actually be able to attain the level of formal operational reasoning (Kohen-Raz 1973), a stage in which the capacity for abstract thinking has been achieved (Piaget 1952a).

In vocational training, it may be advantageous to offer these adolescents, especially the lower-class adolescent, opportunities for remunerative jobs as early as possible. Having experienced considerable humiliation in lower-class, materialistically oriented families as awkward, useless children, the achievement of economic productivity is an important corrective emotional experience.

The lower socioeconomic level, low mental level, minimal organic brain damaged child is for all practical purposes educationally similar to the educable mentally retarded. On the other hand, the medium brain injured type of low socioeconomic background is a rather serious challenge to the educator, especially during adolescence. In this case, socioeconomic deprivation, restricted cognitive, perceptual and motor functioning, disturbed social communication, and affective imbalance result in considerable ego weakness which, at adolescence, may lead to temporary loss of reality control and psychotic or pseudopsychotic episodes.

Clinically, these mental and affective states manifest themselves in aggressive (and sometimes dangerous) outbursts, in stubborn reluctance to communicate with the educator, and in complete indifference to the teaching materials presented. Transient depressive states may appear. Sometimes bizarre behavior can be observed, such as clinging to objects, exhibitionism, and the uttering of incoherent and unsubstantiated statements. They are generally unable to adjust to educational settings for the retarded (because of their aggression, unpredictable outbursts, and resistance to remaining in class), but on the other hand, they are not admitted to psychiatric institutions since they are diagnosed primarily as organic and retarded rather than psychiatric patients. Consequently, they may end up loitering in the streets, endangering themselves and the public, ready victims to drug addiction and delinquency.

Prospects of reasonable vocational rehabilitation are dim. The best solution seems to be sheltered workshops under psychiatric supervision with systematic training in work habits and stimulation of socially competent behavior. Placement in residential treatment centers has the obvious disadvantage of reinforcing their already prevailing tendency to withdraw from confrontation with reality and their reluctance to perform productive work. Transfer to foster families in agricultural settings may be another possibility, provided families are available and able to deal with such grave educational problems. Psychotherapy with both the adolescent and his parents is feasible. Administration of tranquilizers is often necessary to check disruptive behavior and to keep the adolescent manageable at school.

Existential expansion for these adolescents is characterized by specific obstacles that impede the attainment of emotional and social independence. These obstacles are produced by the following circumstances: (1) In contrast to the mentally retarded, who possesses limited insight, the organically impaired adolescent is fully aware of his weakness, awkwardness, and failures to adjust to routine demands of reality, and thus tends to withdraw. (2) Parents are inclined to overprotect the adolescent. They are struck by despair, as hopes and illusions for recovery of their offspring seem to be lost forever once he has reached adolescence. (3) The organic adolescent had great difficulty in joining the normal labor force. In contrast to the mentally retarded, whose vocational skill for a certain job once developed is adequate, the organically handicapped, even with higher intelligence, often remains seriously handicapped in his capacity and efficiency, as he may fail to overcome his unstable muscular tonicity, his tendency to rapid exhaustion, his effective lability, and his sensory deficits.

The Acoustically Handicapped Adolescent

The educational problems of the deaf and acoustically handicapped adolescent are among the most neglected areas in special education. Unable to develop an adequate system of abstract symbols and concepts, he cannot master high school, college, and university curriculums in spite of a normal and often above normal intelligence. More specifically, two higher cognitive functions, which are indispensable for academic studies, are deficient; formal reasoning (Inhelder and Piaget 1959) and the understanding of metaphorical language (proverbs, fables, anecdotes). As these higher mental functions develop intensively at preadolescence and early puberty, the gap between the scholastic achievements of normal and acoustically handicapped adolescents widens considerably at this age period. Consequently, even if integrated in normal schools, the hard of hearing and deaf adolescents will tend to stay at the lower streams and levels of the high school system. Special high schools for this type of handicap have the definitive advantage of exploiting fully the intellectual potential of the acoustically impaired adolescent. Isolation from the normal peer group can be easily overcome by providing an integrated program of extracurricular activities.

The impoverished language inventory of hard of hearing adolescents creates difficulties in verbalizing their feelings, tensions, needs, and inner conflicts. This may result in bizarre gestures, temper tantrums, outbursts of physical aggression, and tears and lamentations.

A still more aggravating situation is created by parents who themselves are deaf or hard of hearing. Sometimes the adolescent who may be superior in his abilities and level of social adjustment, by virtue of the more advanced education offered him by modern special education methods, will dominate the handicapped parent who is unable to handle the problems of his adolescent son or daughter to a much greater extent than normal hearing parents.

Compensating for the loss or loosening of parental emotional relations and support by creating intensive peer relationships is not an easy option for the acoustically handicapped adolescent because of his difficulty in establishing deep ties with his social environment. Vocational rehabilitation is also difficult since even semiskilled occupations require rapid information processing, which is seriously impeded by impaired hearing.

The curriculum should also focus on the development of higher level symbol systems. Sign language, in contrast to other methods of verbal interaction for the deaf (such as lip reading and letter signs) can be used to express abstract concepts and complex syntactic relationships (Stokoe 1965). Training in ballet and pantomime is useful, but traditional methods of teaching reading and writing must not be abandoned.

The area of vocational training for the hard of hearing and deaf still needs to be further developed and refined. Although conspicuous progress has been made and additional, alternative channels of communication have been put at the disposal of the acoustically handicapped by means of new technological and electronical devices, more educational efforts must be invested to exploit fully the intellectual and vocational potential hidden and impeded by the hearing loss.

The problem of existential expansion of the acoustically handicapped also depends on his restricted universe of symbols which limits hopes for the future. From a socioeconomic point of view, his vocational choice is relatively restricted and he is unable to compete with normal persons in almost any field. Regarding family life, he is confronted with many obstacles. If the partner is not handicapped, she will have to possess considerable tolerance because of difficulties in communication. If both partners are deaf because of genetic defects, having children may be contraindicated since the hearing impairment may be inherited. If their children are normal, this will also present problems since the parents will not be able to relate to them linguistically or react to their auditory stimuli.

Behavior Disorder

The behaviorally disturbed adolescent, amply described in the literature (Aichorn 1955, Frankenstein 1957, Ophjuisen 1950), is characterized by a pronounced overdependency, a lack of inner resources, weak affective control, and absence of inhibitions resulting in acting out of his inner tensions and conflicts. One frequently finds severe educational neglect, deficient maternal care, and physical or psychological absence of the father under circumstances of socioeconomic stress and deprivation. Oedipal relationships are weak and preoedipal fixations dominate. Although his intellectual potential may be normal, the child suffering from behavior disorder is poorly motivated and pseudoretardation is often found, characterized by a conspicuous lag in language development. In most cases, the child fails to adapt to school and shows typical learning difficulties, especially in reading, writing, and to a lesser degree in arithmetic. Marginal and ineffective schooling generally leads to dropping out and delinquency.

The failure to meet the educational needs of the behaviorally disturbed adolescent has serious consequences. Some are placed in training schools and institutions. There they pass their adolescence under stress and tension, while the basic adolescent need for expansion is frustrated by the restriction of physical and psychological freedom. They are unable to attain the educational status of secondary school pupils or apprentices. They cannot look forward to a vocation owing to the inadequate educational and vocational programs of the residential treatment centers. In addition, the institutionalized adolescent is barred from contact with peers of the other sex which may result in fixation to autoerotic and homoerotic drive organization.

The establishment of an educational setting which enables the adolescent to stay in school and to reach a level of optimal development requires a carefully designed curriculum. Subject matters must be related, at the beginning at least, to the deeply rooted materialistic interests of the behaviorally disturbed pupil, and scholastic progress must be linked with immediately attainable rewards. All techniques of behavior modification, amply applied to these populations, are based on this principle. However, our own experiments have shown that intrinsic reward systems may also be feasible (Kohen-Raz 1973). In such cases, it is imperative that the objectives of training or acquiring knowledge are intrinsically motivating and enjoy high status. Examples of these experiences include manipulation of machines, understanding of simplified scientific information, the use of communication media, and participation in social events.

Regarding social learning, the behaviorally disturbed adolescent needs a meaningful relationship with an educator who may become a substitute for his weak or absent father. The most successful educators of these adolescents are not necessarily those with academic or semiacademic degrees and specialization in teaching, but rather artisans, craftsmen, or farmers who have a firm and clear position in their respective occupations and possess natural pedagogical talent to deal with such adolescents.

The curriculum for the behaviorally disturbed adolescent must have direct and visible links with a vocational career. Even before reaching a level of qualification in his prospective vocation, the behaviorally disturbed youth should be given opportunities to perform remunerative work during his training. He should earn money and be taught to save and spend wisely. In this way he may sometimes support—in fact or symbolically—his economically disadvantaged family. This may be therapeutically meaningful, as the adolescent now feels, in part at least, to have taken over the role of the weak and inefficient father.

Within the framework of the educational program some room should be left for environmental, group, and individual therapy. Care should be taken, however, not to let these therapeutic interventions serve as an opportunity to withdraw from reality of the educational program and to neglect the tasks put before the adolescent.

The behaviorally disturbed adolescent should be coeducated with peers of the other sex. This poses some difficulties as the behaviorally disturbed girl is in many cases sexually delinquent and not perceived by boys as a peer and partner, but as a depreciated object of sexual aggression. The practical solution consists in mixing classes of behaviorally disturbed boys either with girls of nondelinquent and non-acting out type, or establishing optimal contact with normal classes (in certain school subjects, such as arts, physical training, crafts, as well as in all types of extracurricular activities). These normal coeducative classes would then provide the opportunities to create social contact between the behaviorally disturbed boys and normal boys and girls.

Residential treatment, if necessary, should be limited to short periods, not exceeding one to two years. As already stated, adolescence is a period of existential expansion, and extension cannot be maximally achieved in educational settings which restrict freedom, bar interaction with the wider society, and create negative self images. The high percentage of recidivism in ex-inmates of institutions for juvenile delinquents in all countries is a sad testimony to the general failure of residential treatment for these youngsters.

The Emotionally Disturbed Adolescent

This category of disturbances is characterized by internalized conflicts, repressed aggression, deep anxiety, and various symptoms. In contrast to the behavior disorder, poverty and sociocultural deprivation are not primary. The psychopathology of the parents is a major source of the child or adolescent's emotional problems. In certain cases, genetic and constitutional determinants may play a role. Emotionally disturbed adolescents are predominantly considered to be psychiatric patients and candidates for psychotherapy, and to a much less extent pupils with scholastic and educational difficulties (Rinsley 1974, Garber 1972, Masterson 1968, 1972a, 1972b).

The effects of early trauma can be overcome by educational intervention or therapeutic manipulation of the environment. These children do not suffer from the usual language difficulties seen in the groups just described, with the exception of stutterers and psychogenic mutism, and their superiority in verbal over nonverbal intelligence is considered a classical criterion of differential diagnosis from behavior disorders. However, their symbol systems are often invaded by unconscious conflicts, creating difficulties in communication and in learning certain subjects. Their lack of school readiness, often manifested during adolescence, is primarily emotional; it manifests itself in an unwillingness to accept the teacher as authority, inability to concentrate, resistance to discipline, and difficulties in social coexistence with peers and classmates.

Not enough attention is given to the fact that the school, the teacher, and the peer group play an important role in the psychodynamics of the emotional disturbance. Often the psychotherapy of disturbed children and adolescents involves treatment of one or both parents (this principle being optimally implemented in family therapy). The importance of active participation of educators and peers in the treatment process of emotionally disturbed pupils is still poorly understood. Furthermore, there has been lack of interest in the decisive significance of the curriculum upon the psychodynamics of the disturbed adolescent. It may serve as a projection screen for the pupil's conflicts, and as a stimulant of hidden anxieties and preoccupations. The recent work of Frankenstein (1970, 1972) and Kubovi (1970) uncovering learning inhibitions rooted in unconscious associations between subject matter and repressed social-emotional conflict is of basic importance in this context.

An important finding is the apparent relationship between scholastic failure at adolescence and a bad prognosis of the adolescent's psychopathology (Masterson 1968). Although good adjustment to school is a predictor of favorable outcome of the disturbance at adulthood, smooth scholastic progress is still no guarantee of emotional equilibrium in the disturbed adolescent. A sudden breakdown of the apparently good adaptation to the demands of the school may be imminent. In these cases, success in studies seems to have operated as a defense mechanism, which crumbles under the pressure of pubertal drives.

It appears that specific learning problems (such as dyslexia, agraphia, acalculia) produced by neurotic conflicts are less frequent than lack of motivation to study. In certain cases, the manipulation of abstract ideas and the preoccupation with notions, relations, and symbols may be threatening to the disturbed adolescent and deter him from dealing with theoretical subjects. Other reasons may be unconscious idiosyncratic relations between a personal conflict and the topic to be studied, leading to defenses that impede learning. In this connection Blos (1962) has described the urge of adolescents, at the threshold of young adulthood, to act out

481

early childhood traumatizations. This acting out is manifested by a sudden interruption of studies.

The importance of extracurricular activities should be stressed. Some emotionally disturbed adolescents typically avoid some or all extracurricular programs for psychological reasons rooted in their inner conflicts. On the other hand, the extracurriculum may become a powerful tool in their therapy and reeducation.

In light of the great instability of the emotionally disturbed adolescent's scholastic performance and the persistent danger of interrupting studies, it is useful to maintain special classes for some of these youngsters. Others may be kept in regular classrooms provided they are given individual lessons and psychotherapy. In both cases, intensive team work between the psychotherapist and the educators must be established. Leeway must be given to shift the emphasis of the rehabilitative process from the therapeutic situation to the classroom and vice versa.

Short term intensive consultation services must be available in the secondary school system in order to clarify and help deal with the emotional scholastic problems of the disturbed adolescent. Decisions must be made as to whether it is advisable to transfer the pupil to another teacher or whether a different career of vocational (not primarily intellectual) training should be recommended.

The introduction of productive manual work as an integral part of the curriculum would be of great help in resolving the educational problems of the emotionally disturbed adolescent. The fluctuation and instability of scholastic interests and motivations of emotionally disturbed adolescents is difficult to handle unless a flexible structure in the school system is created. The mentally healthy adolescent is able to choose a more or less realistic program of high school studies, often characterized by rich and multidirectional interests (Kohen-Raz 1962). The more disturbed the adolescent, the stronger his inability to make stable and rational choices.

In this discussion of principles of educational programs, no attempt has been made as to the educational problems of the neurotic, character neurotic, personality disorder, or psychotic borderline type of emotionally disturbed adolescents. The psychodynamics of these subcategories are substantially different. Still, from the point of view of special education practice, the diagnostic label is of minor importance. Obviously teaching the borderline case is essentially more difficult than the neurotic type. But except in extreme cases (when the borderline type has to be hospitalized), neurotic, character neurotic, personality disturbed, and psychotic borderline cases should by no means be kept in different scholastic settings.

These various types of psychopathology should be treated and educated together.

The problem of existential expansion for emotionally disturbed adolescents is, in first line, a struggle for freedom from overdependency on parents or parental figures. In contrast to other clinical types for whom existential expansion is symbolized by external, materialistic achievements, the emotionally disturbed strives for internal autonomy of attitudes, ideas, and principles, as well as for the establishment of social relationships which symbolize independence (Frankenstein 1957, 1959). Typically, he joins groups whose ideologies are dissonant with those of his parents. The educator may help the disturbed adolescent sublimate his strivings for autonomy (for instance, by delegating important decisions to him, by letting him take over leadership in classroom activities and by stimulating him to initiate projects). In many cases there will be inner, unconscious inhibitions to the urge for expansion which may be accessible only to psychotherapeutic intervention. These neurotic inhibitions, if unresolved, will lead to states of anxiety whenever life situations offer or stimulate expansion (such as travel or taking over roles and tasks of higher responsibility) or to counter phobic acting out in the form of irresponsible bravado endangering the adolescent and his environment.

Conclusions

The educational problems of deviant adolescents are multiple, complex, and of considerable variety. These adolescents, lacking appropriate educational facilities, are creating grave problems for society. Experimental projects have often been premature and have not yielded results which could be used to construct a well-elaborated special education program. In this chapter I have described and enumerated some principles which should be the essence of such programs.

Great attention must be paid to the etiology and the dynamics of the disturbance, and its typical features at adolescence. The program must be based on the assumption that adolescence is not a period of stagnation and growing irreversibility of mental and emotional aberrations, but can be used to provoke motivation in the adolescent to proceed in studies and vocational training. It is imperative to present a realistic future perspective, incorporating all the specific aspects and limitations linked with the particular handicap. Sex education and preparation for family life is another indispensable part of the curriculum. Finally, the delicate issue of existential expansion from its economic, social, psychological, and philosophical aspects must be seriously considered by those who wish to guide and to reeducate the deviant adolescent toward a human adult life of freedom, independence, and dignity.

NOTES

1. In this discussion we implicitly include all those disadvantaged types who show a more or less irreversible lag of two or three years of mental age.

2. Synkinetic movements are, from an adaptive point of view, disturbing and superfluous motor responses appearing chiefly in the form of radiation of a motor impulse which involuntarily activates a motor organ generally symmetrical and contralateral to that part of the body which is voluntarily stimulated—for instance, the involuntary closure of one eyelid while trying to keep the other closed.

3. For an extensive discussion of the impact of socioeconomic stress on the biological structure of the organism, see Willerman (1972).

REFERENCES

Aichhorn, A. (1955). *Wayward Youth*. New York: Meridian.

Alcorn, D. A. (1974). Parental views on sexual development and education of the trainable retarded. *Journal of Special Education* 8: 19-30.

Arnan, C. (1973). *Education Towards Family Life*. (In Hebrew). Jerusalem: Ben Yehuda School.

Blos, P. (1962). *On Adolescence*. Glencoe, Illinois: Free Press.

Chiva, M., and Rutschmann, Y. (1971). L'etiologie de la debilite mentale. R. Zazzo, ed., *Les Debilites Mentales*. Paris: Arman Colin.

Cook, R. (1974). Sex education program service model for the multihandicapped adult. *Rehabilitation Literature* 35: 264-267.

Cruickshank, W. M. (1966). *The Teacher of Brain Injured Children*. Syracuse, N.Y.: Syracuse University Press.

Cratty, B. J. (1969). *Movement, Perception and Thought*. Palo Alto, Calif.: Peek.

——— (1972). *Physical Expressions of Intelligence*. Englewood Cliffs, New Jersey: Prentice-Hall.

——— (1974). *Motor Activity and the Education of the Retarded*. Philadelphia: Lea and Felbiger.

De La Cruz, F. F., and Laveck, G. D. (1973). *Human Sexuality and the Retarded*. New York: Brunner-Mazel.

Eisenstadt, S. N. (1958). The new revolt of youth. (In Hebrew). *Megamoth* 9: 95-102.

Fernald, G. M. (1943). *Remedial Techniques in Basic School Subjects.* New York: McGraw-Hill.

Fischer, H. L., and Krajicek, M. J. (1974). Sexual development of the moderately retarded child. *Mental Retardation* 12: 28-30.

Frankenstein, C. (1957). The psychodynamics of social behavior disturbances. *Archives of Criminal Psychodynamics* 2: 82-106.

—— (1959). *Psychopathy.* New York: Grune and Stratton.

—— (1970). *Impaired Intelligence. Pathology and Rehabilitation.* New York: Gordon and Breach.

—— (1972). *They Think Again.* Jerusalem: Hebrew University, School of Education.

Fromm, E. (1950). *Psychoanalysis and Religion.* New Haven: Yale University Press.

Frostig, M. (1964). *The Frostig Program for the Development of Visual Perception.* Chicago: Follett.

Garber, B. (1972). *Follow Up Study of Hospitalized Adolescents.* New York: Brunner-Mazel.

Gold, M. V. (1973). Research on the vocational habilitation of the retarded. N. R. Ellis, ed., *International Review of Research in Mental Retardation,* Vol. 6. New York and London: Academic Press.

Hall, J. (1973). Sexual knowledge and attitudes of mentally retarded adolescents. *American Journal of Mental Deficiency* 77: 706-709.

The Illinois Plan for Special Education of Exceptional Children. (1958). Danville, Illinois: Interstate Printers and Publishers.

Inhelder, B., and Piaget, J. (1959). *The Growth of Logical Thinking from Childhood to Adolescence.* New York: Basic Books.

Johansson, B. A. (1965). *Criteria of School Readiness.* Stockholm: Almquist and Wiksell.

Kafafian, H. (1970). *Study of Man-Machine Communication Systems for the Handicapped.* Washington, D.C.: Cybernetics Research Institute and Office of Education, Bureau of the Handicapped.

Keogh, B. K. (1969). Pattern walking under three conditions of available visual cues. *American Journal of Mental Deficiency* 74: 376-381.

Kephart, N. C. (1971). *The Slow Learner in the Classroom.* Columbus, Ohio: Merrill.

Kohen-Raz, R. (1962). A group Rorschach tool of differentiating between high school students of different streams. (In Hebrew). *Megamoth* 12: 110-119.

—— (1965). Movement representations and their role in the development of concept formation at early school age. *Scripta Hierosolymitana,* Vol. 14. Jerusalem: Magnes Press.

————— (1972). *From Chaos to Reality: An Experiment of Re-education of Disturbed Immigrant Youth in a Kibbutz.* New York and London: Gordon and Breach.

————— (1973). Growth and acquisition of formal reasoning in culturally disadvantaged adolescents as related to physiological maturation. Final Report. Dallas, Texas: Zale Foundation.

————— (1974). Developmental patterns of higher mental functions in culturally disadvantaged adolescents. *This Annual* 3: 152-167.

Kraus, J. (1972). Supervised living in the community and residential and employment stability of retarded male juveniles. *American Journal of Mental Deficiency* 77: 283-290.

Kubovi, D. (1970). *Therapeutic Teaching.* (In Hebrew). Jerusalem: Hebrew University, School of Education.

Long, J. S. (1963). *The Sign Language.* Washington, D.C.: Gallaudet College.

Mackenberg, E. J., Broverman, D. M., and Klaiber, E. L. (1974). Morning to afternoon changes in cognitive performances and in the EEG. *Journal of Educational Psychology* 66: 238-246.

Masterson, J. F. (1968). The psychiatric significance of adolescent turmoil. *American Journal of Psychiatry* 124: 1549-1554.

————— (1972a). Psychiatric treatment of adolescents. A. M. Freeman and H. I. Kaplan, eds., *The Child: His Psychological and Cultural Development.* New York: Atheron.

————— (1972b). *Treatment of the Borderline Adolescent: A Developmental Approach.* New York: Wiley.

Miller, A. S. (1973). The sex education program for teen-agers at Clarke School. *Volta Review* 75: 493-503.

Morganstern, M. (1973). Sexuality, marriage and parenthood among the retarded. *Journal of Clinical Child Psychology* 2: 27-28.

Muchov, H. H. (1962). *Jugend und Zeitgeist.* München: Rohwolt.

Nordquist, I. (1972). *Life Together—the Situation for the Handicapped.* Bromma, Sweden: Swenska Central Kommitten for Rehabilitating.

Olson, D. R. (1970). *Cognitive Development: The Child's Acquisition of Diagonality.* New York: Academic Press.

Ophjusen, J. H. W. van (1950). Primary conduct disturbances. N. D. C. Lewis, ed., *Modern Trends in Child Psychiatry.* New York: International Universities Press.

Parsons, T. (1955). *Family, Socialization and Interaction Processes.* Glencoe, Illinois: Free Press.

Piaget, J. (1952a). *The Origins of Intelligence.* New York: International Universities Press.

—— (1952b). *The Child's Concept of Numbers.* London: Routledge and Kegan Paul.

—— (1956). *The Child's Concept of Space.* London: Routledge and Kegan Paul.

Rey, A. (1952). *Monographies de Psychologie Clinique.* Neuchatel: Delachaux and Niestle.

Rinsley, D. B. (1974). Special education for adolescents in residential psychiatric treatment. *This Annual* 3: 294-418.

Sali, J., and Amir, M. (1971). Personal factors influencing the retarded person's success at work. *American Journal of Mental Deficiency* 76: 42-47.

Sex Education for the Retarded. (1972). Fifth International Congress on Mental Retardation. Bruxelles: Publications of the International League of Societies for the Mentally Handicapped.

Stokoe, W. C. (1965). *A Dictionary of American Sign Language on Linguistic Principles.* Washington, D.C.: Gallaudet College.

Werner, H., and Wapner, S. (1949). Sensori-tonic field theory of perception. *Journal of Personality* 18: 88-107.

——, and Kaplan, B. (1963). *Symbol Formation.* New York: Wiley.

Willerman, L. (1972). Biosocial influences on human development. *American Journal of Orthopsychiatry* 42: 452-462.

CONTENTS OF VOLUMES 1-4

ABERASTURY, A.
The Adolescent and Reality (1973)　　　　　　2:415-423

AMERICAN SOCIETY FOR ADOLESCENT PSYCHIATRY
Position Statement on Training in Adolescent
　　Psychiatry (1971)　　　　　　　　　　　1:418-421

ANTHONY, E. J.
Self-Therapy in Adolescence (1974)　　　　　3: 6-24
Between Yes and No; The Potentially Neutral Area
　　Where the Adolescent and His Therapist
　　Can Meet (1976)　　　　　　　　　　　4:323-344

BAITTLE, B., & OFFER, D.
On the Nature of Male Adolescent
　　Rebellion (1971)　　　　　　　　　　　1: 139-160

BALIKOV, H., see COHEN & BALIKOV (1974)

BARGLOW, P., ISTIPHAN, I., BEDGER, J.,
　　& WELBOURNE, C.
Response of Unmarried Adolescent Mothers to
　　Infant or Fetal Death (1973)　　　　　　2: 285-300

BARISH, J., see KREMER, PORTER, GIOVACCHINI,
LOEB, SUGAR, & SCHONFELD (1971)

489

————, & SCHONFELD, W. A.
Comprehensive Residential Treatment
of Adolescents (1973)   2: 340-350

BEDGER, J. E., *see* BARGLOW, ISTIPHAN, BEDGER,
& WELBOURNE (1973)

BERNS, R. S., *see* KREMER, WILLIAMS, OFFER, BERNS,
MASTERSON, LIEF, & FEINSTEIN (1973)

BERGER, A. S., & SIMON, W.
Sexual Behavior in Adolescent Males (1976)   4: 199-210

von BERTALANFFY, L.
The Unified Theory for Psychiatry and
the Behavioral Sciences (1974)   3: 43-48

BETTELHEIM, B.
Obsolete Youth: Toward a Psychograph
of Adolescent Rebellion (1971)   1: 14-39
Discussion of Alfred Flarsheim's Essay (1971)   1: 459-463

BLOS, P.
The Generation Gap: Fact and Fiction (1971)   1: 5-13
The Overappreciated Child: Discussion of
E. James Anthony's Chapter (1976)   4: 345-351

BOROWITZ, G. H.
Character Disorders in Childhood
and Adolescence: Some Consideration of
the Effects of Sexual Stimulation in Infancy
and Childhood (1971)   1: 343-362
The Capacity to Masturbate Alone
in Adolescence (1973)   2: 130-143
See also GIOVACCHINI AND BOROWITZ (1974)

BOYER, L. B.
Interactions Among Stimulus Barrier, Maternal
Protective Barrier, Innate Drive Tensions,
and Maternal Over-Stimulation (1971)   1: 363-378
Meanings of a Bizarre Suicide Attempt
by an Adolescent (1976)   4: 371-381

BRULL, H. F.
The Psychodynamics of Drug Use:
A Social Work Perspective (1976)   4: 309-317

BUCKY, S. F., *see* SCHULLER & BUCKY (1974)

CARSON, D. I., *see* LEWIS, GOSSETT, KING, & CARSON (1973)

CHIGIER, E.
Adolescence in Israel: Thoughts on
the Middle-Class Urban Adolescent (1973)   2: 435-444

COHEN, R. S., & BALIKOV, H.
On the Impact of Adolescence
Upon Parents (1974)   3: 217-236

COHLER, B. J.
New Ways in the Treatment of
Emotionally Disturbed Adolescents (1973)   2: 305-323

COONS, F. W.
The Developmental Tasks of
the College Student (1971)   1: 256-274

COOPER, B. M., *see* SOLOW & COOPER (1974)

COPELAND, A. D.
Violent Black Gangs:
Psycho- and Socio-Dynamics (1974)   3: 340-353
An Interim Educational Program
for Adolescents (1974)   3: 422-431

DAVIDSON, H.
The Role of Identification in the
Analysis of Late Adolescents (1974)   3: 263-270

EKSTEIN, R.
The Schizophrenic Adolescent's Struggle
Toward and Against Separation
and Individuation (1973)   2: 5-24

From the Language of Play to
Play with Language (1976)   4: 142-162
A Note on the Language of Psychotic
Acting Out: Discussion of
L. Bryce Boyer's Chapter (1976)   4: 382-386

ESCOLL, P. J., *see* SMARR & ESCOLL (1973);
SMARR & ESCOLL (1976)

FARNSWORTH, D. L.
Adolescence: Terminable and Interminable (1973)   2: 31-43

FEINBERG, H. B., *see* REICH & FEINBERG (1974)

FEINER, A. H., *see* LEVENSON, FEINER, & STOCKHAMER (1976)

FEINSTEIN, S. C.
In Memoriam: William A. Schonfeld (1971)   1: v-vi

————, GIOVACCHINI, P. L., & JOSSELYN, I. M.
Introduction (1974)   3: 99-102
See also: FEINSTEIN, GIOVACCHINI, &
MILLER (1971); FEINSTEIN & GIOVACCHINI
(1973); KREMER, WILLIAMS, OFFER, BERNS,
MASTERSON, LIEF, & FEINSTEIN (1973);
KNOBEL, SLAFF, KALINA, & FEINSTEIN (1973);
FEINSTEIN & GIOVACCHINI (1974); FEINSTEIN,
GIOVACCHINI, & JOSSELYN (1974)

FLARSHEIM, A.
Resolution of the Mother-Child Symbiosis
in a Psychotic Adolescent (1971)   1: 428-458
See also BETTELHEIM (1971)

FREEDMAN, D. X.
On the Use and Abuse of LSD (1971)   1: 75-107

GIOVACCHINI, P. L.
Fantasy Formation, Ego Defect, and
Identity Problems (1971)   1: 329-342

The Adolescent Process and Character Formation:
Clinical Aspects—With Reference to
Dr. Masterson's "The Borderline Adolescent" (1973) 2: 269-284
Character Development and the
Adolescent Process (1973) 2: 402-414
The Difficult Adolescent Patient:
Countertransference Problems (1974) 3: 271-288
Madness, Sanity, and Autonomy (1976) 4: 46-59
Productive Procrastination: Technical Factors in
the Treatment of the Adolescent (1976) 4: 352-370

———, & BOROWITZ, G.
An Object Relationship Scale (1974) 3: 186-212
See also: KREMER, PORTER, GIOVACCHINI,
LOEB, SUGAR, & BARISH (1971); FEINSTEIN,
GIOVACCHINI, & MILLER (1971); FEINSTEIN &
GIOVACCHINI (1973); FEINSTEIN &
GIOVACCHINI (1974); FEINSTEIN, GIOVACCHINI,
& JOSSELYN (1974)

GODENNE, G. D.
From Childhood to Adulthood:
A Challenging Sailing (1974) 3: 118-127

GOLDBERG, A.
On Telling the Truth (1973) 2: 98-112

GOSSETT, J. T., *see* LEWIS, GOSSETT,
KING, & CARSON (1973)

GREENACRE, P.
Differences Between Male and Female
Adolescent Sexual Development as Seen
From Longitudinal Studies (1976) 4: 105-120

GREENBERG, R.
Psychiatric Aspects of Physical Disability
in Children and Adolescents (1974) 3: 298-307

GREENWOOD, E. D.
The School as Part of the Total
Hospital Community: A Summary (1974)   3: 435-438

GRINBERG, L.
Identity and Ideology (1973)   2: 424-434

GRINKER, R. R., Sr.
In Memoriam: Ludwig von Bertalanffy (1974)   3: 41

———, GRINKER, R. R., Jr., & TIMBERLAKE, J.
"Mentally Healthy" Young Males: Homoclites (1971)   1: 176-255

ISTIPHAN, I., *see* BARGLOW, ISTIPHAN, BEDGER,
& WELBOURNE (1973)

JOSSELYN, I. M.
Etiology of Three Current Adolescent
Syndromes: An Hypothesis (1971)   1: 125-138
Implications of Current Sexual Patterns:
An Hypothesis (1974)   3: 103-117
See also FEINSTEIN, GIOVACCHINI,
& JOSSELYN (1974)

KALINA, E.
The Adolescent Aspect of
the Adult Patient (1976)   4: 387-392
See also KNOBEL, SLAFF, KALINA, & FEINSTEIN (1973)

KALOGERAKIS, M. G.
The Sources of Individual Violence (1974)   3: 323-339

KENISTON, K.
Youth as a Stage of Life (1971)   1: 161-175

KERNBERG, O. F.
Cultural Impact and Intrapsychic Change (1976)   4: 37-45

KHAN, M. M. R.
To Hear with Eyes: Clinical Notes on
Body as Subject and Object (1974)   3: 25-40

KING, J. W.
Teaching Goals and Techniques
  in Hospital Schools (1974)   3: 419-421
See also: LEWIS, GOSSETT, KING, & CARSON (1973)

KLUMPNER, G. H.
On the Psychoanalysis of Adolescents (1976)   4: 393-400

KNOBEL, M., SLAFF, B., KALINA, E.,
  & FEINSTEIN, S. C.
Introductions from The First Pan-American
  Congress on Adolescent Psychiatry (1973)   2: 391-401

KOHEN-RAZ, R.
Developmental Patterns of Higher Mental
  Functions in Culturally Disadvantaged
    Adolescents (1974)   3: 152-167

KREMER, M. W., PORTER, R., GIOVACCHINI, P. L.,
  LOEB, L., SUGAR, M., & BARISH, J. I
Techniques of Psychotherapy in Adolescents:
  A Panel (1971)   1: 510-539

———, WILLIAMS, F. S., OFFER, D., BERNS, R. S.,
  MASTERSON, J. F., LIEF, H. I., & FEINSTEIN, S. C.
The Adolescent Sexual Revolution (1973)   2: 160-194

LAUFER, M.
Studies of Psychopathology in Adolescence (1973)   2: 56-69

LEVENSON, E. A., FEINER, A. H., & STOCKHAMER, N. N.
The Politics of Adolescent Psychiatry (1976)   4: 84-100

LEVI, L. D., *see* STIERLIN, LEVI, & SAVARD (1973)

LEWIS, J. M., GOSSETT, J. T., KING, J. W.,
  & CARSON, D. I.
Development of a Protreatment Group Process
  Among Hospitalized Adolescents (1973)   2: 351-362

LIEF, H. I., *see* KREMER, WILLIAMS, OFFER, BERNS,
  MASTERSON, LIEF, & FEINSTEIN (1973)

LIFTON, R. J.
Proteus Revisited (1976)   4: 21-36

LOEB, L.
Intensity and Stimulus Barrier
    in Adolescence (1976)   4: 255-263
See also: KREMER, PORTER, GIOVACCHINI,
LOEB, SUGAR, & BARISH (1971)

LOONEY, J. G., *see* MILLER & LOONEY (1976)

MAROHN, R. C.
Trauma and the Delinquent (1974)   3: 354-361

MASTERSON, J. F.
The Borderline Adolescent (1973)   2: 240-268
See also: KREMER, WILLIAMS, OFFER, BERNS
MASTERSON, LIEF, & FEINSTEIN (1973)

MEEKS, J. E.
Adolescent Development and Group Cohesion (1974)   3: 289-297

MILLER, A. A.
Identification and Adolescent Development (1973)   2: 199-210
See also FEINSTEIN, GIOVACCHINI, & MILLER (1971)

MILLER, D. H.
The Drug-Dependent Adolescent (1973)   2: 70-97

————, & LOONEY, J. G.
Determinants of Homicide in Adolescents (1976)   4: 231-254

NAGERA, H.
Adolescence: Some Diagnostic, Prognostic,
    and Developmental Considerations (1973)   2: 44-55

NEFF, L.
Chemicals and Their Effects on
    the Adolescent Ego (1971)   1: 108-120

NEWMAN, K.
Bonnie and Clyde: A Modern Parable (1971)   1: 61-74

NEWMAN, L. E.
Transsexualism in Adolescence:
Problems in Evaluation and Treatment (1973)   2: 144-159

NEWMAN, M. B., & SAN MARTINO, M. R.
Adolescence and the Relationship
Between Generations (1976)   4:60-71

NICHTERN, S.
Introduction: The Educational Needs of
Adolescents in Psychiatric Hospitals (1974)   3: 389-390
The Therapeutic Educational Environment (1974)   3: 432-434

OFFER, D., & OFFER, J. B.
Three Developmental Routes Through
Normal Male Adolescence (1976)   4: 121-141

OFFER, J. B., see OFFER, D., & OFFER, J. B. (1976)

OFFER, D., & VANDERSTOEP, E.
Indications and Contraindications for
Family Therapy (1974)   3: 249-262
See also: BAITTLE & OFFER (1971); KREMER,
WILLIAMS, OFFER, BERNS, MASTERSON,
LIEF, & FEINSTEIN (1973)

PALGI, P.
Death of a Soldier:
Socio-Cultural Expressions (1976)   4: 174-198

PHILIPS, I., & SZUREK, S. A.
Youth and Society: Conformity, Rebellion, and
Learning (1974)   3: 140-151

POLIER, J. W.
The Search for Mental Health Services
for Adolescents (1974)   3: 313-322

POLLAK, O.
Youth Culture, Subcultures, and Survival (1974)   3: 49-53

PORTER, R., *see* KREMER, PORTER, GIOVACCHINI,
LOEB, SUGAR, & BARISH (1971)

POTOK, C.
Rebellion and Authority: The Adolescent
Discovering the Individual in Modern
Literature (1976)   4: 15-20

RASCOVSKY, A.
Filicide and the Unconscious Motivation
for War (1974)   3: 54-67

REDL, F.
Emigration, Immigration and
the Imaginary Group (1976)   4: 6-12

REICH, R., & FEINBERG, H. B.
The Fatally Ill Adolescent (1974)   3: 75-84

RINSLEY, D. B.
Theory and Practice of Intensive Residential
Treatment of Adolescents (1971)   1: 479-509
Special Education for Adolescents in
Residential Psychiatric Treatment (1974)   3: 394-418

ROSE, G. J.
Maternal Control, Superego Formation,
and Identity (1971)   1: 379-387

ROTHSTEIN, D. A.
On Presidential Assassination: The Academia
and the Pseudo-Community (1976)   4: 264-298

SALZMAN, L.
Adolescence: Epoch or Disease (1974)   3: 128-139

SAN MARTINO, M. R., *see* NEWMAN
& SAN MARTINO (1976)

SARGENT, D. A.
A Contribution to the Study of
the Presidential Assassination Syndrome (1976)   4: 299-308

SAVARD, R. J., *see* STIERLIN, LEVI, & SAVARD (1973)

SCHILDKROUT, M. S.
The Pediatrician and the Adolescent
Psychiatrist (1974)   3: 68-74

SCHONFELD, W. A.
Foreword (1971)   1: vii-viii
Adolescent Development: Biological,
Psychological, and Sociological Determinants (1971)   1: 296-323
See also: FEINSTEIN (1971); BARISH
& SCHONFELD (1973)

SCHULLER, A. B., & BUCKY, S. F.
Toward Prediction of Unsuccessful
Adaptation in the Military Environment (1974)   3: 85-95

SEIDEN, A. M.
Sex Roles, Sexuality, and the
Adolescent Peer Group (1976)   4: 211-225

SHIELDS, R. W.
Mutative Confusion at Adolescence (1973)   2: 372-386

SIMON, W., *see* BERGER & SIMON (1976)

SINGER, M.
Family Structure, Disciplinary Configurations,
and Adolescent Psychopathology (1974)   3: 372-386

SLAFF, B., *see* KNOBEL, SLAFF, KALINA,
& FEINSTEIN (1973)

SMARR, E. R., & ESCOLL, P. J.
The Youth Culture, Future Adulthood,
and Societal Change (1973)   2: 113-126

The Work Ethic, the Work Personality,
and Humanistic Values (1976)   4: 163-173

SOLOW, R. A.
Planning for Education Needs (1974)   3: 391-393

————, & COOPER, B. M.
Therapeutic Mobilization of Families Around
Drug-Induced Adolescent Crises (1974)   3: 237-248

STIERLIN, H.
The Adolescent as Delegate of
His Parents (1976)   4: 72-83

————, LEVI, L. D., & SAVARD, R. J.
Centrifugal versus Centripetal Separation in
Adolescence: Two Patterns and Some of
Their Implications (1973)   2: 211-239

SUGAR, M.
Network Psychotherapy of an Adolescent (1971)   1: 464-478
Adolescent Confusion of Nocturnal Emissions
as Enuresis (1974)   3: 168-185
Group Process in the Management of
a High School Crisis (1974)   3: 362-371
Introduction to Chaim Potok's Address (1976)   4: 13-14
See also KREMER, PORTER, GIOVACCHINI,
LOEB, SUGAR, & BARISH (1971)

SZUREK, S. A., *see* PHILIPS & SZUREK (1974)

TOLPIN, P. H.
Some Psychic Determinants of
Orgastic Dysfunction (1971)   1: 388-413

VANDERSTOEP, E., *see* OFFER & VANDERSTOEP (1974)

WELBOURNE, C., *see* BARGLOW, ISTIPHAN, BEDGER,
& WELBOURNE (1973)

WILLIAMS, F. S.
Discussion of Rudolf Ekstein's Chapter (1973)   2: 25-30
Family Therapy: Its Role in Adolescent Psychiatry (1973) 2: 324-339
See also KREMER, WILLIAMS, OFFER, BERNS,
   MASTERSON, LIEF, & FEINSTEIN (1973)

WILSON, M. R., Jr.
A Proposed Diagnostic Classification of
   Adolescent Psychiatric Cases (1971)   1: 275-295

WINNICOTT, D. W.
Adolescence: Struggling Through the
   Doldrums (1971)   1: 40-50
Delinquency as a Sign of Hope (1973)   2: 363-371

WOLF, E. S.
Sigmund Freud: Some Adolescent Transformations
   of a Future Genius (1971)   1: 51-60

INDEX

Abel, G. G., 324

Abraham, K., 169, 170

acoustically handicapped adolescents, special education needs of, 477-478

Adatto, C. P., 390

Adler, R., 83

adolescence

depression in, 257-274 (*see also* adolescence, normal depressive states of, pathological depression in, symptomatic depression in)

  conclusions, 273-274

  natural cure treatment, 273

  syndromes, 262

  treatment of, 272-273

as developmental phase or cultural artifact, 143-150

  conclusions, 149-150

end of, structural criteria of, 5-16

  conclusions, 15

  ego continuity, 12-14

  residual trauma, 14-15

  second individuation process, 10-12

  sexual identity, 15

filial obligation in, 151-171

  conclusions, 171

  discordant, 159-162

  disentanglement from parents, 152-157

  narcissistic factors, 162-165

  persistant tie to parents, 157-159

  requiting, 165-166

  theoretical issues, 166-171

and final sexual organization, 245-247

intervention in, 254-255

nature of, and schizophrenia in, 278-283

normal depressive states of, 262-264

  emancipation mourning, 262-263

  endogenous depressive-like states, 263-264

pathological depression in, 264-270

  anaclitic depression, 268-270

  anhedonic or pleasureless depressions, 267-268

  endogenous depression, 264-265

  reactive depression, 265-267

psychiatry of, and changing social values, 35-38

and psychic development and narcissism, 113-140

  conclusions, 140

  developmental stages and narcissism, 115-122

  dimensions of psychoanalytic treatment, 122-124

  psychopathology and character structure, 113-115

  technical principles and developmental fixation, 134-135

schizophrenia in, 276-289

  aspects, 283-289

  nature of adolescence, 278-283

special education needs at, 460-484

  acoustically handicapped, 477-478

  behavior disorder, 478-480

  conclusions, 483-484

  educable mentally retarded, 463-469

  emotionally disturbed, 480-483

  minimal and medium organic brain damage, 474-476

  physically handicapped, 471-474

  systematic approach to, 461-463

  trainable mentally retarded, 469-471

symptomatic depression in, 270-272

  depressive manifestations of physical illness, 271-272

  drug induced or released, 271

  occurring in course of other emotional disorders, 271

termination of treatment in, 390-410

  criteria for beginning of terminal phase, 397-401

  conclusions, 408-410

  goals of termination, 407-408

  preconditions for emergence of terminal phase, 391-396

  technical questions on start of terminal phase, 401-402

  terminal phase in, 402-407

adolescents

and adoption, 54-66

  adoptee, 57-64

  birth parents, 56-57

  conclusions, 65-66

  future trends, 64-65

hapless, group approach with, 429-440
  conclusions, 439-440
  population, 429-431
  process, 434-439
  program, 431-434
impulse ridden, self-destructive behavior
    of, influence of anomie on, 73-79
and parents, empathy and vicissitudes of
    development in, 175-184
  conclusions, 184
  effect on parents of children's adoles-
    cent development, 177-184
  task of therapist, 177
as patients, self-disclosure by therapist to
    (see therapists)
psychoanalysis of communication in, 442-
    447
  conclusions, 447
sexuality in males, 96-106
  conclusions, 101-102
  discussion, 100-101
  normal adolescent project, 97-99
  Offer self-image questionnaire, 97
adoptee, adolescent, 54-66
  and adoption, 57-64
    birth parents and, 56-57
    conclusions, 65-66
    future trends, 64-65
  continuation of childhood developmental
    difficulties in, 57-59
  intensification of typical adolescent con-
    flicts in, 59-61
  unique symptomatology associated with
    experience of, 61-64
adults, stress and change in, and empathy
    and vicissitudes of development in
    parents and adolescents, 175-177
Agras, W. S., 298, 324, 353
Aichorn, A., 75, 77, 187, 188, 189, 192, 203,
    210, 390, 478
Alcorn, D. A., 468
Alves, F., 442
Amir, M., 467
anaclitic depression, 268-270
Andrews, R. G., 56
Anglim, E., 60
anhedonic depression, 267-268
anomie, influence of, on impulse ridden
    youth and their self-destructive be-
    havior, 73-79
  conclusions, 79
  and impulse-freeing values and urban-
    industrial ethos, 75-76

and nature and functions of values from
    sociological and psychoanalytical
    perspectives, 76-78
anorexia nervosa, 293-302
  atypical, 297
  behavior therapy in, 323-349
    case reports, 331-347
    conclusions, 347-349
    criteria, 325-326
    methodology, 323-349
  conclusions, 301-302
  family therapy in, input and outcome of,
    313-322
    conclusions, 320-322
  in males, 297-298
  narcissistic disturbances in, 304-312
    conclusions, 311-312
  primary, 294
    body image disturbances, 295
    family transactions, 296-297
    ineffectiveness, 296
    misperceptions of bodily functions, 295-
      296
  significance of therapists's feeling in
      treatment of, 352-378
    case of exacerbation of treatment and
      first experiences with psychiatric
      treatment, 366-369
    case family background and early
      childhood, 360-362
    case syndrome and treatment, 359-360
    case of transference and empathy in
      inpatient setting, 369-378
    conclusions, 378
    countertransference in, 353-356
    dieting as expression of symbiosis in
      mother-daughter illness, 362-366
    early childhood development of symbi-
      osis and conflict regarding control,
      356-359
  treatment of, 298-300
Anthony, E. J., 182, 258, 273, 363
Aponte, H., 317
Aponte, J. F., 58
Aristotle, 144
Arnan, C., 468
artifact, cultural. See cultural artifact

Bachrach, A., 353
Bacon, Roger, 171
Bar, E. S., 422
Baker, L., 241, 299, 313, 323
Balikov, H., 182

Index

Balint, E., 170

Balint, M., 407

Balkoura, A., 390, 397, 398

Balla, D., 54

Banfield, E., 74, 77

Banham, K. M., 167

Baran, A., 4, 54-66

Barcai, A., 299

Barinbaum, L., 60, 61

Barlow, D. H., 324

Barret-Lennard, G. T., 450

Barthell, C., 287

Beach, F. A., 149

Becker, H., 74

behavior, self-destructive, of impulse ridden youth, influence of anomie on, 73-79

behavior disorder, and special education needs at adolescence, 478-480

behavior therapy. *See* therapy, behavior

Benedek, T., 171

Bender, L., 287

Berg, I., 265

Berger, A. S., 101

Berlin, I. N., 353

Berman, S., 144

Bernstein, R., 56

Bettelheim, B., 76, 123, 138, 368

Betz, B. J., 449

Bhanji, S., 324

Birney, R., 89

Blatt, S. J., 269

Blinder, B. J., 298, 299, 324, 353

Bliss, E., 352, 373

Block, J., 281

Blos, P., 3, 5-16, 30, 60, 96, 152, 157, 186 204, 208, 247, 481

Blum, L., 75

Blumer, H., 74

Boatman, M. J., 353

body

and anorexia nervosa

disturbance of image, 295

misperceptions of functions, 295-296

physically mature, ownership of, and central masturbation fantasy, 247-249

Bohman, M., 58

Borgatta, E. F., 59

Boston, J. A., 54

Boszormenyi-Nagy, I., 160, 162, 170, 415, 417

Boyar, R. M., 294

Boyer, L. B., 122

Brachelmanns, W. E., 183

Brady, J. P., 323, 324, 348

brain damage, minimal and medium organic, and special education needs at adolescence, 474-476

Branch, C. H., 352, 373

Brandes, N. S., 266

Brekstad, A., 287

Breuer, J., 218

Bridger, H., 407

Brien, R. L., 450

Brierley, M., 18

Briscoe, C. S., 176

Bromet, E., 286

Bruch, H., 240-241, 293-302, 304, 305, 306, 308, 319, 323, 352, 353, 361, 372

Burt, R. A., 4, 39-52

Buxbaum, E., 407

Carkhuff, R. R., 450

Carlson, P., 59, 63

Carney, R., 58

Carpenter, W. T., 271

Carson, L., 241

Casey, T. M., 176

Cebiroglu, R., 257

Cellini, B., 159

Chapin, H. N., 324

character structure, and psychopathology, 113-115

Charcot, J.-M., 368

childhood

continuation of developmental difficulties in, and adolescent adoptee, 57-59

rights of, and therapeutic institutions, 39-52

conclusions, 51-52

techniques of intervention in adolescent maladjustment in, 40-51

Chiva, M., 464

Chwast, J., 262

Clayton, P. J., 176

Clothier, F., 56, 58, 61, 63

Cloward, R., 74

Cody, V. F., 450

Cohen, A., 74

Cohen, D., 30

Cohen, M., 226

Cohen, R. S., 182

Cohler, B. J., 241-242, 352-378

Colby, K., 116

Combrinck-Graham, L., 316

Comfort, A., 19

communication
  in adolescents, psychoanalysis of, 442-447
    conclusions, 447
  empathic breakdown of, and effect of children's adolescent development on parents, 180-182
conflicts, typical adolescent, intensification of, in adolescent adoptee, 59-61
confusion
  integration as response to, 86-87
  as theme, 87-88
Conklin, E. S., 58
control
  conflict regarding, and development of symbiosis in early childhood, and therapist's treatment of anorexia nervosa, 356-359
  gain of, through acceptance of weakness, and treatment of adolescent runaways, 420
Cook, B., 87
Cook, R., 473
countertransference, in treatment of anorexia nervosa, 353-356
Cratty, B. J., 466, 467, 475
Cressey, D., 74
Crisp, A. H., 305, 323
Cross, L. A., 58
Cruickshank, W. M., 474
cultural artifact or developmental phase, adolescence as, 143-150
  conclusions, 149-150
Cunningham, S., 324, 348
cure, natural, as treatment for depression in adolescence, 273
Cytryn, L., 260

Dalle-Molle, D., 206
Dally, P. J., 323
Davis, K. E., 101
Dawkins, S., 55
de Ajuriaguerra, J., 265
delegated runaways. See runaways, adolescent
delinquency, as narcissistic pathology, 192-202
  clinical material on, 193-202
  discussion, 203-209
  and juvenile imposter, 186-210
    conclusions, 209-210
depression in adolescence, 257-275
  conclusions, 273-274

natural cure treatment of, 273
normal states of, 262-264
  emancipation mourning, 262-263
  endogenous depressive-like states, 263-264
pathological depression, 264-270
  anaclitic depression, 268-270
  anhedonic or pleasureless depressions, 267-268
  endogenous depression, 264-265
  reactive depression, 265-267
social manifestations of, 261-262
symptomatic, 270-272
  depressive manifestations of physical illness, 271-272
  drug induced or released, 271
  occurring in course of other emotional disorders, 271
symptoms of, 258-261
  mood, 259
  psychomotor effects, 260
  self-esteem and self-concept, 259-260
  somatic manifestations of, 260-261
syndromes of, 262
treatment of, 272-273
Derdeyn, A. P., 112, 175-184
despair, integrity versus, Erikson's crisis of, 179
Deutsch, A., 21
Deutsch, F., 294, 366
Deutsch, H., 55, 96, 126, 158, 171
development, adolescent
  and changing values, 21-27
  effect on parents, 177-184
    breakdown of empathic communication, 180-182
    empathy as therapeutic goal, 182-184
  difficulties of, continued in adolescent adoptee, 57-59
  factors of, in Kohut's theory of narcissism, 221-228
  fixation in, and technical principles in adolescence, 134-135
    discussion, 135-140
  phase of, or cultural artifact, 143-150
    conclusions, 149-150
  psychic, and narcissism, 113-140
    conclusions, 140
    developmental stages and narcissism, 115-122
    dimensions of psychoanalytic treatment, 122-124

psychopathology and character structure, 113-115

technical principles and developmental fixation, 134-135

stages of, in family, 177-178

vicissitudes of, and empathy, 175-184

    conclusions, 184

    effect on parents of children's adolescent development, 177-184

    stress and change in adult, 175-177

Dienelt, M. N., 176

dieting, as expression of symbiosis of illness in mother and daughter, anorexia nervosa and, 362-366

Diggory, J., 74

disorders, emotional, symptomatic depression in adolescence occurring in course of, 271

Dodge, J. A., 58

Donian, S., 176

drugs, symptomatic depression in adolescence induced or released by, 271

Du Bois, E., 366

Dukette, R., 64

Durkheim, E., 73

Dyrud, J. E., 388, 422-427

Easson, W. M., 59, 206, 240, 257-274

education, special, adolescent needs for, 460-484

    acoustically handicapped, 477-478

    behavior disorder, 478-480

    conclusions, 483-484

    educable mentally retarded, 463-469

    emotionally disturbed adolescent, 480-483

    minimal and medium organic brain damage, 474-476

    physically handicapped, 471-474

    systematic approach to, 461-463

    trainable mentally retarded, 469-471

ego continuity in end of adolescence, 12-14

Eiduson, B. T., 58

Eisenstadt, S. N., 76, 86

Eisler, R. M., 314, 324

Eissler, I. R., 75

Eissler, K. R., 187, 231, 353, 390, 409

Ekstein, R., 123

Eldred, C. A., 63

Elkin, T. E., 324

Ellenberg, J., 21

Ellis, J. W., 41

Elonen, A. S., 59

Elson, M., 157

emancipation mourning, as normal depressive state in adolescence, 262-263

Emerson, Ralph Waldo, 151, 169

emotionally disturbed, special education needs for, 480-483

empathy

    case of, and transference in inpatient setting in treatment of anorexia nervosa, 369-378

    and fairness, need for multigenerational, in treatment of runaways, 419

    as therapeutic goal, 182-184

    and vicissitudes of development, in parents and adolescents, 175-184

    breakdown of communication, 180-182

    conclusions, 184

    as therapeutic goal, 182-184

endogenous depression, and pathological depression in adolescence, 264-265

endogenous depressive-like states, normal, as normal depressive state in adolescence, 263-264

Epstein, E., 78

Erikson, E. H., 6, 30, 60, 89, 96, 152, 162, 176, 177-178, 183, 279, 309

    crisis of integrity versus despair, 179

Erikson, K. T., 176

Erikson, M. T., 58

Erwin, W., 353

Escalona, A., 29

Esman, A. H., 4, 18-32

    discussion by R. C. Marohn of, 35-38

Evans, B. W., 56

experience, gap of, bridging, in treatment of adolescent runaways, 420

Fairbairn, R. W. D., 116

families

    bound up, unbinding of, in treatment of runaways, 415

    developmental stages of, 177-178

    and primary anorexia nervosa, 296-297

family therapy. *See* therapy, family

Fanshel, D., 58, 59, 63

fantasy, central masturbation, and ownership of physically mature body, and adolescent pathology, 247-249

Faris, E., 426, 427

Federn, P., 121

Feiner, A. H., 157

Feinstein, S., 272

Feldman-Toledano, Z., 353
Ferenczi, S., 224, 407
Fernald, G. M., 475
Ferrell, R. B., 311, 323
Feuer, L., 82
Fields, M., 136
filial obligation. *See* obligation, filial
Firstein, S. K., 397, 401, 402, 406
Fish, B., 287
Fisher, F., 63
Fisher, S., 427
fixation, developmental, and technical prin-
    ciples in adolescence, 134-135
    discussion of, 135-140
Flarsheim, A., 136, 356
Fletcher, J., 77
Fliess, R., 355
Flugel, J. C., 171
Ford, C. S., 149
Forgotson, J. H., 450
Framo, J. L., 157
Frankenstein, C., 478, 481
Freedman, A. M., 287
Freedman, D., 353
Freedman, L., 78
Freeman, D. M. A., 298, 324
French, L., 176
Freud, A., 10, 27, 36, 60, 77, 96, 152, 158,
    186, 187, 248, 390
Freud, S., 18, 19, 29, 31-32, 58, 112, 113, 115-
    116, 117, 118, 119, 120, 122, 133, 140,
    164, 167, 169, 187, 188, 190, 203, 213,
    214, 215, 216, 218, 219, 220, 222, 223,
    224, 225, 227, 229, 245, 246, 254, 305,
    354, 355, 394, 400, 407, 408, 427, 449
Friedlander, K., 75, 206
Friedenberg, E. Z., 91
Frisk, M., 61, 62
Fromm, E., 463
Frommer, E. A., 257, 261
Frosch, W., 25
Frostig, M., 475
Furer, M., 170

Gadpaille, W. J., 112, 143-150
Gagnon, J. H., 26, 97, 98, 101
Gallagher, V. M., 56
Gallemore, J. L., 258
Gallup, G., 89
Garber, B., 480
Gardner, G., 20
Garfinkel, P. E., 294
Gartner, M., 83

Gasbarro, D. T., 57
Gaylin, W., 77
Gedo, J. E., 37, 203, 209
Geleerd, E. R., 390
generational theory, and silent generation of
    Fifties college students, 85-86
Gifford, S., 352, 360
Ginsberg, G., 25, 101
Giovacchini, P. L., 52, 112, 113-140, 128,
    213-233
Gitelson, M., 175, 402
Glaser, K., 266
Glatzer, H. T., 59
Glover, E., 75, 116, 226, 397, 398, 406
Gluck, M. R., 57
Goffman, E., 74
Gold, M. V., 467
Goldberg, A., 209
Goldsen, R., 82, 88-89, 91
Goldstein, M. J., 287
Goodman, J., 57, 58
Goodsitt, A., 241, 304-312, 352, 356
Gore, R., 54
Gould, R. L., 152
Gradolph, P., 310
Green, M., 58
Greenacre, P., 29
Grinker, R. R., Jr., 281
Grinker, R. R., Sr., 78, 240, 276-289
Groen, J. J., 353
Gross, S. Z., 58
Grossman, W., 31
group approach, with hapless adolescent,
    429-440
    case population of, 429-440
    case process of, 434-439
    case program of, 431-434
    conclusions, 439-440
Guntrip, H., 170

Haggard, E. A., 287
Hagin, R., 287
Halikas, J. A., 176
Hall, J., 468
Hallsten, A., Jr., 353
Hallsten, E. A., 323
Halmi, K. A., 241, 323-349, 352
handicapped adolescents, special education
    needs of
    acoustically handicapped, 477-478
    physically handicapped, 471-474
Harley, M., 390
Harriman, M., 59

Harrow, M., 286
Hartmann, H., 9, 18, 28, 164
Harvin, D. D., 59
Havens, L. L., 449
Heath, D., 281
Heilbronner, R., 27, 31
Heiman, M., 352, 369
Heinicke, C. M., 390
Hendin, H., 27, 267
Hendrickson, W. J., 207
Heraclitus, 11
Hersen, M., 324
Herskovitz, H. H., 59
Herzog, E., 56, 58
Hill, E., 89
Hoedemaker, F. S., 271
Hoffer, W., 189, 400, 407
Hoffman, L, 317
Hofstadter, R., 89
Hollon, T. H., 260
Holmes, C., 82, 87
Holmes, D., 287
Holmes, D. H., 450, 456
Holzman, P. S., 240, 276-289
Hoopes, J. L., 56
Horn, J. M., 58
Howard, K. I., 97
Hubbard, G. L., 63
Humphrey, J. A., 176
Humphrey, M., 55, 58
Hurn, A. T., 406

identity, sexual, in end of adolescence, 15
illness, physical, depressive manifestations of, in adolescence, 271-272
image, body, disturbances of, and primary anorexia nervosa, 295
impulsiveness, adolescent, and self-destructive behavior, influence of anomie on, 73-79
    conclusions, 78-79
    impulse-freeing value, urban-industrial ethos, 75-76
    and nature and functions of values from sociological and psychoanalytical perspectives, 76-78
individuation process, second, in end of adolescence, 10-12
ineffectiveness, and primary anorexia nervosa, 296
institutions, therapeutic, and children's rights, 39-52
    conclusions, 51-52

and techniques of intervention in adolescent maladjustment, 40-51
integration
    educational system as vehicle of, 90-92
    as response to confusion by silent generation, 86-87
    as theme of silent generation, 90
integrity, vs. despair, Erikson's crisis of, 179
intervention
    in adolescence, and adolescent pathology, 254-255
    techniques of, in adolescent maladjustment, and children's rights and therapeutic institutions, 40-51

Jackson, L., 58
Jacob, P., 82, 84, 90-91
Jacobson, E., 165
Jaffee, B., 58, 63
Jameson, G. K., 57
Johnson, A. M., 23, 58
Jones, E., 164, 166, 169, 215
Jourard, S. M., 449
juvenile imposter, and narcissism and delinquency, 186-210
    conclusions, 209-210
    discussion, 203-209

Kangas, J. A. 450
Kaplan, B., 466
Kaplan, H. B., 267
Kapp, F. T., 176
Kardiner, A., 116
Kasl, S., 286
Kaufman, Judge Irving, 51, 52
Kaufman, M. R., 294, 352, 366, 369
Keniston, K., 6, 144
Keogh, B. K., 467
Kephart, N. C., 467
Kernberg, O., 24, 121, 229, 230, 364
Kety, S. S., 286
Khan, M. M. R., 393
Kiell, N., 144
King, J. W., 388, 449-458
King, L. J., 271
King, S., 152
Kirk, H. D., 54, 62
Klein, M., 31, 116-117, 119, 120, 121, 140, 161, 168, 170, 217, 354, 364, 407, 427, 442
Klickstein, M., 55
Klumpner, G. H., 37, 205
Knesper, D. J., 40

Knoblich, H., 57
Kohen-Raz, R., 388-389, 460-484
Kohlsaat, B., 58
Kohrman, R., 390
Kohut, H., 24, 31, 36, 96, 112, 121, 164, 170, 190-192, 193, 203, 205, 207, 208, 209, 210, 213-228, 229-233, 355
Kornitzer, M., 60, 62
Krakowski, A. J., 259
Kraus, J., 467
Kubovi, D., 481
Kusnetzoff, J. C., 443

La Barre, W., 147, 148, 150
Lacan, J., 422, 427
Landauer, E., 390, 392
Lang, P., 353
La Rochefoucald, 166
Larson, L., 323-349
Lauder, E. A., 56
Laufer, M., 239, 243-256, 390
Laurence, M., 60
Lawton, J. J., 58
Leitenberg, H., 324, 353
Lemon, E. M., 63
Levenson, E. A., 157, 162
Levi, L. D., 179
Levin, B., 57, 59
Levine, E. M., 4, 73-79
Levine, M., 59
Lewin, K. 54
Lewis, D. O., 54, 58
Lewis, H. 56, 62
Lewis, M., 54
Lieberman, M. A., 450
Liebman, R., 241, 299, 313-322, 323
Lifton, R. J., 176
Linde, L., 62
Lindemann, E., 176
Lipset, S. M., 89
Litman, R., 74
Livermore, J. B., 58, 60
Loewald, H., 29
Long, R. L., 456
Lorand, S., 262
Lower, K. D., 56

McClelland, D. C., 287
McCranie, M., 54, 56
McGlashan, T. H., 271
McKnew, D.H., 260
McPherson, S. R., 183
McWhinnie, A. M., 58, 59, 60, 63

Mahler, M. S., 10, 29, 356
maladjustment, adolescent, techniques of intervention in, and children's rights and therapeutic institutions, 40-51
males, anorexia nervosa in, 297-298. *See also* sexuality
Malmquist, C. P., 257
Mandell, W. 57, 58
Mannheim, K. 85
Manning, B. E., 54
Mannoni, M. 422
Marohn, R. C., 35-38, 97, 112, 186-210, 222, 225, 233
  "juvenile imposter" of, 213-221
Martimor, E., 259
Maskin, M. 422
Masterson, J. F., 257, 267, 480, 481
masturbation, central fantasy of, and ownership of physically mature body and adolescent pathology, 247-249
Massarik, F., 56
Maurice, W. L., 176
Maxmen, J. S., 311, 323
Mayer-Gross, W. 276
Mead, G. 74
Mead, M., 144
Mech, E. V., 60
Mecklenburg, R. S., 296
mediator, importance of third party, in treatment of runaways, 419
Meeks, J. E., 450
Mendell, F., 427
Menlove, F. L., 58
Menninger, K. A., 406
mentally retarded, special education needs for
  educable, 463-469
  trainable, 469-471
Merton, R., 74
methodology, of behavior therapy in anorexia nervosa, 323-349
Mikawa, J. K., 54
Miller, D., 4, 39-52
Miller, H., 417
Milman, L., 314
Milner, M., 407
Minuchin, S., 241, 299, 313-322, 323
Modell, A., 158
Mohr, J., 353
mood, as symptom of adolescent depression, 259
Morgan, H. G., 348, 349
Muchov, H. H., 465

Muensterberger, W., 147
Murawski, B., 352, 360
Murray, H., 355
Myers, J. K., 176

Nagel, E., 226
Nameche, G. H., 287
narcissism
  and adolescence and psychic develop-
    ment, psychoanalytic perspectives
    on, 113-140
    conclusions, 140
    and developmental stages, 115-122
    dimensions of psychoanalytic treat-
      ment, 122-124
    discussion, 135-140
    fixation on prementational stage, 124-
      134
    psychopathology and character struc-
      ture, 113-115
    technical principles and developmental
      fixation, 134-135
  and delinquent, juvenile imposter, 186-210
    conclusions, 209-210
    delinquency as narcissistic pathology,
      192-202
    discussion, 203-209
  disturbances of, in anorexia nervosa, 304-
    312
    conclusions, 311-312
  Kohut's theory of, critique of, 221-233
    concepts about psychopathology, 229-
      230
    developmental factors, 221-228
    technical considerations, 230-233
  in struggle against filial obligation, 162-
    165
    clinical example, 162-165
  See also pathology, narcissistic
Nemiah, J., 352
Neubauer, P., 30
Newell, H. W., 162
Newman, K., 208
Newman, L. E., 183
Nietzsche, F., 19
Niswander, G. D., 176
Nordquist, I., 473
Noshpitz, J. D., 162, 368
Novick, J., 387-388, 390-410

obligation, filial, in adolescence, 151-171
  conclusions, 171

and disentanglement from parents, 152-
  157
narcissistic factors in struggle against, 162-
  165
  clinical example, 162-165
and persistent tie to parents 157-159
requiting of, 165-166
theoretical issues of, 166-171
O'Donnell, J., 78
Offer, D., 21, 26, 36, 96-106, 206, 281, 283
Offer, J. B., 96-106, 281, 283
Offer self-image questionnaire
  results of, 100
  and sexuality in adolescent males, 97
Offord, D. R., 58
Ohlin, L., 74
Olsen, T., 265
Olson, D. R., 466
Ophjuisen, J. H. W. van, 478
Ornstein, P., 222, 232
Ortega y Gasset, J., 85
Osorio, L. C., 388, 442-447
Ostrov, E., 97, 206
Otstott, R. L., 450
Ounsted, C., 55, 58

Palazzoli, M. S., 353, 354, 357, 358
Pannor, R., 54-66
parents
  and adolescents, empathy and vicissitudes
    of development in, 175-184
    conclusions, 184
    stress and change in adult, 175-177
  birth, and adoption and adolescent, 56-57
  disentanglement from, and filial obliga-
    tion, 152-157
    clinical example, 154-157
  effect on, of adolescent's development,
    177-184
    breakdown of empathic communica-
      tion, 180-182
    development stages of family, 177-178
    empathy as therapeutic goal, 182-184
    Erikson's crisis of integrity vs. despair,
      179
  persistent tie to, and filial obligation in
    adolescence, 157-159
Parsons, A., 359
Parsons, T., 74, 463
Pasamanick, B., 57
pathology, adolescent
  clinical examples of, 251-254

defined, 249-251
M. Laufer's view of, 243-256
conclusions, 255-256
final sexual organization, 245-247
intervention in adolescence, 254-255
narcissistic, delinquency as, 192-202
clinical material on, 193-202
Paton, J. M., 63
Pauker, J. D., 56
Paul, N. L., 182
Paykel, E. S., 176
Payne, S., 407
Peller, L. E., 58
Pfeffer, A. Z., 390, 397
Phillipson, H., 363
physically handicapped adolescents, special
educations needs of, 471-474
Piaget, J., 40, 446, 466, 475
Piccoli, B., 442
Piers, Maria, 122
Pilot, M., 352, 360
pleasureless depression. *See* anhedonic depression
Pokarny, A. D., 267
Poluan, O., 257
Pope, H., 56
Powers, P., 324, 348
prementational phase
clinical example of, 128-134
fixation on, 124-28
principles, technical, and developmental
fixation, 134-135
discussion of, 135-140
Pringle, M. L. K., 54, 55, 56, 57, 63
Prusoff, B. A., 176
psychoanalysis
of communication in adolescents, 442-447
conclusions, 447
ideas of, and changing social values, 18-21,
27-32, 35-38
psychomotor effects, as symptom of adolescent depression, 260
psychopathology
and character structure, 113-115
concepts about, and Kohut's theory of
narcissism, 229-230
Pumpian-Mindlin, E., 179-181

Rado, S. 284
Rafferty, F. T., 388, 429-440
Raitt, G. E. 390, 397, 398, 406
Rangell, L., 390, 397, 398, 406

Rapaport, D., 28-29
Rautinan, E., 63
Rautman, A., 63
Ravenscroft, K., Jr., 414
reactive depression, 265-267
Redl, F., 162, 431
Reece, S., 57, 58
Rees, K., 30
Reese, H., 162
Reeves, A. C., 58
Reich, A., 390
Reich, C., 28
Reik, T., 355
Reisen, A., 117
Rey, A., 466
Reynolds, W. F., 61
Rickman, J., 407
Ricks, D. F., 287
Rieger, W., 324, 348
Riesman, D., 75, 76, 77, 91
Rinsley, D. B., 206, 480
Riviere, J., 170
Robins, S., 287, 288
Rodnick, E. H., 287
Rogers, R., 57, 60, 62, 449
Rosen, B., 450
Rosenberg, M., 82, 88-89
Rosenthal, D., 286
Rosenthal, M. J., 112, 151-171
Rosman, B. L., 241, 313-322
Rossell, F., 347
Roth, M., 276
Rovera, C. G., 260
Rowland, C., 352, 360, 366
runaways, treatment perspectives on, 413-
421
and bridging experience gap, 420
conclusions, 420-421
and gain of control through acceptance of
weakness, 420
and importance of third party mediator,
419
and need for multigenerational fairness
and empathy, 419
treatment of delegated, 415-417
and unbinding of bound-up families, 415
of wayward expellees, 417-419
Russell, G. F. M., 323, 348, 349
Rutschmann, Y., 464

Sabshin, M., 97
Sali, J., 467
Salzman, L., 144

Sants, H. J., 62
Sargent, W., 323
Savard, R. J., 179
Schachter, M. 257
Schafer, R., 31, 233, 355
Schaflander, J., 89
Schechter, M. D., 55, 57, 58, 59, 63, 183
schizophrenia in adolescence, 276-289
  and nature of adolescence, 278-283
  some aspects of, 283-289
Schoenberg, C., 60
Schulsinger, F., 286
Schwartz, E. M., 58, 59, 60
Scrutchins, M. P., 450
Searles, H. 170
Seglow, J., 54, 56, 57
self-concept, as symptom of adolescent
    depression, 259-260
self-destruction, and impulsiveness of youth,
    influence of anomie in, 73-79
self-disclosure, by therapist, to adolescent
    patient, 449-458
  conclusions, 457-58
  and ego-strength of patient, 453-454
  and goal of treatment, 451
  and indications and contraindications,
    457
  and nature of patient-therapist alliance,
    454-455
  and patient's feelings about therapist, 455
  and real relationship between therapist
    and patient, 451-453
  therapist's feelings about patient, 455-457
self-esteem, as symptom of adolescent
    depression, 259-260
Selvini, M. P., 296, 300
Senn, M., 63
Senturia, A., 57, 59
Settlage, C. F., 143
sexuality, in adolescent males, 96-106
  conclusions, 101-102
  discussion, 100-101
  and normal adolescent project, 97-99
  and Offer self-image questionnaire, 97
sexual organization, final, and adolescent
    pathology, 245-247
Shaiova, C. H., 4, 73-79
Shane, M., 390
Shapiro, T., 25
Sheimo, S., 353
Sherfey, M., 25
Sherman, E. A., 56
Silberfarb, P. M., 311, 323

Silberstein, M. R., 57, 58
silent generation
  and confusion theme, 87-88
  defined as term for college students of
    Fifties, 83-85
  and educational system as vehicle of
    integration, 90-92
  and integration theme, 90
  in theoretical perspective, 85-92
    existential adaptation as integration in
      response to confusion, 86-87
    generational theory, 85-86
  and withdrawal theme, 88-90
Silverman, M., 30
Simmons, J. Q., 59, 63
Simon, B., 31
Simon, N., 57, 59
Simon, W., 97, 98, 101
Sinclair, K., 347
Skard, A. G., 287
Slater, E., 276
Smith, E., 54, 56, 63
Smith, R., 64
Solnit, A., 63
Solomon, M. A., 177, 178
somatic manifestations, as symptom of
    adolescent depression, 260-261
Sontag, L. W., 58
Sorosky, A. D., 4, 54-66
Sours, J. A., 304, 352, 354, 356, 374
Spark, G., 162, 170, 415, 417
Spiegel, J., 419
Spiegel, L. A., 170, 390
Spitz, R., 117, 269
Spivak, G., 59
Steffek, J. C., 388, 429-440
Stierlin, H., 158, 162, 179, 388, 413-421
Stockhammer, H., 157
Stolorowrd-Lubensky, A. W., 287
Stott, D. H., 58
Strachey, J., 123, 218
students, college, as silent generation in
    Fifties, 82-92
  conclusions, 92
  defining silent generation, 83-85
  silent generation in theoretical perspec-
    tive, 85-92
Stunkard, A. J., 298, 324, 353, 358
Suchman, I., 82, 88-89
Sullivan, M. E., 58
Sutherland, E., 74
Sweeny, D. M., 57
Sylvester, E., 368, 464, 470

symbiosis, anorexia nervosa and early childhood development of, and conflict regarding control, 356-359
dieting as expression of, in mother-daughter illness, 362-66
Szurek, S., 353

Taheri, A., 59
Taichert, L. C., 59
Tec, L., 59
technical principles, and developmental fixation in adolescence, 134-135
Teicher, J. D., 257
Terman, D. M., 37, 203
termination of treatment, 390-410
conclusions, 408-410
criteria for beginning terminal phase, 397-401
and goals, 407-408
and preconditions for emergence of terminal phase, 391-396
technical questions on start of terminal phase in, 401-402
terminal phase in, 402-407
criteria for beginning, 397-401
preconditions for emergence, 391-396
technical questions on start, 401-402
Thander, S., 352
therapist
self-disclosure by, to adolescent patient, 449-458
conclusions, 457-458
ego strength of patient, 453-454
goal of treatment, 451
indications and contraindications, 457
nature of patient-therapist alliance, 454-455
patient's feelings about therapist, 455
real relationship between therapist and patient, 451-453
therapist's feelings about patient, 455-457
significance of feeling of, in treatment of anorexia nervosa, 352-378
case of exacerbation of treatment and first experiences with psychiatric treatment, 366-369
case family background and early childhood, 360-362
case syndrome and treatment, 359-360
case of transference and empathy in inpatient setting, 369-378

conclusions, 378
countertransference, 353-356
dieting as expression of symbiosis in mother-daughter illness, 362-366
early childhood development of symbiosis and conflict regarding control, 356-359
task of, 177
therapy
behavior, in anorexia nervosa, 323-349
case reports, 331-347
conclusions, 347-349
criteria, 325-326
methodology, 326-331
empathy as goal of, and effect on parents of children's adolescent development, 182-184
family, input and outcome of, in anorexia nervosa, 313-322
conclusions, 320-322
institutions for, and children's rights, 39-52
conclusions, 51-52
techniques of intervention in adolescent maladjustment, 40-51
Thoma, H., 352
Thompson, J., 324
Thompson, L. E., 324, 353
Ticho, E. A., 402, 407
Ticho, G., 28
Tillich, Paul, 84
Timberlake, I., 281
Titchener, J. L., 176
Todd, T., 314
Toffler, A., 20
Tolpin, M., 164
Toolan, J., 260
Torre, M., 260
Toussieng, P. W., 59, 62
transference, case of, and empathy in inpatient setting, and therapist's feelings in treatment of anorexia nervosa, 369-378
trauma, residual, in end of adolescence, 14-15
treatment
of adolescent runaways, 413-421
bridging experience gap, 420
conclusions, 420-421
delegated, 415-417
gain of control through acceptance of weakness, 420

importance of third party mediator, 419
need for multi-generational fairness and empathy, 419
unbinding of bound-up families, 415
wayward expellees, 417-419
of anorexia nervosa, significance of therapist's feelings in, 298-300
case of exacerbation of treatment and first experiences with psychiatric treatment, 366-369
case family background and early childhood, 360-362
case syndrome and treatment, 359-360
case of transference and empathy in inpatient setting, 369-378
conclusions, 378
countertransference, 353-356
dieting as expression of symbiosis in mother-daughter illness, 362-366
early childhood development of symbiosis and conflict regarding control, 356-359
of depression in adolescence, 272-273
natural cure, 273
psychoanalytic dimensions of, and adolescence, 122-124
termination of, in adolescence, 390-410
conclusions, 408-410
criteria for beginning terminal phase, 397-401
goals of termination, 407-408
preconditions for emergence of terminal phase, 391-396
technical questions on start of terminal phase, 401-402
terminal phase, 402-407
Trilling, L., 19, 20, 35, 83-84
Triscliotis, J., 63
Truax, C. B., 449, 450
truth, telling of, in retrospect, 422-427
Tsai, S. Y., 267

Unwin, J. R., 263, 273

Vaillant, G. E., 281
values
changes in
and adolescent development, 18-27
and psychoanalysis and adolescent psychiatry, 35-38
and psychoanalytic ideas, 18-21, 27-32
impulse-freeing, and urban-industrial ethos, impulse-ridden, self-

destructive youth and, 75-76
nature and function of, from sociological and psychoanalytic perspectives, anomie and, 76-78
Van Dam, A. H., 390

Waelder, R., 75, 77
Waller, J. V., 294, 366
Walters, P. A., 267
Wapner, S., 466
Waters, D. B., 112, 175-184
Watson, Thomas, 84
Watt, N. F., 287
wayward expellees. *See* runaways
weakness, gain of control through acceptance of, and treatment of adolescent runaways, 420
Weaver, L., 176
Wedge, P., 54, 56, 57
Weiner, M. F., 388, 449-458
Weinstein, E. A., 58
Wellisch, E., 62
Wender, P. H., 286
Werble, B., 281
Werman, D., 30
Werner, H., 466
Whitehorn, J. C., 449
Wilden, A., 422
Williams, E. S., 180
Williams, J. B., 324
Williams, R., 82, 88-89, 93
Wilmuth, L. F., 176
Wilson, J., 78
Wilson, W. P., 258
Wineman, D., 162
Winnicott, D. W., 29, 123, 127, 137, 138, 168, 210, 228, 354, 394, 402
withdrawal, as theme of silent generation, 88-90
Witmer, H. L., 58
Wolensky, R. P., 4, 82-92
Wolf, E. S., 37, 203
Wolpe, J., 299, 324
Work, H., 59, 63
Wulheimer, F., 347

Young, I. L., 59
Young, L., 56
Yalom, I., 431

Zachry, C. S., 158
Zetzel, E., 116